S0-ABB-538

UTERINE ARTERY EMBOLIZATION AND GYNECOLOGIC EMBOLOTHERAPY

UTERINE ARTERY EMBOLIZATION AND GYNECOLOGIC EMBOLOTHERAPY

Editors

JAMES B. SPIES, MD

Professor of Radiology and Chief of Service
Department of Radiology
Georgetown University Hospital
Washington, District of Columbia

JEAN-PIERRE PELAGE, MD, PhD

Associate Professor of Radiology
Université Paris Ouest
Garches, France
Department of Body and Vascular Imaging
Hôpital Lariboisière
Paris, France

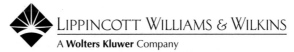

LIPPINCOTT WILLIAMS & WILKINS
A **Wolters Kluwer** Company
Philadelphia • Baltimore • New York • London
Buenos Aires • Hong Kong • Sydney • Tokyo

Acquisitions Editor: Lisa McAllister
Senior Marketing Manager: Sara Bodison
Managing Editor: Lisa R. Kairis
Production Manager: Dave Murphy
Senior Manufacturing Manager: Ben Rivera
Compositor: Graphic World Publishing Services
Printer: Maple Press

Copyright © 2005 by Lippincott Williams & Wilkins.

This book is protected by copyright. No part of it may be reproduced, stored in a retrieval system, or transmitted, in any form or by any means—electronic, mechanical, photocopy, recording, or otherwise—without prior written permission of the publisher, except for brief quotations embodied in critical articles and reviews and testing and evaluation materials provided by publisher to instructors whose schools have adopted its accompanying textbook. Printed in the United States of America. For information write Lippincott Williams & Wilkins, 530 Walnut Street, Philadelphia PA 19106.

Materials appearing in this book prepared by individuals as part of their official duties as U.S. Government employees are not covered by the above-mentioned copyright.

9 8 7 6 5 4 3 2 1

Library of Congress Cataloging-in-Publication Data
Uterine artery embolization and gynecologic embolotherapy / editors, James B. Spies, Jean-Pierre Pelage.
    p. ; cm.
    Includes bibliographical references and index.
    ISBN 0-7817-4532-2 (hardcover)
    1. Uterine fibroids—Treatment.   2. Therapeutic embolization.   I. Spies, James B.   II. Pelage, Jean-Pierre.
    [DNLM: 1. Uterine Neoplasms—therapy.   2. Embolization, Therapeutic—methods.   3. Leiomyoma—therapy.   WP 458 U89 2005]
RC280.U8U733 2005
616.99′366—dc22

                                                          2004015390

Care has been taken to confirm the accuracy of the information presented and to describe generally accepted practices. However, the authors, editors, and publisher are not responsible for errors or omissions or for any consequences from application of the information in this book and make no warranty, express or implied, with respect to the content of the publication.

The authors, editors, and publisher have exerted every effort to ensure that drug selection and dosage set forth in this text are in accordance with the current recommendations and practice at the time of publication. However, in view of ongoing research, changes in government regulations, and the constant flow of information relating to drug therapy and drug reactions, the reader is urged to check the package insert for each drug for any change in indications and dosage and for added warnings and precautions. This is particularly important when the recommended agent is a new or infrequently employed drug.

Some drugs and medical devices presented in this publication have Food and Drug Administration (FDA) clearance for limited use in restricted research settings. It is the responsibility of the health care provider to ascertain the FDA status of each drug or device planned for use in his or her clinical practice.

To my beautiful wife, Vivian, and daughters, Vivian and Ana Cristina, for their unwavering love, support, and forbearance. Without them, this project would not have been possible. Without them, this project would not have mattered.
James B. Spies, MD

This book is dedicated to my family
To my cherished son, Pierre-Antoine, and my lovely wife, Delphine, for their extraordinary love and support
To my parents, for their love and encouragement
To my sister Catherine, to Francis and Elisa,
To Edith and Laurent,
Your support was truly appreciated.
Jean-Pierre Pelage, MD, PhD

Contributors

Sandra J. Allison, MD
Division of Abdominal Imaging
Department of Radiology
Georgetown University Hospital
Washington, District of Columbia

Susan M. Ascher, MD
Professor, Department of Radiology
Georgetown University Medical Center
Director, Division of Abdominal Imaging
Georgetown University Hospital
Washington, District of Columbia

Joseph Bonn, MD
Associate Professor of Radiology
Jefferson Medical College
Chief, Cardiovascular and Interventional Radiology
Thomas Jefferson University Hospital
Philadelphia, Pennsylvania

Michael L. Douek, MD, MBA
Resident, Department of Radiology
UCLA School of Medicine
Los Angeles, California

Uche Ezeh, MD
Instructor, Department of Obstetrics and Gynecology and
    Reproductive Sciences
University of California, San Francisco
Clinical Fellow in Reproductive Endocrinology and
    Infertility
UCSF Center for Reproductive Health
San Francisco, California

Jackeline Gomez-Jorge, MD
Assistant Professor, Department of Radiology
Vascular/Interventional Section
University of Miami, Jackson
Memorial Medical Center, Jackson Memorial Hospital
Miami, Florida

Scott C. Goodwin, MD, FSIR
Professor and Vice Chairman, Department of Radiological
    Sciences
David Geffen School of Medicine at UCLA
Los Angeles, California

David M. Hovsepian, MD
Associate Professor of Radiology and Surgery
Washington University School of Medicine
Attending Radiologist, Mallinckrodt Institute of Radiology
Barnes-Jewish Hospital
Attending Radiologist
St. Louis Children's Hospital
St. Louis, Missouri

Keith Isaacson, MD
Associate Professor of Obstetrics, Gynecology, and
    Reproductive Biology
Harvard Medical School
Director, Minimally Invasive Gynecologic Surgery Center
Newton Wellesley Hospital
Boston, Massachusetts

Denis Jacob, MD
Vice Chairman, Department of Obstetrics and
    Gynecology
Hôpital Lariboisière
Paris, France

Reena C. Jha, MD
Assistant Professor, Department of Radiology
Georgetown University
Director of MRI, Department of Radiology
Georgetown University Hospital
Washington, District of Columbia

Pascal Lacombe, MD
Professor of Radiology
Université Paris Ouest
Garches, France
Chief, Department of Radiology
Hôpital Ambroise Paré
Boulogne, France

Alexandre Laurent, MD, PhD
Associate Professor of Radiology
Université Paris
Department of Neuroradiology
Hôpital Lariboisière
Paris, France

Olivier Le Dref, MD
Cardiovascular and Interventional Radiologist
Department of Body and Vascular Imaging
Hôpital Lariboisière
Paris, France

Hsin-Yi Lee, MD
Assistant Professor, Department of Radiological Sciences
David Geffen School of Medicine at UCLA
Section Chief, Interventional Radiology
VA Greater Los Angeles Healthcare System
Los Angeles, California

Margaret H. Lee, MD
Assistant Professor, Department of Radiological Sciences
David Geffen School of Medicine at UCLA
Los Angeles, California
Director of Vascular and Interventional Radiology
Olive View–UCLA Medical Center
Sylmar, California

Jeffrey Y. Lin, MD
Associate Professor, Department of Obstetrics and
  Gynecology
George Washington University
Director, Divisions of Gynecologic Oncology and General
  Obstetrics and Gynecology
Chief Gynecologic Surgeon
Vice Chairman, Department of Obstetrics and
  Gynecology
Washington, District of Columbia

Jean-Jacques Merland, MD
Professor of Radiology
Université Paris
Chief, Department of Neuroradiology
Hôpital Lariboisière
Paris, France

Jean-Pierre Pelage, MD, PhD
Associate Professor of Radiology
Université Paris Ouest
Garches, France
Department of Body and Vascular Imaging
Hôpital Lariboisière
Paris, France

Antoinette Roth, MD
Resident, Department of Radiology
UCLA Hospital
Los Angeles, California

Gary Siskin, MD
Associate Professor of Radiology, Department of
  Radiology
Albany Medical College
Vice Chairman, Department of Radiology
Medical Director, Vascular and Interventional Radiology
Albany Medical College
Albany, New York

James B. Spies, MD
Professor of Radiology and Chief of Service, Department
  of Radiology
Georgetown University Hospital
Washington, District of Columbia

Elizabeth A. Stewart, MD
Associate Professor, Department of Obstetrics,
  Gynecology, and Reproductive Biology
Harvard Medical School
Clinical Director, Center of Uterine Fibroids
Brigham and Women's Hospital
Boston, Massachusetts

Suresh Vedantham, MD
Assistant Professor of Radiology and Surgery, Mallinckrodt
  Institute of Radiology
Washington University School of Medicine
Attending Interventional Radiologist
Barnes-Jewish Hospital
St. Louis, Missouri

Woodruff Walker, MBBS, FRCR
Consultant Radiologist
Department of Radiology
The Royal Surrey County Hospital
Guildford, United Kingdom

Michel Wassef, MD
Associate Professor of Pathology
Université Paris
Department of Pathology
Hôpital Lariboisière
Paris, France

Foreword

Jean-Jacques Merland, MD

When one looks at the place that uterine embolization has in the current management of uterine fibroids, it seems a long way from the genesis of the procedure in 1974, when the first embolization for fibroids was performed. In April of that year, I was Assistant Professor of Radiology in the Department of Neuroradiology (Pr Bories) of Hôpital de la Salpétrière in Paris, France. In those days, the majority of vascular procedures were performed by neuroradiologists who were trained with all types of catheters and embolization materials. A 38 year old woman with intractable fibroid-related menorrhagia was referred to us by the gynecologists. Surgery and general anesthesia were considered too risky, because she was a spastic paraplegic resulting from carbon monoxide anoxia. This was during the early days of embolization, and we were asked to perform uterine arterial embolization as a last resort treatment for this woman.

Femoral access was not possible because of the irreducible contractures of the lower limbs, and a left brachial artery approach was used. A 5-French catheter was used to successively catheterize both hypogastric arteries and both uterine arteries. Bilateral uterine artery embolization was achieved using gelatin sponge pledgets. She suffered from severe pelvic pain during the post-procedural course, but bleeding ceased in a few days. Six months after the embolization, although the patient was markedly improved, we performed a repeat angiogram to evaluate the persistence of the occlusion of the embolized arteries. A flush pelvic aortogram showed that the uterine arteries were still occluded, but two enlarged ovarian arteries originating from the infrarenal aorta were discovered supplying the embolized fibroids. The largest ovarian artery was selectively catheterized and embolized using gelatin sponge pledgets. The patient had an eventful recovery and no recurrence of symptoms was observed during the follow-up period. The images obtained during the procedure were used for our book titled *Arterial Anatomy of the Pelvis* that we published with our clinical fellow, Dr Chiras, in 1981 (Springer-Verlag ed., Heidelberg, Germany).

In 1977, I moved to the Department of Neuroradiology of Hôpital Lariboisière, Paris (Pr Djindjian). Fifteen years later, I mentioned the case of the patient with fibroids treated with embolization to Dr. Ciraru-Vigneron, a gynecologist in the Obstetrics and Gynecology Department chaired by Professor Ravina. She was intrigued by this concept and subsequently referred several patients with intractable fibroid-related menorrhagia over the next two years. Then I started to offer embolization of the uterine arteries to women with contraindications to surgery (HIV patients, cardiovascular history contraindication to general anesthesia, etc.). During the same time period, Dr. Ravina began to request preoperative embolization in a group of patients scheduled to undergo myomectomy in order to reduce blood loss at the time of surgery. Embolization significantly reduced bleeding at the time of surgery and reduced or avoided the need for transfusion.

In 1993, we developed a French multicenter trial of uterine fibroid embolization as an alternative to hysterectomy. This registry was supported by unrestricted grants from the company Nycomed, which supplied the embolization particles (Ivalon, polyvinyl alcohol particles). Two seminal papers were published as a result of this early experience. The results of the first 16 women treated by embolization as a sole treatment were reported in *Lancet* in 1995 by our group (1). The results of the first patients embolized preoperatively were published a year earlier in a French journal (2). Thanks to Professor Ravina, who quickly published our results in both French and English journals, the diffusion of the technique started all over the world.

This is the true story of the serendipitous discovery of uterine fibroid embolization, first used as a desperate attempt to help one woman in 1974. With the collaboration of Dr. Ravina and Dr. Ciraru-Vigneron, we were able to take this therapy beyond concept to reality. As the procedure became available on a wider scale, results obtained in the United Kingdom (Dr. Walker and Dr. Reidy) and the United Stated (Dr. Goodwin) confirmed our initial findings. With additional studies published over the years, this procedure has become accepted as an effective therapy for fibroids. All this has developed from the application of the known tools of embolization to a new patient problem, an example of the true essence of medical innovation.

I am pleased to introduce this text to you, which documents the extent of our knowledge of uterine embolization to date. It will help providers caring for patients undergoing this procedure to understand the technique and patient care associated with this therapy.

Jean-Jacques Merland
Paris, 30 le Janvier 2004

REFERENCES

1. Ravina JH, Merland JJ. Arterial embolization to treat uterine myomata. *Lancet* 1995;346:671–672.
2. Ravina JH, Merland JJ. Preoperative embolization of uterine fibroma: preliminary results. *Presse Med* 1994;23:1540.

Preface

In planning a text, one must first identify the potential reader. When the subject is uterine embolization for fibroids, the audience is larger than might be expected. While we believe that this text will be an important guide for those interventional radiologists or trainees in the field interested in learning of this therapy, it may have broader appeal. Because this treatment and the care of this group of patients crosses into the field of gynecology, physicians and trainees in that field might have interest in a comprehensive text on this subject. In addition, because endovascular interventions are now becoming multi-specialty in scope, other specialists may also want to learn about this type of therapy.

In this information age, many other parties may have interest in such a text, most importantly potential patients. Many women conduct extensive online research regarding embolization, both before and after consulting with a physician. While the accessibility of information on the Internet is a great advantage, its accuracy varies. The advantage of a textbook is that it is a referenced review of the topic, and thus the reliability of its information can be verified from the original sources. As a therapy matures and additional data accrues, a text becomes a first source for those new to the subject. We wrote this text with all its potential readers in mind.

This text summarizes the current state of our scientific knowledge on uterine embolization and we hope that it will be considered one definitive source for those with interest in the procedure. It includes background on the pathophysiology of fibroids, their diagnosis, and gynecologic management; as well as a comprehensive review of pre-procedure evaluation, technique, peri-procedural care, complications and outcome of uterine embolization. While the primary audience is likely to be medical practitioners, we hope it is both informative and readable for those without formal medical training.

We would like to thank all our contributors for their outstanding efforts in reviewing their topics. Further, we would like to thank other key individuals who have been instrumental in our own understanding of this procedure and the associated patient care. They include Drs. Woody Walker, James Benenati, Robert Worthington Kirsch, John Lipman, Mahmood Razavi, Robert Vogelzang, Richard Shlansky-Goldberg, Howard Chrisman, Robert Andrews, Vivian Fraga, Anthony Scialli, Linda Bradley, Evan Myers, and too many others to mention. In our scientific sessions and meetings, the discussions with these experts have helped shape the development and refinement of this treatment and our own understanding of the theory behind it. Finally, we are equally indebted to our best teachers, our patients, from whose experience all our knowledge is ultimately derived.

We hope this text will be a definitive summary of our current knowledge on this exciting, minimally-invasive treatment and that it will meet our goal of reaching all interested parties.

James B. Spies, MD
Jean-Pierre Pelage, MD, PhD
July 2004

Contents

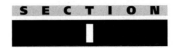

UNDERSTANDING UTERINE FIBROIDS

UTERINE FIBROIDS AND FIBROID EMBOLIZATION

JAMES B. SPIES
JEAN-PIERRE PELAGE

Uterine embolization has become accepted as an effective and safe therapy for fibroids. This minimally invasive procedure requires a recovery of days rather than weeks but has results similar to those of other uterine-sparing therapies. This advantage has led to intense interest among potential patients and rapid acceptance of this new therapy.

What have we learned about this procedure? For physicians interested in this therapy, there is much to master before starting a practice. Patient selection, embolization technique, periprocedural care, and follow-up considerations all need to be learned, because the procedure is just one step in the continuum of care for a woman with fibroids. We will see patients who have undergone prior medical therapies or surgery for their fibroids, who may have symptoms caused by conditions other than fibroids, and who will have recurrences of their symptoms months to years after our treatment. More so than many of our procedures, uterine embolization requires an understanding of the range of clinical presentations of uterine fibroids.

In this text, we hope to present the state of the art on this procedure, as well as the clinical context of this therapy. Not only must the physician understand the technique of embolization, he or she must also learn the natural history of uterine fibroids, the symptoms they cause, and the other therapies used in the management of this condition. For those with the interest, we hope this text will serve as a comprehensive guide to all aspects of fibroids and their therapy. First, however, it is important to understand the origins of this procedure and the events that led to its acceptance as a treatment of fibroids.

THE EARLY REPORTS

As related by Dr. Jacques Merland in this book's introduction, the first uterine embolization for fibroids was performed in 1974 on a patient with life-threatening hemorrhage. The patient was a poor candidate for surgery, and the procedure was performed in a desperate attempt to control the bleeding. It was successful.

This remained the sole experience with this procedure for more than a decade. It wasn't until 1989 that a collaboration to further evaluate this method began between Dr. Merland and Dr. Ciraru-Vigneron, a gynecologist in the Hospital Lariboisiere in Paris. They were subsequently joined in this effort by Dr. Jacques Ravina. The results of these treatments formed the basis for the first published report of the English medical literature by Dr. Ravina in 1995 (1).

In that initial report, 16 patients were treated. Polyvinyl alcohol particles were used as the embolic agent and were injected through catheters placed selectively in the uterine arteries. At a mean follow-up of 20 months, symptoms had resolved in 11 of 16 patients. Three patients had partial improvement, and their residual heavy bleeding was subsequently controlled with progestins. There were two failures: one required hysterectomy 6 weeks after the procedure, and the other required myomectomy 6 months after the procedure.

That initial report led others in the United Kingdom and the United States to begin to investigate this therapy. The first published report in the United States was by Goodwin et al. (2) at UCLA. The embolization procedure used by Goodwin was very similar to that of Ravina, although Goodwin used a larger polyvinyl alcohol particle (500–710 μm). Of the 11 patients treated, bilateral embolization was successful in ten patients and unilateral embolization in one. Within 3 weeks of the procedure, one patient developed endometritis and pyometrium that required hysterectomy. Among the ten other patients, the dominant symptom was noticeably improved in eight. One patient was lost to follow-up, and another (the patient with the unilateral embolization) had no improvement. The mean decrease in uterine volume was 40%, and dominant fibroid volume decreased 60% to 65% at 3-month follow-up. This report led to an explosion of interest among other interventionalists, the lay press, and the public.

Ravina's group reported on a larger group of patients in February 1997 (3). Eighty-eight women underwent attempted embolization. Of these patients, the procedure was not completed successfully in five, and three others were lost to follow-up or required luteinizing hormone-releasing hormone analogue for other reasons. Their paper reports on the results of the remaining 80 women. Eighty-nine percent (60/67) of these patients had resolution of their menorrhagia. There were seven failures. Fibroid volume was reduced by 55% at 2 months and 69% at 6 months. One patient required a hysterectomy for severe ischemic injury.

Bradley et al. (4) in the United Kingdom next reported the results of this therapy in eight patients with large fibroids. Menorrhagia was controlled in four of five patients who presented with that symptom; bulk-related symptoms improved in all patients. These authors reported that most of their patients experienced an intermittent nonpurulent vaginal discharge, which was presumed to be necrotic fibroid tissue debris. One patient spontaneously passed a substantial portion of a submucosal fibroid 6 weeks after the procedure. In addition, the authors had one patient, aged 41 years, who became amenorrheic following the procedure. Serum follicle-stimulating hormone was measured at 59.8 IU/L.

A brief report of two patients in Melbourne, Australia, detailed the experience of two patients treated with uterine fibroid embolization (5). One patient did not have adequate control of symptoms and underwent supracervical hysterectomy 26 weeks after her embolization procedure. The pathologic specimen revealed aseptic necrosis of two of the fibroids, with hyaline change of the others.

Burn et al. (6) also have published their results in 14 patients treated at the Chelsea and Westminster Hospital in London. No complications were encountered, and in follow-up of 6 patients, all were significantly improved. There was a mean fibroid volume reduction of 43%.

All of these early studies suggested that this procedure was an effective treatment that was generally well tolerated. Almost overnight, there was rapid growth in interest in this procedure. The story of that growth represents the coming together of technology, public access to information, and interest among patients for an alternative to hysterectomy.

THE GROWTH OF UTERINE EMBOLIZATION FOR FIBROIDS

That this procedure became so rapidly accepted as a part of fibroid therapy is surprising and yet potentially predictable. What is needed for the acceptance of any therapy are providers with the skills to administer it, data showing positive outcomes, and an interest among patients for a new

approach to treatment. Interventional radiologists had the requisite skills for the procedure; in fact, many had experience with a nearly identical procedure used to control postpartum hemorrhage or vaginal bleeding from pelvic malignancies. Thus, the growth of this procedure was not hindered by skills or knowledge in the broad medical community. The procedure can be performed in a standard angiographic suite, and it does not require any new or complex equipment. Most interventionalists could complete their first procedure with materials off their own shelves. Nonetheless, it takes much more than availability to explain the growth.

Another key component was the desire among patients for some alternative to hysterectomy for relief of symptoms from fibroids. Long the mainstay of therapy, hysterectomy suffers from what makes it a successful procedure: the uterus is removed, which completely eliminates menstrual bleeding, the ability to have children, and the chance of recurrence of fibroids. Although very appealing to some patients, this prospect does not meet the hopes of a growing number of women. A new mood has developed over the last decade among some women—that hysterectomy is too final, too radical a solution for them. The long recovery required after surgery also is a problem for a growing number of professional women who juggle work and families. Several widely publicized studies of the overuse of hysterectomy and the variation in the frequency of hysterectomy in this country have fueled a suspicion among some women that when their doctor recommended hysterectomy, there was more to the story. Was it really necessary in their case? Why weren't less invasive alternatives offered or available? Many patients began to seek more information before consenting to hysterectomy.

As this groundswell of interest in alternatives arose, there were no answers from many individual gynecologists or from national organizations such as the American College of Obstetricians and Gynecologists. Patients sought other sources, and the essential tool for that search appeared in the form of the Internet. Very soon after public access to the Internet became widespread, patients began to search the Web for answers to their questions. Web sites became available, first from UCLA, then from Robert Worthington-Kirsch in Philadelphia, Carlos Forcade in New York, and the Georgetown University group. These Web sites explained and, in some cases, promoted this new procedure. The information no longer had to be filtered by a physician but could be accessed directly. Almost as rapidly, chat groups about this procedure arose and served as a vital source of information, referrals, and support for patients interested in this procedure. It is fair to say that the availability of information for patients is in large part responsible for the rapid rate with which this procedure grew.

It is important to understand the distinction between

how the procedure grew so rapidly and why it did so. This procedure never would have grown if there had not been a demand among patients for an alternative to hysterectomy. Patients did not have this procedure because of its merits alone but rather because it did not have all the disadvantages of hysterectomy.

It is important for all involved in fibroid therapies to understand this distinction. The patients of today will accept any proven procedure (even if only proven in the short run) if it meets their goals of less invasive treatment, with less impact on their day-to-day lives. It is particularly important for interventionalists to understand. We have succeeded not because of the intrinsic attractiveness of what we offer but because it is more acceptable than the alternative. Thus, it must be our goal to perfect our technique and patient management skills to optimize our outcomes, because patients continue to see even easier alternatives such as high-frequency ultrasound ablation or new medical therapies currently under development. We have shown that innovation can revolutionize treatment, and it is important that we don't forget that innovation continues.

We describe all the steps necessary for the practitioner to learn about uterine embolization and uterine fibroids. The first section provides a review of the basic science and natural history of fibroids, along with an overview of the anatomy relevant to treatment, the gynecologic evaluation of the patient, pelvic imaging relevant to fibroids, and finally the surgical approach to fibroids. In the second section, we introduce the procedure, preprocedural and postprocedural care, and a review of the pitfalls of the procedure. The third section provides a comprehensive review of the outcome of the procedure, including symptom control, complications,

and pregnancy outcomes. We conclude with a review of two related topics, postpartum hemorrhage and gynecologic hemorrhage, in which many of the techniques used in uterine embolization can be applied.

With this text, the reader is introduced to the state of the art in uterine embolization. This exciting procedure has had a dramatic impact on the management of patients with fibroids and on the practice of interventional radiology. We now provide comprehensive management of a clinical condition in a way that we previously have not. The interventionalist needs to have a comprehensive understanding of this condition to provide the best care. We hope that this text meets that challenge and will become a key tool for those interested in entering this practice.

REFERENCES

1. Ravina, J, Herbreteau D, Ciraru-Vigneron N, et al. Arterial embolisation to treat uterine myomata. *Lancet* 1995;346: 671–672.
2. Goodwin S, Vedantham S, McLucas B, et al. Preliminary experience with uterine artery embolization for uterine fibroids. *J Vasc Interv Radiol* 1997;8:517–526.
3. Ravina J, Bouret J, Cirary-Vigneron N, et al. Application of particulate arterial embolization in the treatment of uterine fibromyomata. *Bull Acad Natl Med* 1997;181:233–243.
4. Bradley E, Reidy J, Forman R, et al. Transcatheter uterine artery embolisation to treat large uterine fibroids. *Br J Obstet Gynaecol* 1998;105:235–240.
5. Kuhn R, Mitchell P. Embolic occlusion of the blood supply to uterine myomas: report of 2 cases. *Aust N Z J Obstet Gynaecol* 1999;39:120–121.
6. Burn P, McCall J, Chinn R, et al. Embolization of uterine fibroids. *Br J Radiol* 1999;72:159–161.

UTERINE FIBROIDS: BACKGROUND AND SIGNIFICANCE FOR UTERINE ARTERY EMBOLIZATION

UCHE EZEH
ELIZABETH A. STEWART

INTRODUCTION

Uterine fibroids (also called *leiomyomas* or *myomata)* are benign tumors arising from the uterine smooth muscle cells and containing significant fibrous connective tissues. Fibroids constitute a major public health care problem. They are the most common gynecologic tumors in women of the reproductive age group, being symptomatic in about 25% to 30% of women but present in as many as 70% to 80% of women by age 50 (1–3). They are a leading indication for surgery in women, accounting for 30% of more than 600,000 hysterectomies performed annually in the United States (4). The economic implications of fibroids are enormous. The annual cost of hysterectomy for fibroids and abnormal uterine bleeding is estimated at $2 billion (5), and the cost for each woman in lost productivity due to menorrhagia amounts to $1,692 per woman per year (6).

Despite the importance and common occurrence of fibroids, research on this disease stalled until recently, probably because fibroids are a common source of morbidity but a rare cause of mortality. However, increasing attention to research on this disorder has brought new insights into the understanding of the biology and has led to the development of novel, less radical alternatives to the traditional treatments of hysterectomy or myomectomy. This chapter reviews this disease with these developments in mind.

PATHOLOGY

Macroscopic Features

Fibroids may grow either as a single tumor or in clusters. Each fibroid is a spherical, firm, bulging tumor. The cut surfaces of a fibroid reveal a tan-white, whorl-like pattern of smooth muscle and fibrous tissues. Although they are not encapsulated, fibroids are well circumscribed so that they can be distinguished or shelled out from the surrounding myometrium.

Each fibroid ranges in size from several millimeters to many centimeters. Sometimes, fibroids can grow to enormous proportions, distorting pelvic anatomy, developing extensive blood supply, and compromising operative fields. Giant fibroids, defined as weighing 25 lb (11.4 kg) or more, are uncommon and can produce pelvic or lower limb thrombosis, respiratory difficulties, secondary polycythemia, or sciatic neuropathy, in addition to distortion of the pelvic anatomy and pressure symptoms (7). The largest-ever reported fibroid weighed 140.2 lb (63.6 kg) (7).

Fibroids are located throughout the uterus. Depending on their locations, they are classified into three main morphologic types: submucosal, subserosal, and intramural, as shown in Figure 2-1. Submucosal fibroids protrude into the uterine cavity, distorting the underlying endometrium, and are more likely to cause abnormal uterine bleeding and reproductive dysfunction rather than pain and pressure symptoms (1). Subserosal fibroids are located on the serosa of the uterus and give the myomatous uterus its characteristic irregular contour. Subserosal fibroids are more likely to cause pressure symptoms, especially if they are large. Intramural fibroids grow wholly within the muscle of the uterus and give it a globular feeling. The intramural type is the most common type, and submucosal variety is the least common. Most women have fibroids that are of the mixed type in terms of their size, number, and location (8). It should be noted that the association between fibroid symptoms on the one hand and the location, size, and growth on the other hand are poorly defined. For example, contrary to earlier thought, a recent study found no association between fibroid location and menorrhagia, although the study relied on ultrasound instead of a technique that more clearly delineates the endometrial cavity (9). Both submucosal and subserosal fibroids can

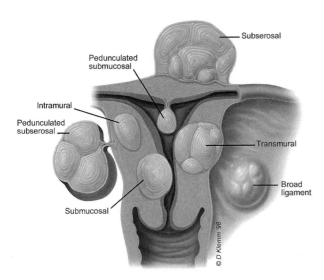

FIGURE 2-1. Nomenclature for fibroids based on location within the uterus.

grow from a stalk to become pedunculated fibroids. Pedunculated subserosal fibroids may attach themselves to adjacent structures such as the bowel, momentum, or mesentery and develop a secondary blood supply, losing its primary uterine blood supply, to become parasitic fibroids, or they may reach into the broad ligament as intraligamentary fibroids, which may be associated with polycythemia. Pedunculated submucosal fibroids may remain sessile or rarely prolapse through the cervical os via the stalk.

Microscopic Features

Microscopically, fibroids, like the adjoining myometrium, consist of uniform spindled-shaped smooth muscle cells arranged in anastomosing fascicles. The cells have abundant eosinophilic cytoplasm and elongated nuclei that are of uniform size, shape, and chromasia. They show no significant mitosis, atypia, or necrosis. These cells, in turn, are surrounded by increased amounts of extracellular matrix. It is the abundance of this extracellular matrix, especially the type I and III collagens, which distinguishes fibroids from the surrounding normal myometrium (10).

Malignant transformation of a fibroid into a leiomyosarcoma is rare at 0.2% to 0.3% if it indeed occurs (11,12). Given the significant differences in karyotypes, some authorities believe that "malignant degeneration" does not occur. Although rare, leiomyosarcomas are clinically important because without a tissue diagnosis, leiomyosarcomas and fibroids can be indistinguishable. In contrast to fibroids, leiomyosarcomas display hypercellularity and a less fascicular pattern, and consist of atypical smooth muscle cells with enlarged nuclei showing hyperchromasia, pleomorphism, increased mitotic activity, and coagulative necrosis. Mitotic index, described as the number of mitosis per 10 high-power fields, is used to distinguish a benign fibroid

from leiomyosarcoma. An index of 10 or more is considered by many to be diagnostic of leiomyosarcoma, but others have disagreed with this critical mitotic count (13,14). Current research is focusing on karyotypic abnormalities and gene expression profile to define malignant potential of fibroids.

It is important to recognize several benign fibroid variants. Both the *cellular* and *symplastic leiomyomas* have one or more of the malignant features noted previously, making prediction of malignant potential of a fibroid difficult. In addition, both *intravenous leiomyomatosis* and *disseminated peritoneal leiomyomatosis* manifest unusual growth patterns. Although these variants have similar histologic features, hormone responsiveness, and cytogenic characteristics similar to benign fibroids, they manifest intraperitoneal and pulmonary metastasis (15).

A number of benign degenerative changes can occur in the fibroid. Hyaline degeneration is the most common type and should not be confused with the coagulative tumor cell necrosis seen in leiomyosarcoma. Red degeneration (necrobiosis) is typically but not exclusively seen in pregnancy. It is often the cause of pain and fever in pregnancy, presenting diagnostic difficulties with other causes of pain such as placenta abruption. Gonadotropin-releasing hormone (GnRH) agonists may lead to substantial degeneration, whereas uterine arterial embolization results in infarction and necrosis (16–18).

Growth

Although large fibroids are more likely to produce morbidity than the small ones, data on fibroid growth are very scanty (19–21). One study followed 31 asymptomatic women with large uteri (greater than 12 weeks' gestation) with magnetic resonance imaging (MRI) and biopsy for 1 year (20). They found that the size of the largest fibroid increased in 50% of the women, 20% of the women had an increase of 50% or more, and growth was related to higher tissue levels of progesterone receptor and higher cellularity of the fibroids. Similarly, a second study reported a greater than 30% increase in fibroid size in 30% of women followed by ultrasound over a 1-year period (19). Earlier studies have reported conflicting reports, ranging from a decline of 15% to an increase of 44% (22,23), but these findings were limited by study design flaws. Given that so many women with fibroids are asymptomatic, why some fibroids grow to produce symptoms in some women but not in others is unknown. This wide variation in fibroid growth among women makes the prediction of the natural history of fibroids very difficult.

The development of myomas appears to entail two critical stages: the transformation of normal myocytes into abnormal myocytes, and their subsequent growth into clinically apparent tumors (24). The high prevalence of microscopic myomas suggests that the first step is quite common (2,25). The subsequent growth occurs via clonal expansion, with each separate myoma growing independently. The independent clonal origin of multiple myomas has been shown by two different polymorphic markers, namely, glucose-6-phosphate dehydrogenase isoenzyme and CAG repeat polymorphism in the X-linked androgen receptor, which demonstrated a random pattern of inactivation among multiple tumors in the same uterus (26,27). These findings confirm the independent origin of each tumor gene.

PATHOPHYSIOLOGY

Steroid Hormones

Little is known about the factors involved in initiation and growth of fibroids. Until recently, the gonadal steroid hormones, especially estrogens, were thought to be the only regulators of fibroid development and growth. The role of estrogens is supported by the clinical observation showing that fibroids arise after menarche, grow, and are common during the reproductive years but regress after menopause or GnRH agonist therapy. Several *in vitro* studies also support the role of these hormones (28–31). The high prevalence of fibroids in the human population raises the possibility of the involvement of environmental toxins in fibroid etiology and pathogenesis. Although direct evidence is lacking in humans, studies using Eker rats suggest that some exogenous estrogen receptor ligands such as organochlorine, pesticides, and dietary flavonoids acting via estrogen receptors could affect fibroid growth (32).

Contrary to the opinion of many clinicians, progesterone appears potentially to be more important than estrogen. This assumption is supported by clinical observations showing that progesterone add-back therapy inhibits GnRH agonist–mediated shrinkage and that antiprogestins such as mifepristone (RU486) cause myoma regression (24,33–35). *In vitro* evidence also supports this contention. Fibroids obtained from patients treated with progesterone show more cellular growth than those from patients without progesterone therapy, and fibroids have higher concentrations of progesterone receptors than normal myometrium (35). Furthermore, it has been proposed that fibroid formation may actually represent an exaggerated and abnormal steroid hormone responsiveness similar to that of a smooth muscle cell response during pregnancy (36). However, many studies on the growth of fibroids coexisting with pregnancy have produced inconsistent findings. Some fibroids were found to be growing, others were shrinking, while others remained unchanged (37). Therefore, it is surprising that even under the same environment that should stimulate fibroid growth, no clear pattern of response is observed.

Recent studies over the last 2 decades have advanced our understanding of the pathogenesis of fibroids beyond ovarian steroid hormones. It now is evident that the growth-promoting, fibrotic, and angiogenesis effects of these hormones are thought to be orchestrated through the activation of many genes for autocrine or paracrine growth factors in the uterus. The critical role of endometrial dysfunction in the pathogenesis of fibroid-related bleeding is also increasingly being appreciated (38). Evidence is emerging that genetic predisposition plays a critical role.

Growth Factors

There is increasing interest in *vascular endothelial growth factor* (VEGF), which causes angiogenesis, because fibroids have an enormous vascular supply and several stages of angiogenesis are dysregulated in fibroids (39,40). It has been shown that steroid hormones regulate uterine VEGF expression at the transcriptional level via the classic nuclear steroid receptor pathway (41). The angiogenic factor *basic fibroblast growth factor* (bFGF) and its type 1 receptor are important in fibroid-related bleeding. They are expressed in higher amounts in fibroids and fibroid-specific extracellular matrix compared with normal controls (42–45).

Both *growth hormone* and *insulin-like growth factors I and II*, which mediate growth hormone function, have been implicated in myoma pathogenesis (46–48). Further support for the role of the growth hormone is the observation that women with acromegaly, a condition characterized by growth hormone excess, have a higher incidence of fibroids (49).

Fibroids can be viewed as a fibrotic process; they demonstrate specific up-regulation of collagens type I and III during specific phases of the menstrual cycle (10). Fibrotic growth factors such as *transforming growth factor-beta* (TGF-β) and *granulocyte-macrophage colony-stimulating factor* (GM-CSF) are elevated in fibroids compared to control. TGF-β3 appears to be significantly involved in the pathophysiology of myomas, being increased at both the RNA and protein levels (50,51). GM-CSF, a TGF-β homologue, differentially stimulates myoma growth relative to the myometrium (52). Dysregulation of the TGF-β receptor/ligand system has been implicated in myoma-associated menorrhagia (40). A novel TGF-β homologue, termed *ebaf* (endometrial bleeding-associated factor), similarly appears to be abnormally expressed in endometrium of women with abnormal uterine bleeding, including those with fibroids (53). Although these findings indicate a central role for these growth factors in fibroid pathology, how they promote fibroid growth is not fully understood.

Genetic Basis

Despite our improved knowledge of the roles of the steroid hormones and growth factors in promoting fibroid growth, the initiators of fibroid development are unknown. However, there is increasing cytogenetic and molecular evidence supporting a genetic basis for fibroids.

There are a number of lines of indirect evidence for the inheritable aspect of fibroids. First, fibroids are about two- to six-fold higher in the first-degree relatives of affected women than in the controls (54). Second, monozygotic twins have twice the rate of concordance for hysterectomy of dizygotic twins, and fibroids are the most common indication for hysterectomy (55). Third, African-American women have twice the incidence of fibroids and have increased severity of disease compared with their Caucasian counterparts (56,57). Fourth, there are a number of inheritable syndromes, such as Reed syndrome, hereditary leiomyomatosis and renal cell cancer (HLRCC), Bannayan-Zonana syndrome, and Cowden disease, of which fibroids are one of the manifestations (58–61).

The neoplastic transformation of myometrium to fibroids may involve somatic mutations of normal myometrium. Karyotypic abnormalities are found in 40% of fibroids (62,63). Four main karyotypic abnormalities are seen: translocation t(12;14), deletion of 3q and 7q, trisomy 12, and rearrangements involving 6p, 10q, and 13q (64). About 20% of karyotypically abnormal fibroids show the characteristic t(12;14), which is the most common abnormality seen. Although age and parity are not related to karyotypic abnormalities, there is a correlation between cytogenetic abnormalities and fibroid size and location (65,66). The incidence of abnormal karyotype varies with fibroid location (intramural 35%, subserosal 29%, submucosal 12%) (66). There also is a correlation between chromosome abnormalities and mean tumor size, suggesting that chromosomal abnormalities associated with individual fibroids enhance fibroid growth or *vice versa* (65). Multiple fibroids from a single uterus harbor different chromosomal changes (64), suggesting multiple gene involvement and supporting the clonal nature of fibroid development. These facts may explain the wide variation in size, growth, and response to hormonal therapy observed among fibroids in the same patient.

Many of the candidate genes identified for fibroids map to the regions involved in the karyotypic groups noted earlier. Disruption of *HMGA2* and *HMGA1* genes by chromosomal rearrangements has been implicated in fibroid formation. These genes normally encode proteins that play a critical role in controlling cell growth by regulating DNA transcription. *HMGA2* (formerly called HMGI-C) is located on chromosome 12, yet most mutations are not intragenic but instead map to the 5' region of this gene (67). *HMGA1* (formerly called HMGI-Y) codes for a related HMG-protein whose gene resides on chromosome 6p (68,69).

Another gene, *RAD51L1* (also called hREC2), located on chromosome 14q23-24, encodes an enzyme that repairs double-stranded DNA breaks, and has also been implicated

in fibroid formation. However, a fusion event involving *HMGA2* and *RAD51L1* via t(12;14)(q15;q23-24) translocation is no longer thought to be a major molecular mechanism for fibroid formation (70–72).

The Multiple Leiomyoma Consortium demonstrated a role for mitochondrial defects in the etiology of myomas. *Fumarase hydratase* (FH), which catalyzes a critical step in the Krebs tricarboxylic cycle, maps to chromosome 1q42.3-43 and appears to act as a tumor suppressor gene. Germline FH mutations were described in individuals with HLRCC and Reed syndrome (61). However, the mechanism by which FH acts as a tumor suppressor gene and its association with fibroid formation are unknown. Another tumor suppressor gene mutation, *PTEN,* has been reported in individuals with Bannayan-Zonana syndrome (59). Although these genes have been found in hereditary fibroid-associated syndromes, it is unknown whether these mutations lead to the development of sporadic fibroids. Current attention is focused on the use of genome wide scan and microarray technology to identify more susceptibility genes for fibroids (73).

EPIDEMIOLOGY

Although the exact cause of fibroids is unknown, several risk factors for fibroids are recognized. Race is an important risk factor. African-American women are at two to three times greater risk for developing fibroids than their Caucasian counterparts (3,56,74). They also are more likely to develop the disease at an earlier age and are disproportionately affected by more multiple and larger fibroids (3,56,74,75). Consequently, they run a greater risk of anemia and surgery and their associated complications (75,76). Although extensive prospective studies in other races have not been conducted, this variation supports the genetic basis of this disease. Overweight or obese women are at a slightly higher risk (74,77). This may be due to extragonadal estrogens, which are stored in body fat. Women with occult obesity and upper body fat distribution are particularly at risk (77).

Reproductive characteristics affect the risk of fibroids. Pregnancy and parity appear to be protective. Baird and Dunson (78) have hypothesized that this protection is due to postpartum tissue remodeling during uterine involution, which eliminated small fibroids. Their observation requires further confirmation. With regard to the use of oral contraceptives, studies suggest that combined pills do not increase the growth of uterine fibroids and may in fact decrease the bleeding and dysmenorrhea associated with fibroids (79,80). Evidence from the Nurses' Health Study suggests that timing of the combined oral contraceptive pill is important with regard to the risk of developing fibroids. Exposure early in reproductive life (13–16 years of age) increases the risk, whereas use in the general population shows protection in relation to the duration of use (80).

Environmental factors may play a role in the risk of fibroid development. Smoking as well as eating fruits and vegetables appear to be protective, whereas excessive consumption of red meat increases risk (81–83). However, there is no evidence that nutritional adjustments or changes in lifestyle result in relief of fibroid size or symptoms.

Presentation

Although about 70% of women with fibroids are asymptomatic, fibroids constitute a major health issue for women. Morbidity includes abnormal uterine bleeding, pelvic pressure and pain, and reproductive dysfunction.

Abnormal Uterine Bleeding

Abnormal menstrual bleeding is the most common symptom associated with fibroids and is the main indication for therapy. This typically presents as menorrhagia (prolonged or excessive uterine bleeding occurring at regular intervals) or polymenorrhea (frequent menstrual bleeding occurring every 21 days or less) often with clot formation. Intermenstrual bleeding or metromenorrhagia (menstrual bleeding that is excessive and irregular in amount and duration) often occur and should be investigated to rule out an endometrial disease such as polyps, hyperplasia, or carcinoma. Abnormal uterine bleeding may lead to iron deficiency anemia and interfere with social, work, and sexual activities. The location, size, and number of fibroids determine the bleeding risk. Bigger and multiple fibroids as well as submucosal fibroids or those intruding into the endometrial cavity produce more bleeding than other types. The exact mechanism by which fibroids result in abnormal menstrual bleeding remains unknown. However, a number of mechanisms have been postulated, including fibroids altering the contraction pattern of the uterus, which in turn prevents the uterus from controlling the degree of bleeding during menstruation, or bulky fibroids compressing veins in the wall of the uterus, causing their dilation and increased bleeding. Evidence is emerging that abnormalities in blood vessels and angiogenic growth factors rather than mechanical factors may in fact be responsible for fibroid-related bleeding (40,84).

Pressure Effects and Pain

Pressure effects arise as the size of the fibroid increases. Such pressure symptoms may feel like heaviness, a dull ache, or bloating. When they compress the nerve supply to the pelvis and the legs, they cause pain in the back, legs, or suprapubic region. They may press on adjacent structures, producing urinary symptoms from anterior fibroids, constipation from the posterior ones, and dyspareunia from general pressure effects. Rarely, acute pain can result from fibroid degeneration or torsion of pedunculated fibroids. Severe dysmenorrhea during a menstrual cycle can occur either with fibroid alone or more commonly when they coexist with other conditions such as pelvic inflammatory disease, adhesions, or endometriosis.

Fibroids and Reproduction

The relationship between fibroids and infertility remains controversial. Advances in fibroid treatment and assisted reproduction have increased tremendously the chances of pregnancy in patients with fibroids. Although distortion of the endometrial cavity by submucosal fibroids can increase the risk of infertility (85), the role of intramural or subserosal fibroids in causing infertility or adversely affecting the outcome of assisted conception therapy remains controversial (86). Therefore, in infertile couples, other factors of infertility should be assessed before addressing the role of uterine fibroids. Fibroids can cause pregnancy complications such as spontaneous abortion, preterm labor, placental previa, malpresentation, or dystocia (87,88). The risk of placental abruption is significantly increased if a myoma is located under the placenta (87,88).

Establishing Diagnosis in Fibroids

The diagnosis of fibroids usually is suspected by the palpation of an enlarged uterus with an irregular contour with or without the symptoms mentioned earlier and confirmed by pelvic ultrasound. Ultrasound is highly accurate for the diagnosis of fibroids and has been reported to be as efficient as MRI in detecting myoma presence (89). Ultrasonography also excludes the possibility of ovarian neoplasm and maps the size and location of the fibroids. MRI provides a better resolution of the individual fibroid and therefore better fibroid mapping. However, for most clinical indications, the cost of MRI can hardly be justified. Contrary to wide belief that a rapid fibroid growth is suggestive of malignant transformation to leiomyosarcoma, this has been found not to be the case (11,90). Age or prior radiation exposure is associated with a high risk of leiomyosarcoma (12). Both endometrial or fibroid biopsy and MRI may occasionally help in distinguishing fibroids and leiomyosarcoma (91,92), but they have their limitations (13).

TREATMENT

Expectant Management

Various factors, including the presence of symptoms, uterine size, fibroid number and location, patient age, proximity to menopause, obstetric intentions, and the surgeon's skills, influence the decision to treat symptomatic women. For example, asymptomatic fibroids usually require no treatment other than surveillance with gynecologic examination or ultrasonography at 6- to 12-month intervals. Similarly, expectant management rather than intervention is adopted in postmenopausal women with fibroids as the tumor size and associated symptoms gradually reduce. However, in women on hormone replacement therapy, the tumor and symptoms may continue or reoccur (93). Nevertheless, if the mass is thought to be a sarcoma rather than uterine fibroids, further evaluation or intervention rather than expectant management becomes necessary. In rare situations, intervention is warranted where renal function is compromised by obstructive uropathy from fibroids, which may not be causing obvious symptoms. The potential risk of compromising fertility by adhesions from surgery must be taken into consideration in patients planning future pregnancy in whom asymptomatic fibroids are found.

Surgical Therapy

Surgery in the form of abdominal hysterectomy or myomectomy has been the traditional treatment for symptomatic fibroids.

Abdominal Hysterectomy

Hysterectomy provides the only cure for symptomatic fibroids and offers increased quality of life. All other alternative forms of treatment allow new fibroids to form or small ones to grow bigger. However, fertility is lost with hysterectomy. Hysterectomy can be in the form of total or supracervical (subtotal). Supracervical hysterectomy is increasingly being performed because of the belief that sexual function is enhanced (94,95). Some studies show that supracervical hysterectomy does not increase sexual function compared to total hysterectomy (96,97). The increasing use of supracervical hysterectomy has some implications for women with fibroids. About 7% percent of women who had supracervical hysterectomy have cyclical bleeding following surgery, but whether the risk is increased in women with myomas requires further clarification (98). Moreover, cervical fibroids may develop in the cervical stump following this type of hysterectomy. Another form of hysterectomy often performed is vaginal hysterectomy after shrinking the fibroid size using GnRH agonists. This has the advantage of avoiding abdominal incisions and allowing a shorter hospital stay.

Abdominal Myomectomy

Abdominal myomectomy (removal of fibroids while preserving the uterus) used to be the only alternative surgery to hysterectomy in women desirous of further childbearing or having a strong aversion to hysterectomy. Interestingly, both share similar morbidity in terms of abdominal incision, operative time, blood loss, and hospital stay (99,100). Although myomectomy offers the main advan-

tage of preserving reproductive function, there is an estimated 11% to 26% risk of subsequent surgery due to recurrent or new fibroids (101,102). Following myomectomy, adhesion formation may compromise future fertility, especially if microsurgical principles are not used and bleeding is not properly controlled. Pregnancy after abdominal myomectomy is safe. Contrary to clinical assumptions, associated scar rupture in labor, even after transmural incisions, is extremely rare at 0.002% compared with 0.1% for previous classical cesarean section (103).

Minimally Invasive Techniques

Traditional surgery entails general anesthesia, long hospital stay and recovery periods, and disruption at work and home. Consequently, many women with symptomatic fibroids are averse to surgery despite their burden of suffering and are actively looking for alternatives to traditional surgical treatment (7). This drive for less invasive forms of therapy and the need to reduce health care costs have led to the development of alternatives to the traditional surgical approaches. These alternatives include laparoscopic myomectomy, myolysis, hysteroscopic fibroid resection, endometrial ablation, and bilateral uterine artery embolization.

Laparoscopic Myomectomy

Laparoscopic myomectomy is the removal of fibroids guided by a telescope placed at the umbilicus and abdominal incisions, usually two to four small ones. Although it involves small incisions and a quicker recovery time, it is limited by the need for high surgical skill and by the number and size of myomas. It is ideal for women with a small number of subserosal or intramural fibroids in whom the uterus is small enough to allow the insertion of a laparoscope in order to obtain an appropriate view of the operating field. Optimal conditions include uterine size equivalent or less than 16 weeks, fibroids measuring 8 cm or less in diameter, and removal of one or two myomas (104). Whether laparoscopic reapproximation of the myometrium gives the same tensile strength as a multilayer technique used at laparotomy remains controversial. There are reports of uterine rupture as early as 33 to 34 weeks of gestation, even when uterine repair is conducted via a minilaparotomy (105,106).

Myolysis

In this technique, electric current is delivered via diathermy needles or lasers in order to coagulate the fibroids during laparoscopy instead of removing them. Experience with this technique is limited (107). Although this technique is easier to master than removal or suturing, localized destruction without repair may increase the chance of rupture and adhesion formation. Use of an electronic morcellator during laparoscopic surgery offers an alternative to myolysis, allows the fibroids to be removed via an incision far smaller than the fibroid size, and permits tissues to be obtained for pathologic examination.

Hysteroscopic Approaches

These include two approaches—hysteroscopic myomectomy and endometrial ablation. Like laparoscopy, the hysteroscopic approach requires highly skilled surgeons but offers the major advantage of being an outpatient procedure and, in many cases, use of regional or local analgesia combined with conscious sedation, which eases recuperation. Severe complications, such as uterine perforation and fluid overload from the distending medium, can occur.

Hysteroscopic Myomectomy.   In this procedure, the fibroids are resected with an operative endoscope placed through the cervix. The primary goal is amelioration of fibroid-related bleeding and, to a lesser degree, reduction in fibroid size. This procedure is mainly indicated for patients with submucosal fibroids. Symptomatic relief is good; fewer than 16% of women undergoing hysteroscopic resection of submucosal fibroids who were treated for menorrhagia required a second procedure within 9 years (108). Subsequent fertility rates are good, with 59% of patients conceiving in another series (109). There has been no case report of uterine rupture during pregnancy after hysteroscopic myomectomy.

Endometrial Ablation.   For women who have completed childbearing and for whom bleeding is the primary problem, endometrial ablation alone or in combination with hysteroscopic myomectomy may give relief by destroying the endometrial lining through various means, including laser, thermal energy, physical resection, or cryotherapy balloon. Endometrial ablation in patients with fibroids is less effective in controlling bleeding than that done for dysfunctional uterine bleeding, with failure rates of 40% versus 5%, respectively (110). Although most case series of endometrial ablations have excluded patients with substantial myomas, one study of endometrial ablation with hysteroscopic myomectomy showed that only 8% of women needed a second procedure after a mean follow-up of 6 years (108).

Uterine Artery Embolization

This is a novel technique for the treatment of fibroids whereby uterine vessels are embolized or occluded in order to decrease blood supply to the fibroids. This technique will be covered in greater detail in subsequent chapters.

Medical Therapy

There is no reliable evidence that the traditional treatment of myoma-related bleeding with oral contraceptive or progestogen therapy is effective. Nonsteroidal antiinflammatory agents or antifibrinologic agents, which are effective for treating idiopathic menorrhagia, have not been properly studied with fibroid-related menorrhagia. The situation is similar with androgenic agents such as danazol and gestrinone. However, a number of new therapies are emerging as the biology of this disease becomes better understood.

Gonadotropin-Releasing Hormone Agonists

GnRH agonists are the most effective medical therapy currently available for the treatment of myomas, but discontinuation of treatment results in rapid return of symptoms and tumor volume. GnRH is the native hypothalamic hormone that, when released in a pulsatile fashion, stimulates the entire reproductive endocrine axis. GnRH agonists disrupt this pulsatile system and lead to initial stimulation, followed by longtime suppression of the entire hormonal system similar to that seen in prepubertal girls. Several formulations are available in the United States, including goserelin acetate implant (Zoladex), leuprolide acetate depot injection (Lupron), and nafarelin acetate nasal spray (Synarel). Leuprolide acetate is US Food and Drug Administration (FDA) approved for use with iron in the preoperative treatment of leiomyomas. Other agents and indications are off-label uses.

GnRH agonists are expensive and cause significant side effects, such as postmenopausal symptoms and osteoporosis if they are used beyond 6 months. Surgically they can make the uterus softer and surgical planes less distinct. However, they produce 30% to 60% volume reduction and amenorrhea in most women over 3 to 6 months of use (111). Consequently, GnRH agonists are used to build up the preoperative hematocrit level and reduce the size of the uterus to enable vaginal hysterectomy, easier abdominal hysterectomy, and a smaller and more cosmetic abdominal incision. The side effects and high cost of GnRH agonists must be weighed against these benefits.

Gonadotropin-Releasing Hormone Agonists and Add-Back Therapy

For many women, 3 to 6 months of therapy with GnRH agonists does not prevent them from undergoing surgery. To prolong the use of GnRH agonists beyond 6 months while minimizing the side effects, two main types of add-back regimens are in use: simultaneous and sequential administration. With simultaneous regimens, both the GnRH agonists and the add-back regimen are started at the same time, whereas in the sequential model, the GnRH agonists are given for 3 to 6 months, after which the add-back therapy is started. Recent studies suggest that both models can be effective if properly given (112,113).

Progestins used in a simultaneous fashion antagonized the fibroid volume reduction effect of GnRH agonists, unlike the sequential regimen (87). It has been shown that the simultaneous add-back therapy with low-dose estradiol produced fibroid volume reduction and amenorrhea without endometrial hyperplasia (87). Recent studies using more modern imaging techniques contradicted earlier studies, which used unreliable outcome measures such as size on bimanual examination to show that progestins induce uterine shrinkage in fibroid uterus (87).

More innovative forms of add-back therapies are being studied. Results similar to those obtained with combined pills were obtained using selective estrogen receptor modulators, such as tamoxifen and raloxifene, in combination with GnRH agonists in a sequential fashion for add-back therapy (114,115). Raloxifene differs from tamoxifen in its lack of agonist activity in the uterine activity. Studies with another selective estrogen receptor modulator, clomiphene, show an increase rather than a decrease in the size of fibroids (116,117). Animal studies with these two modulators show a 40% to 60% reduction in tumor incidence without the use of GnRH agonists (118). In a study of postmenopausal women receiving raloxifene, there was a decrease in uterine and myoma size but no change in bleeding patterns (119). This is not surprising because raloxifene lacks agonist activity in the uterus. However, studies in premenopausal women show that raloxifene is not effective for management of fibroids without GnRH agonists (120).

Tibolone, a synthetic steroid, has estrogenic, progestational, and androgenic activities. In postmenopausal women with fibroids, it is associated with alleviation of climacteric symptoms and prevention of osteoporosis without endometrial stimulation and produced a higher rate of amenorrhea than conventional hormone replacement therapy (121). In premenopausal women with fibroids, tibolone used as sequential add-back therapy with GnRH agonists preserved bone density and lipid profiles without reversal of uterine shrinkage (122); therefore, tibolone has good potential as a single-agent add-back therapy in the future.

Gonadotropin-Releasing Hormone Antagonists

GnRH antagonists, including ganirelix acetate (Antigone) and cetrorelix acetate (Cetrotide), currently are FDA approved for use in superovulation. Although not approved for the treatment of fibroids, GnRH antagonists have several advantages over GnRH agonists. They have no flare effect, so the rare instance of heavy bleeding that is seen with the agonist at the start of therapy is absent. They have a rapid onset of action, with a decrease in steroidal levels seen within 48 hours and significant clinical effects in less than 1 month (123,124); therefore, they are very suitable for preoperative fibroid volume reduction.

Progesterone Antagonists

Mifepristone (RU486) is a steroid that binds and primarily inhibits progesterone receptors. The resulting 48% reduction in fibroid volume seen at 12 weeks and the induction of amenorrhea are equivalent to that seen with GnRH agonists (34,125). Unlike therapy with GnRH agonists, the follicular concentrations of estradiol are maintained. Mifepristone produced mild hot flushes in 20% of patients during the first month of use and may produce simple endometrial hyperplasia without atypia (126). However, a recent study suggests that mifepristone in doses of 5 or 10 mg produces comparable fibroid regression, improvement in symptoms, and fewer side effects than the 25-mg dose previously used or GnRH agonists (127). The prototype of a new generation of selective progesterone receptor modulators, J867 (Asoprisnil), is currently undergoing clinical trials for the treatment of myomas (128).

Growth Factor-Directed Treatments

Growth factor manipulation provides another avenue to treat fibroids. Recent studies have shown that antagonists against the angiogenic factor *bFGF*, the fibrotic growth factor *TGF-β*, and *insulin-like growth factors I* and *II*, which mediate the effect of growth hormone (GH), are effective against fibroids. Angiogenic factor bFGF and its type 1 receptor are important in fibroid-related bleeding. It has been shown that interferon-α reverses the proliferative action of bFGF and can produce clinically significant myoma reduction while maintaining regular menses throughout treatment (129). The observation that women with acromegaly have a high incidence of myomas gave rise to growth hormone manipulation as novel way to treat fibroids. Lanreotide, a long-acting somatostatin analogue, has been shown to produce temporary reduction of 24% to 42% in fibroid volume after 3 months of therapy and permanent reduction of 17% to 29% (130). Levels of estradiol remain unaffected during therapy. Manipulation of the fibrotic growth factor system and other growth factors is still being investigated.

Image-Guided Approaches

The gold standard for assessing both the safety and accuracy of surgical techniques has been direct visualization, which in open procedures can be augmented by palpation. However, the traditional surgical approach allows only one view. In minimally invasive surgeries, the three-dimensional view is absent, and the visualization of structures is often restricted by limitations of the equipment, such as the angle of the endoscope. In contrast, image-guided therapy offers several advantages for the treatment of fibroids. It allows the operator to view the operating structure in three dimensions and to visualize from the serosal to mucosal surface and the intramural portion of the uterus. In addition, image-guided therapy can identify other relevant tissues, such as the bladder or bowel. Both ultrasound and MRI can direct image-guided therapy.

Although ultrasound has the advantages of ease and less expense, MRI is preferable in certain circumstances. First, the ability of MRI to delineate and characterize lesions in the uterine wall is superior to that of ultrasound. Therefore, MRI-guided therapy may be preferable in instances where it is important to distinguish between multiple individual intramural fibroids versus one large myoma, or where the lesion is suggestive of adenomyosis instead of a fibroid. Second, with the increasing use of thermally ablative therapies, the capacity of MRI to measure temperature shifts in real time allows for both accuracy in targeting and complete tissue destruction. Using assessment of the proton shift capacity, very small temperature shifts can be detected. This allows the initial use of energy too low to cause tissue destruction to be delivered and detected to confirm targeting accuracy. In addition, by monitoring peak temperature during treatment, it allows confirmation of the completeness of tissue destruction without concern about injury to surrounding tissue. It is this combination of accuracy and safety that may make image-guided therapy far more cost effective and safer than surgical therapy. With these image techniques, therapy for fibroids can be performed using laser ablation, cryomyolysis, or high-density focused ultrasound.

Percutaneous Laser Ablation, Cryomyolysis, and High-Density Focused Ultrasound

In percutaneous laser ablation, percutaneously placed laser fibers placed under MRI guidance are used for the treatment of fibroids. The fibroid volume decreased by 37.5% after 3 months of therapy and a significant reduction in menorrhagia after 12 months (131,132). In cryomyolysis, this thermal ablation technique (guided by MRI instead of laparoscopy) is used to freeze fibroid tissue, resulting in its destruction. A case report of image-guided cryomyolysis involving two patients showed a mean reduction in fibroid size of 53% to 65% at 8 weeks (133,134). Like laser, ultrasound can be amplified and collated into a therapeutic modality capable of delivering a large amount of energy to target tissues in a noninvasive way. Treatment may be accomplished by placing a transducer against the abdomen as is currently done for diagnostic ultrasound, targeting an intraabdominal fibroid without breaching the skin. The intensity of high-density focused ultrasound used for treatment is significantly higher than that used for diagnostic ultrasound and can rapidly increase the temperature at the focal point in excess of 70°C to produce coagulative necrosis of the fibroids. Preliminary studies in humans reveal significant reduction in fibroid volume and

symptoms, and the therapy is associated with minimal morbidity (135).

CONCLUSION

Fibroids are the most common gynecologic tumors, produce significant morbidity, and constitute the most common indication for hysterectomy. Health care costs and the impact on quality of life are enormous. Abdominal hysterectomy and myomectomy are the traditional treatments for this disorder.

The quest for less invasive forms of treatment has given rise to a number of minimally invasive techniques, including laparoscopic and hysteroscopic myomectomy, myolysis, and endometrial ablation. Image-guided therapy may offer advantages over the traditional or minimally invasive approaches in that it allows a more detailed and three-dimensional view of the structures of interest. This may provide a more targeted approach to therapy. Recent years have also seen progress in medical therapies and the development of potentially very effective alternatives to procedures for some patients. A better understanding of the biology of fibroids has allowed the developments of antagonists to growth factors and the steroid hormones. Limitations in the duration of therapy due to side effects and subsequent tumor regrowth remain a major impediment to the broad use of these medical therapies to date, but newer alternatives are on the horizon. In the longer term, discovery of the genetic basis of fibroids may provide novel preventive and permanent therapeutic modalities.

REFERENCES

1. Buttram VC Jr, Reiter RC. Uterine leiomyomata: etiology, symptomatology, and management. *Fertil Steril* 1981;36:433–445.
2. Cramer SF, Patel A. The frequency of uterine leiomyomas. *Am J Clin Pathol* 1990;94:435–438.
3. Baird DD, Dunson DB, Hill MC, et al. High cumulative incidence of uterine leiomyoma in black and white women: ultrasound evidence. *Obstet Gynecol* 2003;188:100–107.
4. Wilcox LS, Koonin LM, Pokras R, et al. Hysterectomy in the United States, 1988-1990. *Obstet Gynecol* 1994;83:549–555.
5. Zhao SZ, Wong JM, Arguelles LM. Hospitalization costs associated with leiomyoma. *Clin Ther* 1999;21:563–575.
6. Cote I, Jacobs P, Cumming D. Work loss associated with increased menstrual loss in the United States. *Obstet Gynecol* 2002;100:683–687.
7. Oelsner G, Elizur SE, Frenkel Y, et al. Giant uterine tumors: two cases with different clinical presentations. *Obstet Gynecol* 2003;101[Pt 2]:1088–1091.
8. Pron G, Cohen M, Soucie J, et al. The Ontario Uterine Fibroid Embolization Trial. Part 1. Baseline patient characteristics, fibroid burden, and impact on life. *Fertil Steril* 2003;79:112–119.

9. Wegienka G, Baird DD, Hertz-Picciotto I, et al. Self-reported heavy bleeding associated with uterine leiomyomata. *Obstet Gynecol* 2003;101:431–437.

10. Stewart EA, Friedman AJ, Peck K, et al. Relative overexpression of collagen type I and collagen type III messenger ribonucleic acids by uterine leiomyomas during the proliferative phase of the menstrual cycle. *J Clin Endocrinol Metab* 1994;79:900–906.

11. Parker WH, Fu YS, Berek JS. Uterine sarcoma in patients operated on for presumed leiomyoma and rapidly growing leiomyoma. *Obstet Gynecol* 1994;83:414–418.

12. Leibsohn S, d'Ablaing G, Mishell DR Jr, et al. Leiomyosarcoma in a series of hysterectomies performed for presumed uterine leiomyomas. *Am J Obstet Gynecol* 1990;162:968–974, discussion 974–966.

13. Kawamura N, Ito F, Ichimura T, et al. Transient rapid growth of uterine leiomyoma in a postmenopausal woman. *Oncol Rep* 1999;6:1289–1292.

14. Kawamura N, Ichimura T, Takahashi K, et al. Transcervical needle biopsy of uterine myoma-like tumors using an automatic biopsy gun. *Fertil Steril* 2002;77:1060–1064.

15. Quade BJ, Dal Cin P, Neskey DM, et al. Intravenous leiomyomatosis: molecular and cytogenetic analysis of a case. *Mod Pathol* 2002;15:351–356.

16. Robboy SJ, Bentley RC, Butnor K, et al. Pathology and pathophysiology of uterine smooth-muscle tumors. *Environ Health Perspect* 2000;108[Suppl 5]:779–784.

17. Colgan TJ, Pendergast S, LeBlanc M. The histopathology of uterine leiomyomas following treatment with gonadotropin-releasing hormone analogues. *Hum Pathol* 1993;24:1073–1077.

18. Colgan TJ, Pron G, Mocarski EJ, et al. Pathologic features of uteri and leiomyomas following uterine artery embolization for leiomyomas. *Am J Surg Pathol* 2003;27:167–177.

19. Tsuda H, Kawabata M, Nakamoto O, et al. Clinical predictors in the natural history of uterine leiomyoma: preliminary study. *J Ultrasound Med* 1998;17:17–20.

20. Ichimura T, Kawamura N, Ito F, et al. Correlation between the growth of uterine leiomyomata and estrogen and progesterone receptor content in needle biopsy specimens. *Fertil Steril* 1998;70:967–971.

21. DeWaay DJ, Syrop CH, Nygaard IE, et al. Natural history of uterine polyps and leiomyomata. *Obstet Gynecol* 2002;100:3–7.

22. Audebert AJ, Madenelat P, Querleu D, et al. Deferred versus immediate surgery for uterine fibroids: clinical trial results. *Br J Obstet Gynaecol* 1994;101[Suppl 10]:29–32.

23. Schlaff WD, Zerhouni EA, Huth JA, et al. A placebo-controlled trial of a depot gonadotropin-releasing hormone analogue (leuprolide) in the treatment of uterine leiomyomata. *Obstet Gynecol* 1989;74:856–862.

24. Rein MS, Barbieri RL, Friedman AJ. Progesterone: a critical role in the pathogenesis of uterine myomas. *Am J Obstet Gynecol* 1995;172[1 Pt 1]:14–18.

25. Stewart EA. Uterine fibroids. *Lancet* 2001;357:293–298.

26. Linder D, Gartler SM. Glucose-6-phosphate dehydrogenase mosaicism: utilization as a cell marker in the study of leiomyomas. *Science* 1965;150:67–69.

27. Mashal RD, Fejzo ML, Friedman AJ, et al. Analysis of androgen receptor DNA reveals the independent clonal origins of uterine leiomyomata and the secondary nature of cytogenetic aberrations in the development of leiomyomata. *Genes Chromosomes Cancer* 1994;11:1–6.

28. Puukka MJ, Kontula KK, Kauppila AJ, et al. Estrogen receptor in human myoma tissue. *Mol Cell Endocrinol* 1976;6:35–44.

29. Pollow K, Geilfuss J, Boquoi E, et al. Estrogen and progesterone binding proteins in normal human myometrium and leiomyoma tissue. *J Clin Chem Clin Biochem* 1978;16:503–511.

30. Sumitani H, Shozu M, Segawa T, et al. In situ estrogen synthesized by aromatase P450 in uterine leiomyomas cells promotes cell growth probably via an autocrine/intracrine mechanism. *Endocrinology* 2000;141:3852–3861.

31. Shozu M, Sumitani H, Segawa T, et al. Inhibition of in situ expression of aromatase P450 in leiomyoma of the uterus by leuprorelin acetate. *J Clin Endocrinol Metab* 2001;86:5405–5411.

32. Hunter DS, Hodges LC, Eagon PK, et al. Influence of exogenous estrogen receptor ligands on uterine leiomyoma: evidence from an in vitro/in vivo animal model for uterine fibroids. *Environ Health Perspect* 2000;108[Suppl 5]:829–834.

33. Carr BR, Marshburn PB, Weatherall PT, et al. An evaluation of the effect of gonadotropin-releasing hormone analogs and medroxyprogesterone acetate on uterine leiomyomata volume by magnetic resonance imaging: a prospective, randomized, double blind, placebo-controlled, crossover trial. *J Clin Endocrinol Metab* 1993;76:1217–1223.

34. Murphy AA, Kettel LM, Morales AJ, et al. Regression of uterine leiomyomata in response to the antiprogesterone RU 486. *J Clin Endocrinol Metab* 1993;76:513–517.

35. Rein MS. Advances in uterine leiomyoma research: the progesterone hypothesis. *Environ Health Perspect* 2000;108[Suppl 5]:791–793.

36. Andersen J, Barbieri RL. Abnormal gene expression in uterine leiomyomas. *J Soc Gynecol Investig* 1995;2:663–672.

37. Strobelt N, Ghidini A, Cavallone M, et al. Natural history of uterine leiomyomas in pregnancy. *J Ultrasound Med* 1994;13:399–401.

38. Stewart EA, Strauss JF. Uterine fibroids, adenomyosis and endometrial polyps. In: Barbieri RL, Strauss JF, eds. *Yen and Jaffe's reproductive endocrinology,* 5th ed. *(in press).*

39. Torry RJ, Rongish BJ. Angiogenesis in the uterus: potential regulation and relation to tumor angiogenesis. *Am J Reprod Immunol* 1992;27:171–179.

40. Stewart EA, Nowak RA. Leiomyoma-related bleeding: a classic hypothesis updated for the molecular era. *Hum Reprod Update* 1996;2:295–306.

41. Hyder SM, Huang JC, Nawaz Z, et al. Regulation of vascular endothelial growth factor expression by estrogens and progestins. *Environ Health Perspect* 2000;108[Suppl 5]:785–790.

42. Vlodavsky I, Folkman J, Sullivan R, et al. Endothelial cell-derived basic fibroblast growth factor: synthesis and deposition into subendothelial extracellular matrix. *Proc Natl Acad Sci U S A* 1987;84:2292–2296.

43. Mangrulkar RS, Ono M, Ishikawa M, et al. Isolation and characterization of heparin-binding growth factors in human leiomyomas and normal myometrium. *Biol Reprod* 1995;53:636–646.

44. Anania CA, Stewart EA, Quade BJ, et al. Expression of the fibroblast growth factor receptor in women with leiomyomas and abnormal uterine bleeding. *Mol Hum Reprod* 1997;3:685–691.

45. Lee BS, Stewart EA, Sahakian M, et al. Interferon-alpha is a potent inhibitor of basic fibroblast growth factor-stimulated cell proliferation in human uterine cells. *Am J Reprod Immunol* 1998;40:19–25.

46. Rein MS, Friedman AJ, Pandian MR, et al. The secretion of insulin-like growth factors I and II by explant cultures of fibroids and myometrium from women treated with a gonadotropin-releasing hormone agonist. *Obstet Gynecol* 1990;76[3 Pt 1]:388–394.

47. Vollenhoven BJ, Herington AC, Healy DL. Messenger ribonucleic acid expression of the insulin-like growth factors

and their binding proteins in uterine fibroids and myometrium. *J Clin Endocrinol Metab* 1993;76:1106–1110.

48. Giudice LC, Irwin JC, Dsupin BA, et al. Insulin-like growth factor (IGF), IGF binding protein (IGFBP), and IGF receptor gene expression and IGFBP synthesis in human uterine leiomyomata. *Hum Reprod* 1993;8:1796–1806.

49. Cohen O, Schindel B, Homburg R. Uterine leiomyomata—a feature of acromegaly. *Hum Reprod* 1998;13:1945–1946.

50. Lee BS, Nowak RA. Human leiomyoma smooth muscle cells show increased expression of transforming growth factor-beta 3 (TGF beta 3) and altered responses to the antiproliferative effects of TGF beta. *J Clin Endocrinol Metab* 2001;86:913–920.

51. Arici A, I S. Transforming growth factor-[beta]3 is expressed at high levels in leiomyoma where it stimulates fibronectin expression and cell proliferation. *Fertil Steril* 2000;73:1006–1011.

52. Chegini N, Tang XM, Ma C. Regulation of transforming growth factor-beta1 expression by granulocyte macrophage-colony-stimulating factor in leiomyoma and myometrial smooth muscle cells. *J Clin Endocrinol Metab* 1999;84:4138–4143.

53. Kothapalli R, Buyuksal I, Wu SQ, et al. Detection of ebaf, a novel human gene of the transforming growth factor beta superfamily association of gene expression with endometrial bleeding. *J Clin Invest* 1997;99:2342–2350.

54. Kurbanova MK, Koroleva AG, Sergeev AS. [Genetic-epidemiologic analysis of uterine myoma: assessment of repeated risk]. *Genetika* 1989;25:1896–1898.

55. Treloar SA, Martin NG, Dennerstein L, et al. Pathways to hysterectomy: insights from longitudinal twin research. *Am J Obstet Gynecol* 1992;167:82–88.

56. Kjerulff KH, Langenberg P, Seidman JD, et al. Uterine leiomyomas. Racial differences in severity, symptoms and age at diagnosis. *J Reprod Med* 1996;41:483–490.

57. Marshall LM, Spiegelman D, Barbieri RL, et al. Variation in the incidence of uterine leiomyoma among premenopausal women by age and race. *Obstet Gynecol* 1997;90:967–973.

58. Reed WB, Walker R, Horowitz R. Cutaneous leiomyomata with uterine leiomyomata. *Acta Derm Venereol* 1973;53:409–416.

59. Marsh DJ, Dahia PL, Zheng Z, et al. Germline mutations in PTEN are present in Bannayan-Zonana syndrome [Letter]. *Nat Genet* 1997;16:333–334.

60. Launonen V, Vierimaa O, Kiuru M, et al. Inherited susceptibility to uterine leiomyomas and renal cell cancer. *Proc Natl Acad Sci U S A* 2001;98:3387–3392.

61. Tomlinson IP, Alam NA, Rowan AJ, et al. Germline mutations in FH predispose to dominantly inherited uterine fibroids, skin leiomyomata and papillary renal cell cancer. *Nat Genet* 2002;30:406–410.

62. Nilbert M, Heim S, Mandahl N, et al. Trisomy 12 in uterine leiomyomas. A new cytogenetic subgroup. *Cancer Genet Cytogenet* 1990;45:63–66.

63. Rein MS, Friedman AJ, Barbieri RL, et al. Cytogenetic abnormalities in uterine leiomyomata. *Obstet Gynecol* 1991;77:923–926.

64. Ligon AH, Morton CC. Leiomyomata: heritability and cytogenetic studies. *Hum Reprod Update* 2001;7:8–14.

65. Rein MS, Powell WL, Walters FC, et al. Cytogenetic abnormalities in uterine myomas are associated with myoma size. *Mol Hum Reprod* 1998;4:83–86.

66. Brosens I, Deprest J, Dal Cin P, et al. Clinical significance of cytogenetic abnormalities in uterine myomas. *Fertil Steril* 1998;69:232–235.

67. Schoenberg Fejzo M, Ashar HR, Krauter KS, et al. Translocation breakpoints upstream of the HMGIC gene in uterine

leiomyomata suggest dysregulation of this gene by a mechanism different from that in lipomas. *Genes Chromosomes Cancer* 1996;17:1–6.

68. Kazmierczak B, Bol S, Wanschura S, et al. PAC clone containing the HMGI(Y) gene spans the breakpoint of a 6p21 translocation in a uterine leiomyoma cell line. *Genes Chromosomes Cancer* 1996;17:191–193.

69. Williams AJ, Powell WL, Collins T, et al. HMGI(Y) expression in human uterine leiomyomata. Involvement of another high-mobility group architectural factor in a benign neoplasm. *Am J Pathol* 1997;150:911–918.

70. Schoenmakers EF, Huysmans C, Van de Ven WJ. Allelic knockout of novel splice variants of human recombination repair gene RAD51B in t(12;14) uterine leiomyomas. *Cancer Res* 1999;59:19–23.

71. Takahashi T, Nagai N, Oda H, et al. Evidence for RAD51L1/HMGIC fusion in the pathogenesis of uterine leiomyoma. *Genes Chromosomes Cancer* 2001;30:196–201.

72. Quade BJ, Weremowicz S, Neskey DM, et al. Fusion transcripts involving HMGA2 are not a common molecular mechanism in uterine leiomyomata with rearrangements in 12q15. *Cancer Res* 2003;63:1351–1358.

73. Tsibris JC, Segars J, Coppola D, et al. Insights from gene arrays on the development and growth regulation of uterine leiomyomata. *Fertil Steril* 2002;78:114–121.

74. Marshall LM, Spiegelman D, Manson JE, et al. Risk of uterine leiomyomata among premenopausal women in relation to body size and cigarette smoking. *Epidemiology* 1998;9:511–517.

75. Unger J, Paul R, Caldito G. Hysterectomy for the massive leiomyomatous uterus. *ACOG* 2002;100:1271–1275.

76. Roth TM, Gustilo-Ashby T, Barber MD, et al. Effects of race and clinical factors on short-term outcomes of abdominal myomectomy. *Obstet Gynecol* 2003;101[5 Pt 1]:881–884.

77. Sato F, Nishi M, Kudo R, et al. Body fat distribution and uterine leiomyomas. *J Epidemiol* 1998;8:176–180.

78. Baird DD, Dunson DB. Why is parity protective for uterine fibroids? *Epidemiology* 2003;14:247–250.

79. Parazzini F, La Vecchia C, Negri E, et al. Epidemiologic characteristics of women with uterine fibroids: a case-control study. *Obstet Gynecol* 1988;72:853–857.

80. Marshall LM, Spiegelman D, Goldman MB, et al. A prospective study of reproductive factors and oral contraceptive use in relation to the risk of uterine leiomyomata. *Fertil Steril* 1998;70:432–439.

81. Ross RK, Pike MC, Vessey MP, et al. Risk factors for uterine fibroids: reduced risk associated with oral contraceptives [published erratum appears in Br Med J (Clin Res Ed) 1986;293:1027]. *Br Med J (Clin Res Ed)* 1986;293:359–362.

82. Parazzini F, Negri E, La Vecchia C, et al. Uterine myomas and smoking. Results from an Italian study. *J Reprod Med* 1996;41:316–320.

83. Chiaffarino F, Parazzini F, La Vecchia C, et al. Diet and uterine myomas. *Obstet Gynecol* 1999;94:395–398.

84. Farrer-Brown G, Beilby JO, Tarbit MH. Venous changes in the endometrium of myomatous uteri. *Obstet Gynecol* 1971;38:743–751.

85. Pritts EA. Fibroids and infertility: a systematic review of the evidence. *Obstet Gynecol Surv* 2001;56:483–491.

86. Garcia CR, Tureck RW. Submucosal leiomyomas and infertility. *Fertil Steril* 1984;42:16–19.

87. Rice JP, Kay HH, Mahony BS. The clinical significance of uterine leiomyomas in pregnancy. *Am J Obstet Gynecol* 1989;160[5 Pt 1]:1212–1216.

88. Coronado GD, Marshall LM, Schwartz SM. Complications in pregnancy, labor, and delivery with uterine leiomyomas: a population-based study. *Obstet Gynecol* 2000;95:764–769.

89. Karasick S, Lev-Toaff AS, Toaff ME. Imaging of uterine leiomyomas. *AJR Am J Roentgenol* 1992;158:799–805.

90. American College of Obstetricians and Gynecologists. *Surgical alternatives to hysterectomy in the management of leiomyomas (ACOG Technical Bulletin No. 16).* Washington, DC: American College of Obstetricians and Gynecologists, 2000.

91. Schwartz LB, Diamond MP, Schwartz PE. Leiomyosarcomas: clinical presentation. *Am J Obstet Gynecol* 1993;168[1 Pt 1]:180–183.

92. Schwartz LB, Zawin M, Carcangiu ML, et al. Does pelvic magnetic resonance imaging differentiate among the histologic subtypes of uterine leiomyomata? *Fertil Steril* 1998;70:580–587.

93. Sener AB, Seckin NC, Ozmen S, et al. The effects of hormone replacement therapy on uterine fibroids in postmenopausal women. *Fertil Steril* 1996;65:354–357.

94. Helstrom L, Lundberg PO, Sorbom D, et al. Sexuality after hysterectomy: a factor analysis of women's sexual lives before and after subtotal hysterectomy. *Obstet Gynecol* 1993;81:357–362.

95. Maas CP, Kenter GG, Trimbos B. Outcomes after total versus subtotal abdominal hysterectomy. *N Engl J Med* 2003;348:856–857, author reply 856–857.

96. Schaeffer J, Word A. Hysterectomy: still a useful operation. *N Engl J Med* 2002;347:1360–1362.

97. Roovers JP, van der Bom JG, van der Vaart CH, et al. Hysterectomy and sexual wellbeing: prospective observational study of vaginal hysterectomy, subtotal abdominal hysterectomy, and total abdominal hysterectomy. *BMJ* 2003;327:774–778.

98. Thakar R, Ayers S, Clarkson P, et al. Outcomes after total versus subtotal abdominal hysterectomy. *N Engl J Med* 2002;347:1318–1325.

99. Ecker JL, Foster JT, Friedman AJ. Abdominal hysterectomy or abdominal myomectomy for symptomatic leiomyoma: a comparison of preoperative demography and postoperative morbidity. *J Gynecol Surg* 1995;11:11–18.

100. Iverson RE Jr, Chelmow D, Strohbehn K, et al. Relative morbidity of abdominal hysterectomy and myomectomy for management of uterine leiomyomas. *Obstet Gynecol* 1996;88:415–419.

101. Malone LJ. Myomectomy: Recurrence after removal of solitary and multiple myomas. *Obstet Gynecol* 1969;34:200–203.

102. Acien P, Quereda F. Abdominal myomectomy: results of a simple operative technique. *Fertil Steril* 1996;65:41–51.

103. Garnet JD. Uterine rupture during pregnancy. *Obstet Gynecol* 1964;23:898–905.

104. Dubuisson JB, Chapron C, Fauconnier A. Laparoscopic myomectomy. Operative technique and results. *Ann N Y Acad Sci* 1997;828:326–331.

105. Arcangeli S, Pasquarette MM. Gravid uterine rupture after myolysis. *Obstet Gynecol* 1997;89[5 Pt 2]:857.

106. Hockstein S. Spontaneous uterine rupture in the early third trimester after laparoscopically assisted myomectomy. A case report. *J Reprod Med* 2000;45:139–141.

107. Goldfarb HA. Laparoscopic coagulation of myoma (myolysis). *Obstet Gynecol Clin North Am* 1995;22:807–819.

108. Derman SG, Rehnstrom J, Neuwirth RS. The long-term effectiveness of hysteroscopic treatment of menorrhagia and leiomyomas. *Obstet Gynecol* 1991;77:591–594.

109. Ubaldi F, Tournaye H, Camus M, et al. Fertility after hysteroscopic myomectomy. *Hum Reprod Update* 1995;1:81–90.

110. Yin CS, Wei RY, Chao TC, et al. Hysteroscopic endometrial ablation without endometrial preparation. *Int J Gynaecol Obstet* 1998;62:167–172.

111. Stewart EA, Friedman AJ, eds. *Steroidal treatment of myomas: preoperative and long-term medical therapy.* New York: Thieme, 1992.

112. Friedman AJ, Daly M, Juneau-Norcross M, et al. Long-term medical therapy for leiomyomata uteri: a prospective, randomized study of leuprolide acetate depot plus either oestrogen-progestin or progestin "add-back" for 2 years. *Hum Reprod* 1994;9:1618–1625.

113. Balance Pharmaceuticals, Inc. *End of phase II report to the FDA.* Santa Monica, CA: Balance Pharmaceuticals, Inc., 2002.

114. Lumsden MA, West CP, Hillier H, et al. Estrogenic action of tamoxifen in women treated with luteinizing hormone-releasing hormone agonists (goserelin): lack of shrinkage of uterine fibroids. *Fertil Steril* 1989;52:924–929.

115. Palomba S, Russo T, Orio F, et al. Effectiveness of combined GnRH analogue plus raloxifene administration in the treatment of uterine leiomyomas: a prospective, randomized, single-blind, placebo-controlled clinical trial. *Hum Reprod* 2002;17:3213–3219.

116. Frankel T, Benjamin F. Rapid enlargement of a uterine fibroid after clomiphene therapy. *J Obstet Gynaecol Br Commonw* 1973;80:764.

117. Felmingham JE, Corcoran R. Rapid enlargement of a uterine fibroid after clomiphene therapy. *Br J Obstet Gynaecol* 1975;82:431–432.

118. Walker CL, Burroughs KD, Davis B, et al. Preclinical evidence for therapeutic efficacy of selective estrogen receptor modulators for uterine leiomyoma. *J Soc Gynecol Investig* 2000;7:249–256.

119. Palomba S, Sammartino A, Di Carlo C, et al. Effects of raloxifene treatment on uterine leiomyomas in postmenopausal women. *Fertil Steril* 2001;76:38–43.

120. Palomba S, Orio F, Morelli M, et al. Raloxifene administration in premenopausal women with uterine leiomyomas: a pilot study. *J Clin Endocrinol Metal* 2002;87:3603–3608.

121. de Aloysio D, Altieri P, Penacchioni P, et al. Bleeding patterns in recent postmenopausal outpatients with uterine myomas: comparison between two regimens of HRT. *Maturitas* 1998;29:261–264.

122. Palomba S, Affinito P, Tommaselli GA, et al. A clinical trial of the effects of tibolone administered with gonadotropin-releasing hormone analogues for the treatment of uterine leiomyomata. *Fertil Steril* 1998;70:111–118.

123. Kettel LM, Murphy AA, Morales AJ, et al. Rapid regression of uterine leiomyomas in response to daily administration of gonadotropin-releasing hormone antagonist. *Fertil Steril* 1993;60:642–646.

124. Gonzalez-Barcena D, Alvarez RB, Ochoa EP, et al. Treatment of uterine leiomyomas with luteinizing hormone-releasing hormone antagonist Cetrorelix. *Hum Reprod* 1997;12:2028–2035.

125. Murphy AA, Morales AJ, Kettel LM, et al. Regression of uterine leiomyomata to the antiprogesterone RU486: dose-response effect. *Fertil Steril* 1995;64:187–190.

126. Murphy AA, Kettel LM, Morales AJ, et al. Endometrial effects of long-term low-dose administration of RU486. *Fertil Steril* 1995;63:761–766.

127. Eisinger SH, Meldrum S, Fiscella K, et al. Low-dose mifepristone for uterine leiomyomata. *Obstet Gynecol* 2003;101:243–250.

128. Chwalisz K, Elger W, McCrary K, et al. Reversible suppression of menstruation in normal women irrespective of the effect on ovulation with the novel selective progesterone receptor modulator (SPRM) J867. *J Soc Gynecol Investig* 2002;9[1S]:82A.

129. Minakuchi K, Kawamura N, Tsujimura A, et al. Remarkable and persistent shrinkage of uterine leiomyoma associated with interferon alfa treatment for hepatitis [Letter]. *Lancet* 1999;353:2127–2128.

130. De Leo V, la Marca A, Morgante G, et al. Administration of somatostatin analogue reduces uterine and myoma volume in women with uterine leiomyomata. *Fertil Steril* 2001;75:632–633.

131. Law P, Gedroyc WM, Regan L. Magnetic-resonance-guided percutaneous laser ablation of uterine fibroids [Letter]. *Lancet* 1999;354:2049–2050.

132. Hindey J, Law P, Hickey M, et al. Clinical outcomes following percutaneous magnetic resonance image guided laser ablation of symptomatic uterine fibroids. *Hum Reprod* 2002;17:2737–2741.

133. Sewell PE, Arriola RM, Robinette L, et al. Real-time I-MR-imaging–guided cryoablation of uterine fibroids. *J Vasc Interv Radiol* 2001;12:891–893.

134. Cowan BD, Sewell PE, Howard JC, et al. Interventional magnetic resonance imaging cryotherapy of uterine fibroid tumors: preliminary observation. *Am J Obstet Gynecol* 2002;186:1183–1187.

135. Stewart EA, Gedroyc WM, Tempany CM, et al. Focused ultrasound treatment of uterine fibroid tumors: safety and feasibility of a noninvasive thermoablative technique. *Am J Obstet Gynecol* 2003;189:48–54.

3

PELVIC ANATOMY RELEVANT IN UTERINE EMBOLIZATION

JACKELINE GOMEZ-JORGE

INTRODUCTION

With the advent of uterine fibroid embolization (UFE), a new procedure for treatment of symptomatic fibroids, interventional radiologists are relearning the pelvic anatomy. To quote Soulen et al. (1): "After 30 years of embolizing the hypogastric arteries, how can we know so little?" Typical of our constantly changing and challenging field, we realize the importance of understanding the anatomy of the pelvis in order to perform UFE safely. The purpose of this chapter is to provide a comprehensive review of the anatomy of the pelvis, preparing interventionalists to feel comfortable when performing UFE procedures. First, the arterial anatomy of the pelvis is reviewed because it is the key to the procedure and its outcome. The venous anatomy is discussed next. This is followed by a review of the anatomy of the uterus and adnexa and, finally, a discussion of how fibroids may distort both the uterine anatomy and its arterial supply.

ARTERIAL ANATOMY OF THE HYPOGASTRIC ARTERY

The internal iliac artery (hypogastric artery) supplies the wall of the pelvis, the pelvic viscera, and the inner aspect of the thigh. In an adult, it is a short vessel, smaller than the external iliac artery. It is approximately 1.5 inches in length. The internal iliac artery passes to the upper margin of the greater sacrosciatic foramen and divides into two trunks: the posterior division and the anterior division. The internal iliac artery is flanked by the peritoneum and ureter anteriorly and by the internal iliac vein, lumbosacral cord, and pyriformis muscle posteriorly. Lateral to the internal iliac artery is the psoas muscle (Fig. 3-1) (2).

The branches of the internal iliac artery are as follows (Fig. 3-2):

Anterior division:

1. Inferior gluteal artery
2. Obturator artery

Plan of the Relations of the Internal Iliac Artery.

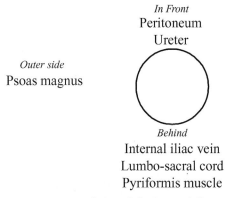

In Front
Peritoneum
Ureter

Outer side
Psoas magnus

Behind
Internal iliac vein
Lumbo-sacral cord
Pyriformis muscle

FIGURE 3-1. Boundaries of the internal iliac artery. (From Gray H. *Gray's Anatomy: The Classic Collector's Edition.* Avenel, NJ: Crown Publishers, 1977:562, with permission.)

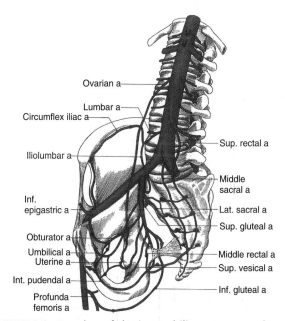

FIGURE 3-2. Branches of the internal iliac artery, anterior and posterior divisions. (From Berek JS, Adashi EY, Hillard PA. *Novak's gynecology, 12th ed.* Baltimore: Williams & Wilkins, 1996:84, with permission.)

Type I

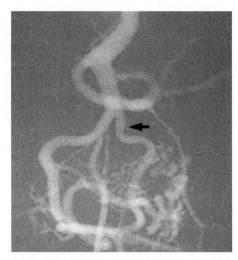

FIGURE 3-3. Type I configuration of the origin of the uterine artery.

Type II

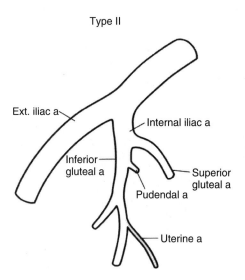
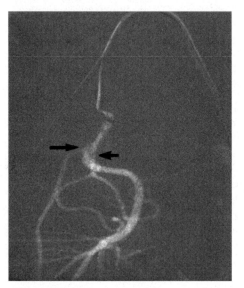

FIGURE 3-4. Type II configuration of the origin of the uterine artery.

3. Internal pudendal artery
4. Visceral branches
    I. Superior vesical artery
    II. Inferior vesical artery
    III. Middle hemorrhoidal artery
    IV. Internal genital arteries *(uterine artery)*
Posterior division:
1. Superior gluteal artery
2. Iliolumbar artery
3. Lateral sacral artery

The Uterine Artery

The key to performing uterine embolization is understanding the anatomy of the uterine artery. This artery usually arises from the inferior gluteal artery, but there is some variability in the site of origin. These variations have been classified as follows, with the frequency of occurrence given in parentheses (3):

Type I (45%): the uterine artery is the first branch off the inferior gluteal artery (Fig. 3-3)

Type II (6%): the uterine artery is the second or third branch off the inferior gluteal artery (Fig. 3-4)

Type III (43%): the uterine artery, the inferior gluteal artery, and the superior gluteal artery arise as a trifurcation off the internal iliac artery (Fig. 3-5)

Type IV (6%): the uterine artery is the first branch off the internal iliac artery, above the level of the inferior gluteal and superior gluteal arteries (Fig. 3-6)

This classification is given in Table 3–1.

Others have reported rare anatomic variants, such as duplicated uterine arteries and unilateral or bilateral absence

Type III

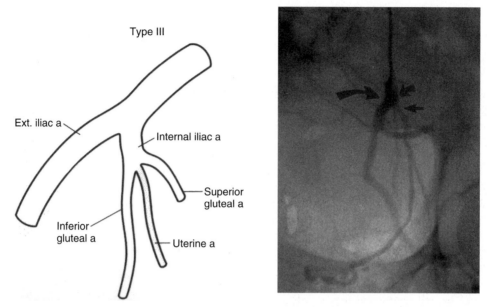

FIGURE 3-5. Type III configuration of the origin of the uterine artery.

Type IV

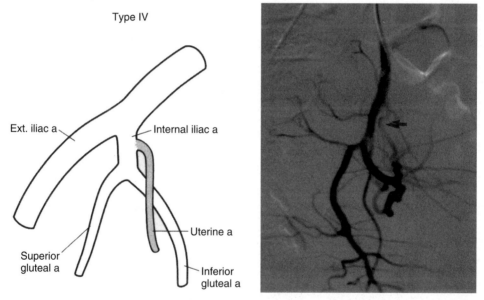

FIGURE 3-6. Type IV configuration of the origin of the uterine artery.

TABLE 3-1. CLASSIFICATION OF VARIATIONS IN THE SITE OF ORIGIN OF THE UTERINE ARTERY

Uterine Artery Classification	Incidence	Anatomic Description
Type I	45%	Uterine artery is the first branch of the inferior gluteal artery
Type II	6%	Uterine artery is the second or third branch of the inferior gluteal artery
Type III	43%	Uterine artery, inferior gluteal artery, and superior gluteal artery are at the same level (trifurcation)
Type IV	6%	Uterine artery is the first branch of the hypogastric artery (proximal to the inferior gluteal and superior gluteal arteries)

of the uterine arteries (4–6). It is important to determine the exact location of the origin of the uterine artery at the time of catheterization. Perhaps the most common reason for a difficult selective catheterization of the vessel is failure to appreciate its origin. The uterine artery is often very tortuous because of increased flow to the fibroids, and it frequently is seen to overlay other vessels when it is imaged in two dimensions, as with a digital arteriographic or "road map" image. The vessel may arise from the medial, anterior, or lateral aspect of the vessel. Only when a true tangential image is obtained may the origin be visible. In addition, proximal kinks or angulation of the vessel may make catheterization difficult, even when the origin is identified. The use of varying degrees of oblique projection will usually identify the best visualization of the vessel origin. In general, the uterine artery origin can be visualized by placing the image intensifier in a contralateral steep oblique position. However, in a type III configuration, where the origin of the uterine artery is high, the ipsilateral steep oblique position is better to visualize the origin of the vessel.

The uterine artery descends along the lateral pelvic wall to the level of the cardinal ligament and then courses medially toward the lateral uterine wall. At the level of the internal os of the cervix it crosses the distal ureter. At the uterine margin, it divides into ascending and descending branches. The ascending branch courses along the uterine margin, at the medial edge of the broad ligament, distributing into the centripetal branches and providing terminal branches to the uterine fundus and the fallopian tube. The branch to the tube communicates with the ovarian artery branches (Fig. 3-7).

The uterine arteries have several branches. Near the origin, the superior vesicle artery arises and courses in a roughly parallel course to the descending uterine artery,

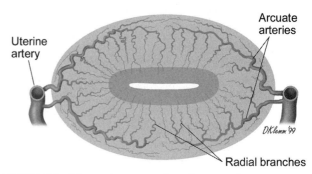

FIGURE 3-8. Schematic cross section of a normal uterus.

leading to the urinary bladder. There is also a branch to the distal ureter, which often arises near the distal transverse portion of the uterine artery proximal to the lateral uterine margin. The cervicovaginal branch also arises in this segment of the artery and is the blood supply to the cervix. The vaginal branches from each side anastomose with the vaginal artery to form the azygos arteries. The azygos arteries are two parallel arteries. They run medially and longitudinally along the vagina. One runs anteriorly while the other runs posteriorly. These branches of the uterine artery that supply other adjacent structures are important to consider during an embolization procedure, as they are potential targets of misembolization. This topic will be discussed in Chapters 9 and 12.

The uterine artery supplies the myometrium via innumerable penetrating arteries. These immediately branch into posterior and anterior arcuate arteries, which course circumferentially around the uterus at approximately the level of the outer third of the myometrium (Fig. 3-8). The arcuate arteries anastomose with similar branches on the opposite side, providing the basis for a rich collateral network. The arcuate arteries branch into peripheral and radial (or centripetal) branches. The peripheral branches course in a roughly parallel course to the arcuate arteries in the outer third of the myometrium, supplying that portion of the uterus. The radial branches are centripetal, running at a right angle to the arcuate arteries toward the endometrial surface.

The presence of leiomyomata will distort the anatomy of the uterine arteries as well as enlarge them. In the early 1900s, Sampson (7) showed that each fibroid is supplied by a few arcuate or peripheral arteries (usually fewer than 6) that are parasitized by the fibroid. These arteries enlarge substantially, and their flow increases correspondingly to supply the tumor (Fig. 3-9). It is this discrepancy in both the size and degree of flow to the fibroid compared to normal that allows uterine embolization to be both safe and effective. As discussed in greater detail in Chapter 9, the embolics used for embolization are sized to occlude the fibroid branches, but the normal branches in general are smaller in diameter than the embolic.

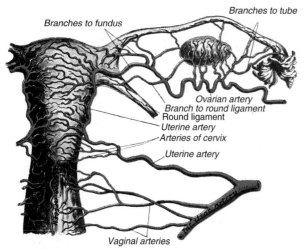

FIGURE 3-7. Branches of the uterine artery. (From Netter FH. *Atlas of human anatomy.* Summit, NJ: Ciba-Geigy Corporation, 1995:379, with permission.)

OVARIAN BLOOD SUPPLY

The ovarian artery can play a significant role in uterine leiomyomata by providing blood supply to the tumors. In addition, there is a rich vascular connection between the uterine artery and the ovarian artery. This blood supply to the adnexa and uterus may explain failed procedures despite proper embolization of the uterine artery. It can also explain the incidence of ovarian failure after embolization reported by some investigators (8).

The ovarian arteries arise from the abdominal aorta in 81% to 91% of cases. Seventy percent of the gonadal arteries arise from the ventral surface of the abdominal aorta a few centimeters below the renal arteries. Up to 20% of the gonadal arteries originate from the renal arteries. Rarely, the blood supply to the ovaries arises from the adrenal, lumbar,

and iliac arteries. The origin is typically off the anterior surface of the aorta, 2 to 3 cm below the superior mesenteric artery (Fig. 3-10). The ovaries are supplied by the ovarian artery in 40% of cases, from both the ovarian and the uterine arteries in 56% of cases, and from the uterine artery alone in 4% of cases. The normal ovarian artery is usually not visualized angiographically because of its small diameter (1 mm), but in the presence of uterine pathology such as fibroids, the vessels enlarge and their flows increase. Some authors recommend the use of flush aortography, before or after uterine artery embolization for fibroids, to rule out possible blood supply from the ovarian arteries (9). The variations in anatomic contributions of the ovarian arteries to the uterus in the presence of fibroids are discussed in detail in Chapter 10.

When additional supply from the ovarian arteries to the fibroids is identified, ovarian embolization has been used to supplement uterine artery embolization. However, the role of ovarian embolization is not well defined; in particular, its potential impact on ovarian function is not known. In some patients, the ovarian artery completely replaces the ipsilateral uterine artery. If that vessel supplies a major portion of the fibroids, then it is likely that embolization will fail to control the symptoms from the fibroids. In this circumstance, many interventionalists will proceed with embolizing that vessel. In the setting of unilateral embolization, it is unlikely that there will be an overall decrease in ovarian function; however, little study has been completed on ovarian function after embolization of the ovarian artery. For this reason, if there is any question about the necessity of ovarian embolization, then the procedure should be deferred. The patient can be reevaluated for outcome 3 months after treatment. If contrast-enhanced magnetic

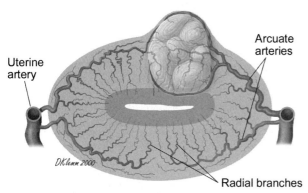

FIGURE 3-9. Schematic cross section of a uterus with a single fibroid. The fibroid has parasitized myometrial arteries, which have enlarged in response to the increased arterial flow.

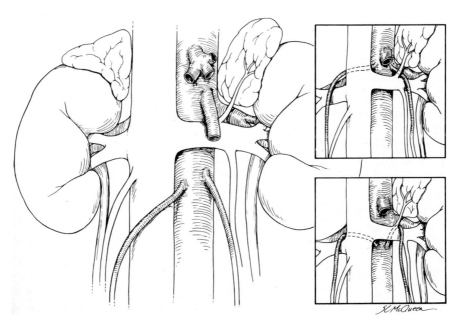

FIGURE 3-10. Origin of the ovarian arteries. (From Kadir S. *Atlas of normal and variant angiographic anatomy.* Philadelphia: WB Saunders, 1991:263, with permission.)

resonance imaging study reveals that viable fibroid tissue is still present in the apparent distribution of the ovarian supply and the patient has not demonstrated a sufficient improvement in symptoms, then ovarian embolization may be considered. If embolization of the ovarian arteries is undertaken, it must be after careful discussion with the patient about the potential for injury to the function of that ovary. This approach is particularly important when a bilateral ovarian artery supply is present (10). Although ovarian failure after ovarian embolization has not yet been reported, it certainly has been reported after uterine embolization, and its likelihood probably is higher in this circumstance. This topic is further discussed in Chapter 10.

VENOUS DRAINAGE OF THE PELVIS

The uterine veins drain the uterus into the iliac veins. The ovarian veins form a plexus near the ovaries and the uterus. Two veins emerge from the plexus and lie next to the ovarian artery. The veins communicate freely with the uterine venous plexus (Fig. 3-11).

The left gonadal vein joins the left renal vein at right angles close to its junction to the inferior vena cava (IVC) but lateral to the junction of the adrenal vein and the superior mesenteric artery (SMA) crossing. If there is a circumaortic renal vein, the gonadal vein may form either the preaortic or the retroaortic renal vein. If there is a duplicated IVC, the left gonadal vein will join the left-sided IVC (Fig. 3-12).

On the right side, accessory channels may drain into the renal vein or the IVC below the junction of the right renal vein in 25% of cases. In 90% of cases, the gonadal veins have

valves at the origin or within 1 to 4 cm below the origin. The gonadal veins communicate with the retroperitoneal veins at the level of the iliac crest with the paravertebral, lumbar, colic, capsular, renal, and ureteric veins.

UTERINE AND ADNEXAL ANATOMY

The uterus is comprised of the body and the cervix. The division between the body and the cervix is delineated by a slight external constriction and internally by narrowing in the internal canal or "internal os." A reflection of the peritoneum from the anterior surface of the uterus onto the bladder completes the anatomic delineation between body and cervix.

The body of the uterus gradually narrows from the fundus to the lower segment just above the cervix. The anterior surface is flattened and covered by peritoneum. The posterior surface is more convex in its transverse axis. It is entirely covered by peritoneum. The pouch of Douglas, posterior to the uterus, is defined as the space within the following boundaries:

Anterior: posterior wall of the uterus/supravaginal cervix
Posterior: rectum and sacrum
Superior: small intestine
Lateral: sacrouterine ligaments

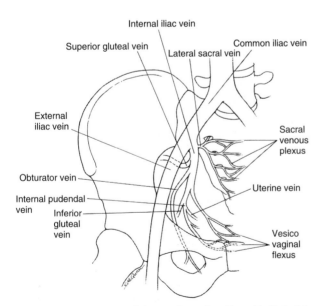

FIGURE 3-11. Drainage of the uterine veins. (From Kadir S. *Atlas of normal and variant angiographic anatomy.* Philadelphia: WB Saunders, 1991:218, with permission.)

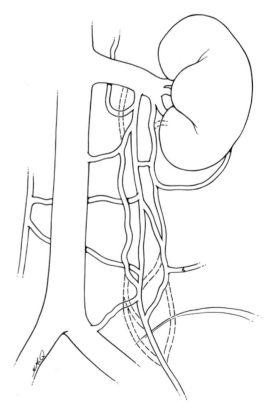

FIGURE 3-12. Drainage of the left gonadal vein. (From Kadir S. *Atlas of normal and variant angiographic anatomy.* Philadelphia: WB Saunders, 1991:272, with permission.)

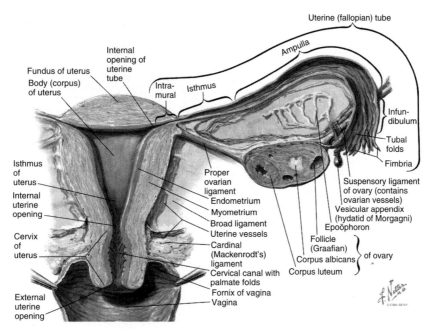

FIGURE 3-13. Appendages from the uterus. (From Netter FH. *Atlas of human anatomy.* Summit, NJ: Ciba-Geigy Corporation, 1995:350, with permission.)

The uterus has several appendages (Fig. 3-13). These include the fallopian tubes, the ovaries and ligaments, and the round ligaments. The fallopian tubes, or oviducts, are located in the upper margin of the broad ligament.

GROSS ANATOMY

The uterus has three coats: serous, muscular, and mucous.

1. The external serous coat derives from the peritoneum. It covers the fundus of the uterus and the whole posterior surface of the uterus. It covers only down to the junction of the body and cervix.

2. The muscular coat is a bundle of smooth muscular fibers disposed in layers. It divides into external fibers that pass transversely across the fundus. The middle fibers are the thickest, run in a longitudinal, oblique, or transverse fashion, and contain most of the vascular structures. The deep (internal) layer is composed of circular fibers in the form of two hollow lines.

3. The endometrium is the lining layer of the uterus and surrounds the potential space of the uterine cavity. The cavity is triangular, with closely approximated walls and the base of the triangle at the fundus (Fig. 3-14). The apex of the triangular cavity, the internal orifice (ostium internum), leads into the cervix cavity, which is fusiform and flattened. The endometrium is lined by columnar ciliated epithelium that connects to the muscularis mucosa. The cervix is lined by a mucous membrane that is sharply differentiated from the uterine cavity. In the upper two thirds of the canal, the mucous membrane has many deep glandular follicles that produce a viscid alkaline substance that provides the barrier at the external cervix os. The upper end of the vagina is attached to the cervical circumference. The supravaginal portion of the cervix is covered by peritoneum (Fig. 3-15).

LIGAMENTOUS ATTACHMENTS OF THE UTERUS

The uterus is suspended in the pelvis by several ligamentous attachments (Fig. 3-15).

1. Vesicouterine ligament (anterior) from the anterior aspect of the uterus to the bladder at the level of the cervix.

2. Rectouterine ligament (posterior) passes from the posterior wall of the uterus over the upper fourth of the vagina to the rectum and sacrum, thus forming the pouch of Douglas.

3. Two lateral or broad ligaments from each side of the uterus to the lateral wall of the pelvis. The broad ligaments divide the pelvis into anterior and posterior segments. The anterior segment includes the bladder, urethra, and vagina. The rectum comprises the posterior segment. Between the two layers of each broad ligaments, the following structures are contained: the fallopian tube within the mesosalpinx, the round ligament, the ovary and its ligament, the paraovarium (organ of Rosenmüller), muscular fibers, blood vessels, and nerves.

4. Two sacrouterine ligaments (from the second and third bones of the sacrum). These ligaments attach on each side of the uterus at the junction of the supravaginal cervix and the body.

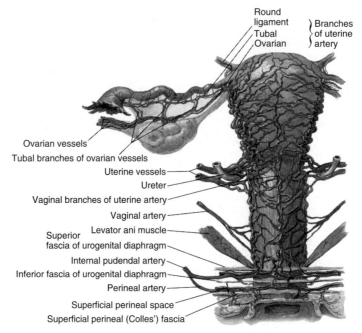

FIGURE 3-14. The body and cervix. (From Netter FH. *Atlas of human anatomy.* Summit, NJ: Ciba-Geigy Corporation, 1995:350, with permission.)

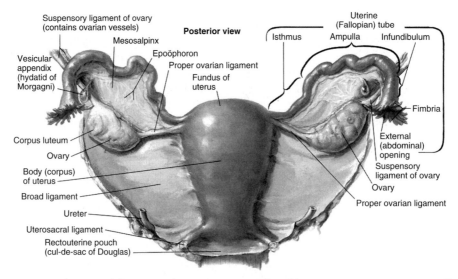

FIGURE 3-15. Ligamentous attachments of the uterus. (From Netter FH. *Atlas of human anatomy.* Summit, NJ: Ciba-Geigy Corporation, 1995:350, with permission.)

5. Two round ligaments. These ligaments are, in essence, an extension of the muscular tissue of the uterus, fibrous and areolar tissue, blood vessels, and nerves.

SUMMARY

Until the advent of uterine embolization, interventionalists needed only a limited knowledge of the anatomy of the female pelvis. Now, to perform a procedure with the potential for both major therapeutic benefit but also the potential injury to adjacent organs, an understanding of the anatomic relationships of the uterus and how these relationships might be altered in the presence of fibroids is essential. This chapter has served as an introduction to that anatomy, and it is hoped that it has provided a basis for the safe and effective embolization of fibroids.

REFERENCES

1. Soulen MC, Fairman RM, Baum RA. Embolization of the internal iliac artery: still more to learn. *JVIR* 2000;11:543–545.
2. Gray H. *Gray's Anatomy: The Classic Collector's Edition.* Avenel, NJ: Crown Publishers, 1977:561–564.
3. Gomez-Jorge J, Keyoung A, Levy EB, et al. Uterine artery anatomy relevant to uterine leiomyomata embolization. *Cardiovasc Intervent Radiol* 2003;26(6):522–527.
4. Pelage JP, Le Dref O, Soyer P, et al. Arterial anatomy of the female genital tract: variations and relevance to transcatheter embolization of the uterus. *AJR Am J Roentgenol* 1999;172:989–994.
5. Andrews RT, Bromley PJ, Pfister ME. Successful embolization of collaterals from the ovarian artery during uterine artery embolization for fibroids: a case report. *JVIR* 2000;11:607–610.
6. Worthington-Kirsh RL, Walker WJ, Adler L, et al. Anatomic variation in the uterine arteries: a cause of failure of uterine artery embolization for the management of symptomatic myomata. *Min Invas Ther Allied Technol* 1999;8(6):397–402.
7. Sampson JA. The blood supply of uterine myomata. *Surg Gynecol Obstet* 1912;3:215–234.
8. Nikolic B, Spies JB, Abbara S, et al. Ovarian artery supply of uterine fibroids as a cause of treatment failure after uterine artery embolization: a case report. *JVIR* 1999;10:1167–1170.
9. Nott F, Riedy JF, Forman RG, et al. Complications of fibroid embolisation. *Min Invas Ther Allied Technol* 1999;8:421–424.
10. Binkert CA, Andrews RT, Kauffman JA. Utility of nonselective abdominal aortography in demonstrating ovarian artery collaterals in patients undergoing uterine artery embolization for fibroids. *JVIR* 2001;12:841–845.

4

GYNECOLOGIC EVALUATION OF PATIENTS WITH FIBROIDS

KEITH ISAACSON

INTRODUCTION

It is essential that physicians interested in uterine embolization understand the gynecologist's approach to patients suspected of having fibroids, particularly when patients are self-referred for evaluation. This chapter reviews the components of the gynecologic examination, the role of imaging and other tests to supplement that evaluation, and the differential diagnosis of symptoms that may be caused by uterine fibroids. Although the knowledge gained from this review does not replace the expertise that the gynecologist's consultation brings to the care of these patients, the greater the understanding the interventionalist has of this process and the logic behind it, the better he or she will be able to enhance the care the patient receives.

THE GYNECOLOGIC EXAMINATION

There are two scenarios in which women with uterine fibroids are evaluated by their gynecologist: during a routine gynecologic visit or during a visit in which there are problematic symptoms that may be related to uterine fibroids. It is the recommendation of the American College of Obstetricians and Gynecologists (ACOG) as well as the American Cancer Society that women in the reproductive and postreproductive years undergo a regular gynecologic visit every 1 to 3 years. The purpose of this visit is primarily to screen for cancerous or precancerous conditions of the breasts, ovaries, uterus, cervix, vagina, and female genitalia. In addition to cancer screening, it is the role of the gynecologist to annually review the family medical history, as well as to perform a complete review of systems that covers in detail any symptoms that may be related to abnormal uterine bleeding, the urogenital tract, the gastrointestinal system, back pain, or pelvic pain. Once the annual history is complete, the gynecologist will perform a physical examination that includes the following:

1. Routine vital signs
2. Head and neck examination
3. Breast examination
4. Auscultation of heart and lungs
5. Abdominal examination
6. Vulva/vaginal examination
7. Cervical examination and Pap smear
8. Bimanual pelvic examination
9. Rectal examination (in patients older than 40 years)

If a patient presents for her annual examination with no current complaints, there are several opportunities during the history and physical examination in which an asymptomatic or symptomatic fibroid can be suspected. Because the gynecologist is aware that 20% to 30% of all women of reproductive age have fibroids, he or she will key in on certain parts of the visit that may lead him or her to make the diagnosis.

Family History

Women at the highest risk for developing uterine fibroids are those of African-American descent and those with a family history of uterine fibroids. In a study by Baird et al. (1), it was shown that 70% of white women and 80% of black women develop fibroids by age 50 and that the fibroid tumors develop at earlier ages in black women.

It is estimated that women who have family members with uterine fibroids have more than a 25% higher risk of developing fibroids than does the general population (2). Knowing this, the gynecologist will routinely ask the patient if anyone in her immediate family has a known history of fibroids. Because hysterectomies have been performed in as many as one in three women by age 60, many patients will tell their gynecologist that their mothers had hysterectomies for bleeding. In light of the fact that the majority of patients suffer these symptoms as a result of uterine fibroids, this will alert the gynecologist to look for fibroids in this patient.

Physical Examination

The first time the gynecologist may suspect the presence of a uterine fibroid is during an abdominal examination. This examination is routinely performed to rule out enlargement of the liver and spleen, as well as to rule out ascites and any abdominal masses such ovarian or uterine tumors. By far the most common tumor palpated is the benign uterine fibroid, which presents as a firm mobile mass palpable in the area above the pubic bone up to and beyond the umbilicus. The characteristics and location will be dependent on the fibroid size and location, as well as its attachment to the uterus. A pedunculated fibroid will feel mobile and separate from the uterus, whereas a large intramural and subserosal fibroid will feel like a single large mass. Most often, palpating the fibroid on abdominal examination will not stimulate pain. The rare exception to this occurs when the fibroid undergoes degeneration or torsion. When an asymptomatic pelvic mass is palpated, the most important step is to rule out a malignant lesion, which is most often ovarian in nature.

It is fairly uncommon to diagnose an asymptomatic fibroid during an abdominal examination. Most often, when the fibroid or uterus has reached the size that it can be palpated by abdominal examination, it is already symptomatic. More commonly, any asymptomatic fibroid that is diagnosed by physical examination is done so during the bimanual examination. Just prior to the bimanual examination, the gynecologist will perform a speculum examination and Pap smear. During this examination, the cervical location will be observed and, if there is significant deviation from the normal position, a uterine fibroid must be ruled out as the cause. For example, a lower uterine segment posterior fibroid will often displace the cervix anteriorly, which can make a Pap smear difficult to perform.

The bimanual examination is performed with two digits from one hand placed into the posterior fornix of the vagina and the other hand on the lower abdomen. In order to best evaluate the uterus, the vaginal hand is moved upward while mild pressure is displaced downward on the abdominal hand place just above the pubic bone. Several characteristics of the uterus should be documented, including the following:

1. Size: measured in estimated weeks of a gestational-size uterus (on average, 1 week = 1 cm). Normal size is 6 weeks for a nulliparous uterus and 6 to 8 weeks for a multiparous uterus. A uterus just reaching the pubic bone is 12 to 14 weeks' size and a uterus at the umbilicus is 20 weeks' size.
2. Position: anterior, mid position, or retrodisplaced
3. Shape: regular, irregular, or nodular
4. Consistency: firm, soft, or hard
5. Fixed or mobile
6. Tender or nontender

On a normal examination, the uterus is typically described as having a size of 6 to 8 weeks, anterior (30% are posterior, which is normal), nontender, smooth, mobile, and firm. A fibroid uterus in an asymptomatic patient will often be slightly enlarged, irregular, hard, and nodular. When this is the case, as will be discussed, further evaluation is indicated.

Once an asymptomatic patient is suspected of having fibroids, either by history, physical examination, or both, it is reasonable to confirm the diagnosis utilizing an imaging modality. Typically, this is done with a combination of abdominal and pelvic ultrasound. The abdominal scan is most useful when there is a large mass and the pathology is located away from the vaginal apex. When the uterus is 12 weeks' size or smaller, or when there is a lateral lesion and ovarian pathology must be ruled out, a vaginal ultrasound utilizing a 7.5-MHz probe is the most useful tool to assess the presence or absence of fibroids and their size. For initial evaluation there is no obvious role for color Doppler imaging or three-dimensional ultrasound imaging. If the abdominal/vaginal scan is inconclusive, magnetic resonance imaging (MRI) can be useful for ruling out other uterine or adnexal pathology such as adenomyosis, adenomyomas, endometriomas, dermoid cysts, uterine sarcoma, or endometrial carcinomas with invasion.

Gynecologic Management of the Asymptomatic Fibroid

When a fibroid is detected in a patient without symptoms, there are several options for management:

1. Watchful waiting
2. Medical therapy
3. Surgical removal (myomectomy)
4. Hysterectomy
5. Ablative therapies
6. Embolization

Prior to the mid-1980s, several misconceptions by gynecologists guided them to recommend one of the therapies other than "watchful waiting." These myths included the following:

1. Because of the fibroids, the ovaries cannot be palpated and there might be an ovarian cancer.
2. Rapid fibroid growth means the fibroid is more likely a sarcoma.
3. If the fibroids grow, they will be too large to remove, and a hysterectomy will be necessary.
4. Fibroids will grow back after a myomectomy, and a hysterectomy will eventually be necessary.
5. Fibroids will impair fertility.
6. Fibroids might damage adjacent organs, such as the bowel, bladder, or ureters.
7. The fibroids may not have symptoms now, but they will in the future.

Unfortunately, 70% of women diagnosed with ovarian cancer already have stage III or IV cancer, whether or not a woman has fibroids. If the fibroids are so large that the ovaries cannot be palpated by physical examination, an annual ultrasound should be ordered to adequately assess ovarian size. Rarely will a small postmenopausal ovary that is not seen by ultrasound be abnormal. However, if there is a personal or family history that places the patient at higher risk for ovarian cancer, pelvic computed tomography (CT) will be useful to rule out an abnormal pelvic mass.

As with many decisions we make in medicine that are not evidence based, recommending a hysterectomy for "rapidly growing" fibroids is without foundation. First of all, the term "rapid growth" has never been adequately defined. Buttram (2a) suggested a growth of 6 weeks within 1 year, but others have used the definition of a fibroid doubling in size over a 6- to 12-month period. The frequency of finding a uterine sarcoma in all patients undergoing surgery for fibroids is 0.07% (3). In a group of 371 women who had surgery for rapidly growing fibroids, only one was found to have a sarcoma. This incidence of 0.27% was not statistically different from that in the general population (3). The typical patient with known fibroids is 43 years old and is most often asymptomatic. The average age of a patient with a uterine sarcoma is 68 years, and most often presents with postmenopausal bleeding.

Patients have been told that if fibroids grow too large, the risks of surgical complications will be excessive. Although it has been shown that patients undergoing hysterectomy for large uteri (>500 g) have a higher blood loss than hysterectomies for small uteri (<500 g), the incidence of complications requiring prolonged hospitalization or readmission or which are life threatening are no different (4).

It has been a long time since I have attended a national gynecologic meeting related to surgery or fertility in which the association between uterine fibroids and fertility was not debated. It will be safe to say that at the time this textbook is published, the issue will still not be resolved. In 2001, Pritts (5) published a meta-analysis looking at 11 studies, none of which were randomized, that included more than 3,900 patients with fibroids. This analysis concluded that fibroids that are not submucosal and do not protrude into the uterine cavity do not impact fertility. The question remains as to whether or not intramural fibroids that cause uterine cavity enlargement or those that are very closely located to the endometrial cavity can impact fertility. Given the lack of definitive evidence, most gynecologists will recommend that patients who have asymptomatic fibroids that do not distort the endometrial cavity try to conceive for 6 to 12 months before considering treatment for fibroids. After 6 to 12 months, other factors that can cause infertility should be ruled out before a myomectomy is recommended. If, on the other hand, a fibroid is submucosal, removal should be discussed prior to attempting conception. These fibroids not only make it more difficult to conceive, they can also lead to early spontaneous miscarriages.

To date, there are no case reports in the English literature of uterine fibroids causing damage to adjacent organs such as the bladder, ureters, or bowel. There is no justification for using this reasoning as a recommendation for fibroid therapy.

If a fibroid is diagnosed and is currently not causing symptoms, should it be treated so that it will not cause problems in the future? Most of the time, the answer is no. Carlson et al. (6) demonstrated that the mental health index, the general health index, and the activity index did not change in women with fibroids after 1 year of watchful waiting. Many of the patients in this study did suffer from pain, bleeding, and fatigue. The only exception to watchful waiting for fibroid removal due to fear of future symptoms would be for patients who have had pregnancy complications due to uterine fibroids. Such complications include pain and premature delivery thought to result from fibroids during pregnancy. These patients should consider therapy prior to the next pregnancy even if they are not symptomatic in the nongravid condition.

In summary, the vast majority of fibroids that are detected in asymptomatic patients should be left untreated. These fibroids should be followed with annual ultrasound screenings and pelvic examinations. Patients with recently diagnosed asymptomatic fibroids should be informed of the various symptoms that could occur as a result of the fibroids. They should be educated to inform their physician if they develop symptoms of pain, pressure, urinary frequency, constipation, or abnormal uterine bleeding. These asymptomatic patients should be aware that many fibroids do not grow, but that approximately half of the fibroids normally will grow at a rate of up to 1 to 2 cm per year. Fibroids grow as a result of estrogen and/or progesterone exposure. Therefore, patients in menopause who are not on hormone replacement therapy should not have enlarging fibroids. This finding, even without the symptom of abnormal uterine bleeding, would require further investigation.

There is one additional scenario in which an asymptomatic fibroid should be treated. This is the rare case in which the fibroid is large enough to cause partial or complete ureteral obstruction leading to hydronephrosis. This is a very rare complication of uterine fibroids. In fact, no case reports of kidney damage could be found in a search of modern English literature.

EVALUATION OF SYMPTOMATIC PATIENTS

Fibroids that require therapy present with one of the following symptoms:

1. Heavy uterine bleeding leading to anemia
2. Symptoms that affect a patient's quality of life
    I. Heavy menses
    II. Pain
    III. Constipation
    IV. Urinary frequency
    V. Enlarged abdomen altering a woman's appearance

We will consider each in turn.

ABNORMAL UTERINE BLEEDING

More than 30% of all nonroutine visits to the gynecologist are made for the complaint of abnormal uterine bleeding. One woman in 20 seeks help from her health care provider for this symptom every year. Abnormal uterine bleeding affects more than 20% of all women older than age 35 and accounts for 12% of all visits (including annual examinations) to the gynecologist. In the United Kingdom, 821,700 prescriptions are written each year for abnormal bleeding alone.

Before we can evaluate abnormal uterine bleeding, we must understand what is normal. A normal cycle length is 28 days, plus or minus 7 days. The average duration of flow is 4 days, with normal being from 2 to 6 days. The average blood loss per cycle is 40 mL. Normal loss is between 20 and 60 mL per cycle. Blood loss greater than 80 mL per cycle will often lead to anemia. Excess uterine bleeding is defined as a cycle length less than 21 days, a duration of flow greater than 7 days, and blood loss greater than 80 mL per cycle, as previously stated.

It has been shown that it is very difficult for women to accurately assess exactly how much blood loss occurs per cycle. In fact, one third of women who lose more than 80 mL per cycle feel their bleeding is normal. Moreover, 15% of women with a flow of less than 15 mL per cycle feel their flow is heavy. For study purposes only, patients can keep a patient blood loss assessment card (PBLAC) record that has been validated to reflect actual blood loss per cycle (Fig. 4-1). A score greater than 150 is considered menorrhagia; a score less than 100 is considered normal.

The gynecologist does not require patients to keep a PBLAC score in order to determine if they are actually having excessive abnormal uterine bleeding. What is asked are clinical indicators of heavy bleeding, such as the following:

- Increase in use of sanitary pads to more than two per day
- Duration of flow lasting 3 days more than usual
- Intermenstrual bleeding
- Cycles more than 2 days shorter than usual
- Blood clots and socially embarrassing bleeding

Abnormal uterine bleeding can result from one of three causes:

1. Dysfunctional (anovulatory) uterine bleeding (DUB)
2. Iatrogenic causes
3. Organic conditions

Dysfunctional Uterine Bleeding

DUB is defined as abnormal uterine bleeding in the absence of uterine pathology. Symptoms associated with DUB include irregular cycles and unexpected breakthrough bleeding throughout a cycle. It is very rare for a woman to

ONE MONTH MENSTRUAL DIARY

PATIENT INITIALS: _RLH_
START DATE (MM/DD/YY): _01/07/98_

New Freedom® Super Maxi Pad	1	2	3	4	5	6	7	8
⬤		I						
▬			I	II				
▬▬		II						
Tampax® Super Plus Tampon	1	2	3	4	5	6	7	8
▭				I	II	HHt	II	
▭		II	IIII	III	HHt II			
▭	HHt I	IIII	II	I				
Kotex® Overnight Pad	1	2	3	4	5	6	7	8
⬤								
▬								
▬▬	I							
Clots	1d, 2n	2d, 3Q						
Flooding	On day 2, flooded tampons & pad, soiled panties & pants. Pants lightly soiled.							
Kotex Lightdays® Pantyliners	1	2	3	4	5	6	7	8
⬤								
▬								
▬▬								

FIGURE 4-1. Example of a patient blood loss assessment card (PBLAC).

have regular heavy cycles and be given the accurate diagnosis of DUB. DUB is most often caused by conditions that lead to irregular ovulation. When a female does not ovulate on a regular basis, she does not produce progesterone and is thus exposed to unopposed estrogen. Depending on the irregularity of ovulation, this condition will lead to a buildup of endometrium, which will break apart at will and lead to unpredictable irregular uterine bleeding. Because the source of the irregular bleeding is inadequate regular exposure of the endometrium to progesterone in patients with DUB, this is the one condition in which medical therapy with progestins or oral contraceptives is effective. DUB is most commonly seen in women just after menarche, women in perimenopause, and women diagnosed with polycystic ovarian syndrome.

Iatrogenic Causes of Abnormal Uterine Bleeding

Iatrogenic causes of abnormal uterine bleeding are usually easy to identify and are most often related to intrauterine device use, steroid contraceptives, or other medications such as certain tranquilizers. Like DUB, abnormal uterine bleeding associated with iatrogenic sources typically will present with unpredictable irregular bleeding rather than heavy regular menses. As with DUB, this is due to an irregular pattern of shedding caused by external hormonal therapy. Why a small percentage of patients on this therapy suffers from irregular bleeding while most do not is not known. By far, steroid contraceptives such as the birth control pill or patch and the long-acting progestins such as Depo-Provera (medroxyprogesterone acetate; Pharmacia and Upjohn Corp, Peapack, NJ, USA) are the most common iatrogenic causes of abnormal uterine bleeding. Patients taking these medications who experience a new onset of abnormal bleeding should first be taken off these drugs before a further workup is warranted. When patients are taking long-acting medications such as Depo-Provera, it may take up to 3 to 4 months for the medication to be metabolized. Intrauterine devices should be removed if abnormal uterine bleeding is present after 2 weeks of use.

Organic Conditions Leading to Abnormal Uterine Bleeding

Organic conditions that can result in heavy menstrual bleeding include the following:

- Complications of pregnancy
- Malignancy
- Infection
- Systemic diseases

  - Coagulopathies
  - Hypothyroidism
  - Liver disease

- Benign pelvic lesions

  - Submucous myomata
  - Intramural myomata (rare)
  - Endometrial and endocervical polyps
  - Adenomyosis

Abnormal bleeding associated with complications of pregnancy is the first condition that must be ruled out because it is the only condition that can be acutely life threatening. The bleeding may range from abnormal spotting to heavy clotting. It may or may not be associated with uterine cramping and abdominal pain. Abnormal uterine bleeding is often seen in the first trimester of pregnant patients who have a normal intrauterine pregnancy, an impending miscarriage, or an ectopic pregnancy. As a general rule, a serum pregnancy test should be obtained from all patients with a new onset of abnormal bleeding who are of reproductive age, regardless of their sexual history or history of contraceptive use. If a pregnancy test is positive and the serum level of human chorionic gonadotropin (hCG) is greater than 1,500 mIU/mL, then a pregnancy outside the uterine cavity must be ruled out by vaginal ultrasound. If an ectopic pregnancy is suspected due to an empty uterine cavity, the patient should immediately be referred to her gynecologist.

Malignancy is a very rare cause of abnormal uterine bleeding and typically presents as unexpected, unpredictable vaginal bleeding in menopause. However, 25% of endometrial cancers are found in patients younger than 50 years; therefore, this condition must also be considered in younger patients with irregular bleeding. A malignancy must be ruled out in any menopausal patient who is not on hormonal therapy and is bleeding. In this population, endometrial cancer is responsible for the bleeding in 3% to 10% of patients. Abnormal vaginal bleeding can also be the presenting symptom in patients with vulvar, vaginal, cervical, or tubal carcinomas. Uterine sarcomas are a rare source of abnormal bleeding, whereas endometrial carcinomas are the most common malignancy associated with postmenopausal bleeding.

Acute infection is an unlikely source of abnormal bleeding. These infections most often occur in women of reproductive age and present with pain, fever, and abnormal vaginal discharge. Chronic endometritis can be a source of irregular bleeding. This condition may have no symptom other than abnormal uterine bleeding.

Up to 20% of adolescents who present with excessive menorrhagia from the onset of menarche will be diagnosed with a coagulopathy (7). The most common coagulopathy is von Willebrand disease, but others may stem from a defect in the following:

- Primary hemostasis (formation of platelet plug)
- Secondary hemostasis (stabilization of platelet plug with fibrin deposition)
- Orderly dissolution of clot (fibrinolysis)

Benign uterine conditions that lead to abnormal uterine bleeding include submucous myomata, intramural myomata (rare), endometrial and endocervical polyps, and adenomyosis. Typically, submucous myomata and adenomyosis will present with regular heavy menses associated with large clots and cramping. Endometrial and endocervical polyps rarely present with heavy bleeding. Instead, they typically cause midcycle spotting or postcoital spotting. Most intramural myomata do not cause abnormal uterine bleeding. Exceptions occur when the intramural myomata are located very close to the endometrium. In this case, patients will complain of heavy regular cycles.

EVALUATION OF ABNORMAL UTERINE BLEEDING

History

As with many medical conditions, a brief medical history will guide the gynecologist to the most likely cause of abnormal uterine bleeding. The key questions in the family history relate to a history of bleeding coagulopathies and uterine fibroids. The patient's personal history should include the following:

- Past medical history (systemic disease)
- Medications
- Contraceptive use
- Age at onset of abnormal uterine bleeding
- Last menstrual period; rule out pregnancy
- Cycle regularity
- Abnormal bleeding from other sites

If the menstrual cycle is regular, there is a 95% chance the patient is ovulating. If the patient is ovulating, there is no need for an extensive hormonal evaluation. Early onset of abnormal bleeding, as well as a history of abnormal bleeding from other sites, would lead one to investigate a coagulopathy. A systemic disease affecting liver function could increase bleeding times and lead to menorrhagia.

If the menstrual cycles are irregular, a hormonal evaluation is indicated. Hormonal evaluation includes serum follicle stimulating hormone, luteinizing hormone, and estradiol measurements to rule out polycystic ovarian disease and hypothalamic oligomenorrhea. A serum prolactin and thyroid profile should be obtained as well.

If an adolescent presents with menorrhagia and a coagulopathy is suspected, the following evaluation is recommended:

- Platelet count
- Prothrombin time: factors II, V, VII, X, fibrinogen
- Activated partial thromboplastin time: factors VIII, IX, XII, II, V, X
- Bleeding time: platelet function, platelet number, von Willebrand factor, vascular integrity
- Platelet function test (replaces bleeding time)

If a patient has regular heavy menses and there is no history suggesting a coagulopathy, the reproductive tract must be evaluated. Malignancy should be ruled out in any patient older than 35 years. This is done with an office endometrial biopsy, a Pap smear, and a stool guaiac test. If the patient is postmenopausal, a vaginal ultrasound to measure endometrial thickness is also indicated. If the thickness is less than 6 mm, the chance of endometrial cancer is very low.

Chronic endometritis as a source of abnormal bleeding is also ruled out with an office endometrial biopsy. The absence of plasma cells in the endometrium rules out chronic endometritis. Cervical cultures are indicated if there is evidence of cervical bleeding on speculum examination.

If a patient has a smooth, boggy, enlarged uterus combined with a history of painful heavy menses, adenomyosis should be ruled out. Adenomyosis is a benign condition in which endometrial glands and stroma are found within the myometrium at least 1 cm from the endometrial basalis. The mechanism causing menorrhagia

and pain is unknown but is thought to be due to increased production of prostaglandins and prostacyclins. The only way to confirm the diagnosis of adenomyosis is with a myometrial biopsy. This is most commonly done in the pathology lab after a hysterectomy. If the uterus is not going to be removed, a T2-weighted MRI has the best sensitivity and specificity for diagnosing this condition with a thickened junctional zone (8). There have been reports of using ultrasound, myometrial needle biopsies, and hysteroscopy for making this diagnosis; however, none of these has proven as predictable as MRI (9,10).

The endometrial cavity should be evaluated in patients who suffer from menorrhagia and fall into one of four categories:

1. Premenopausal and ovulatory (regular cycles)
2. Premenopausal and anovulatory (irregular cycles) and do not respond to hormonal therapy
3. Any postmenopausal bleeding if not on hormonal therapy
4. Unexpected bleeding in menopause on hormonal therapy

In these groups of patients, an anatomic source of bleeding will be found in more than 50% of patients. Primary evaluation of the uterine cavity has been performed most commonly by a blind dilation and curettage (D&C). Other instruments for evaluation include a hysterosalpingogram, abdominal and vaginal ultrasound, sonohysterography, and office hysteroscopy.

There is an ongoing trend in gynecology to eliminate the blind D&C as the sole mechanism for evaluating the endometrial cavity. Loffer (11) has demonstrated that the D&C will miss up to 40% of focal lesions such as endometrial polyps and fibroids, which are often the cause of abnormal uterine bleeding. When a direct view with the hysteroscope was added to the evaluation, none of 90 lesions was missed in his series. The blind D&C is adequate for diagnosing diffuse and microscopic endometrial disease such as endometrial hyperplasia or carcinoma, which involves the entire cavity; however, most lesions that cause regular heavy menses are focal. A D&C can also be of value in stopping acute hemorrhage from the uterus. However, the effect on reducing bleeding rarely lasts longer than 3 months.

The specificity and sensitivity of the hysterosalpingogram, the abdominal ultrasound, and the vaginal ultrasound for diagnosing abnormalities of the uterine cavity are not in the same 90% and above category as the sonohysterogram and the office hysteroscope. As a result, these tests are rarely used today to evaluate the uterine cavity. The vaginal ultrasound is an excellent tool to evaluate myometrial and subserosal lesions as well as the endometrial thickness in postmenopausal women.

Sonohysterography is a technique in which 15 to 20 mL of saline are injected into the uterine cavity in order to distend the cavity while a vaginal ultrasound is performed. This is an excellent tool to demonstrate intrauterine abnormalities (Fig. 4-2) and has a very high rate of sensitivity. Because one cannot visualize the lesion or biopsy the lesion in the uterine cavity, the specificity of sonohysterography is not as high as a direct view with the hysteroscope (12).

The most common uterine lesion in ovulatory patients who suffer from menorrhagia is the submucous fibroid. The gold standard for diagnosing a submucous fibroid is the

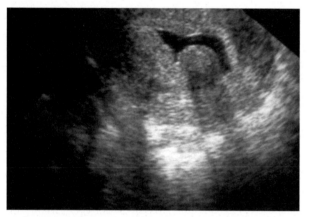

FIGURE 4-2. Sonohysterogram of a submucous myoma.

office hysteroscope. This instrument allows for direct visualization of the uterine cavity lesion and does not require interpretation of a radiologic image. Office hysteroscopy can be performed with a 5-mm rigid rod lens system using CO_2 gas or saline for uterine distention. This instrument requires that a paracervical block be placed in the cervix for anesthesia and a tenaculum be placed on the anterior lip of the cervix in order to straighten a curved cervical/uterine canal. This technique typically takes 15 to 20 minutes to complete. Alternatively, diagnostic office hysteroscopy can be performed with a 3.5-mm flexible fiberoptic hysteroscope using saline for distention. Using this instrument, the diagnostic procedure takes less than 1 minute and is most often tolerated with no local or oral anesthesia (13). The flexible hysteroscope is an excellent tool to diagnose most of the intrauterine lesions that cause abnormal uterine bleeding (Fig. 4-3).

When diagnosing a submucous myoma as a cause of menorrhagia, it is important to classify the myomas as type 0 (100% of the fibroid within the uterine cavity), type I (>50% of the fibroid within the uterine cavity), or type II (>50% of the fibroid is intramural) (Fig. 4-4). It is necessary to make this classification when advising women on management strategies. De Block et al. demonstrated that more than 90% of type 0 and type I submucous fibroids can be resected with a single hysteroscopic procedure. However,

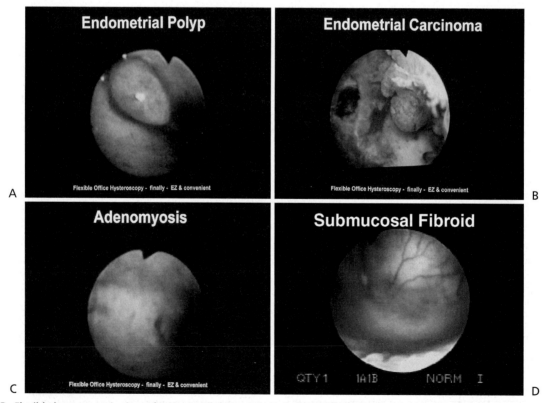

FIGURE 4-3. Flexible hysteroscopic view of intrauterine lesions. **A:** Endometrial polyp. **B:** Focal endometrial carcinoma. **C:** Adenomyosis with pitting endometrium. **D:** Type I submucous myoma.

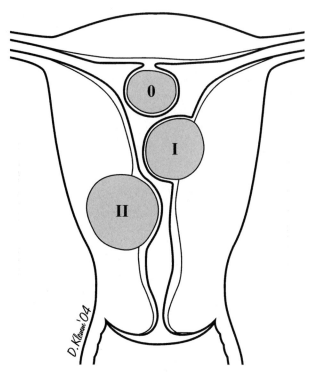

FIGURE 4-4. Line drawing of submucous fibroid classification.

most type II submucous fibroids require at least two procedures to complete the resection (14). It is important to relate this information to the patient when she is deciding among several treatment options for her menorrhagia.

Evaluation of Pelvic Pressure

When a patient presents to the gynecologist with a complaint of pelvic pressure, it is important to again take a thorough history, perform an abdominal pelvic examination, and order the appropriate radiologic examinations. A lesion such as a uterine fibroid typically grows at a slow pace, and the patient will describe a pressure symptom that worsens over a period of 6 to 24 months. If the pressure is in the lower back and the fibroid is located in the posterior lower uterine segment, the patient will often admit to dyspareunia as well as back pain. Other sources of pelvic pressure include ovarian masses or musculoskeletal abnormalities, which typically present more acutely with a recent onset.

The physical examination will begin with abdominal palpation and include a bimanual examination. A bimanual examination will likely differentiate a uterine from an ovarian mass unless the mass is adhered to the uterus. In this case, a large uterine fibroid may make it impossible to palpate the ovary. Likewise, a large ovarian mass will make it difficult to accurately assess the uterine size and position.

When any pelvic mass is palpated, the next appropriate step is to obtain an abdominal and pelvic ultrasound. This examination will usually be sufficient to assess the ovaries and the uterus as the source of the abdominal or pelvic mass.

When the ultrasound is insufficient to evaluate the abdominal and pelvic organs, an abdominal/pelvic CT scan or MRI is ordered. If an ovarian mass is diagnosed by ultrasound, CT, or MRI, it is advisable to order a serum cancer antigen 125 (CA-125) measurement to help approximate the risk of a malignancy. Even with suboptimal sensitivity and specificity, this test may be helpful in determining the best management approach for an abnormal pelvic mass.

URINARY FREQUENCY

For women 40 years of age and older, urinary frequency and stress incontinence are common problems, as is the presence of uterine fibroids. The primary question is whether or not the fibroid is responsible for the urinary symptoms. Patients with fibroids and urinary symptoms should have complete urodynamic testing before one can conclude the fibroid is causing the urinary problems. Urodynamic testing will assess bladder capacity, bladder irritability, urethral sphincter integrity, and pelvic support. When the bladder symptoms are caused by a reduced bladder capacity from a large fibroid, urodynamic testing will demonstrate normal bladder contractions, normal urethral pressures, and normal pelvic support. The scenario that the gynecologist and the patient wish to avoid is removal of an asymptomatic fibroid with subsequent continuation of the bladder symptoms.

CONSTIPATION

As is the case with bladder symptoms, other more common causes of constipation should be ruled out before one can conclude that a fibroid, no matter how large, is the cause of this symptom. As a general rule, the gynecologist will not perform this evaluation. Rather, a thorough evaluation by a gastroenterologist is indicated prior to removal of a fibroid for the sole symptom of constipation.

SUMMARY

Uterine fibroids are very common benign smooth muscle tumors. The symptoms they can create range from none to debilitating uterine bleeding leading to anemia as well as significant pelvic pressure and bulk symptoms. The workup for uterine fibroids is dependent on the primary presenting symptom. If a patient is unaware the fibroid is present and the fibroid is found during a routine pelvic examination, no treatment is necessary and appropriate follow-up includes annual pelvic ultrasounds. On the other hand, if a patient presents with fibroids and menorrhagia, it is imperative to determine the fibroid location within the uterus to evaluate the causal relationship. As well, if the fibroid is determined to cause the menorrhagia, knowledge of the type of fibroid is essential when consulting the patient on management options. Just as sources other than fibroids need to be excluded as the cause of menorrhagia, the same holds true for bladder, bowel, and pain symptoms thought to be related to uterine fibroids. With a thorough history, abdominal and pelvic examinations, and appropriate imaging test, the likelihood that the fibroid is causing the symptom can be accurately determined. As in the treatment of abnormal uterine bleeding due to uterine fibroids, when the fibroid causes the symptom and the fibroid is removed, the symptom(s) will resolve in nearly 90% of patients (14).

REFERENCES

1. Day Baird D, Dunson DB, Hill MC, et al. High cumulative incidence of uterine leiomyoma in black and white women: ultrasound evidence. *Am J Obstet Gynecol* 2003;188(1):100–107.
2. Luoto R, Kaprio J, Rutanen EM, et al. Heritability and risk factors of uterine fibroids: the Finnish Twin Cohort study. *Maturitas* 2000;37:15–26.
2a. Buttram VC Jr, Reiter RC. Uterine leiomyomata: etiology, symptomology, and management. *Fertil Steril* 1981;36:433–445.
3. Parker WH, Fu YS, Berek JS. Uterine sarcoma in patients operated on for presumed leiomyoma and rapidly growing leiomyoma. *Obstet Gynecol* 1994;83:414–418.
4. Hillis SD, Marchbanks PA, Peterson HB. Uterine size and risk of complications among women undergoing abdominal hysterectomy for leiomyomas. *Obstet Gynecol* 1996;87:539–543.
5. Pritts EA. Fibroids and infertility: a systematic review of the evidence. *Obstet Gynecol Surv* 2001;56:483–491.
6. Carlson KJ, Miller BA, Fowler FJ Jr. The Maine Women's Health Study: II. Outcomes of nonsurgical management of leiomyomas, abnormal bleeding, and chronic pelvic pain. *Obstet Gynecol* 1994;83:566–572.
7. Claessens EA, Cowell CA. Acute adolescent menorrhagia. *Am J Obstet Gynecol* 1981;139:277–280.
8. Togashi K, Ozasa H, Konishi I, et al. Enlarged uterus: differentiation between adenomyosis and leiomyoma with MR imaging. *Radiology* 1991;180:81–83.
9. Reinhold C, McCarthy S, Bret PM, et al. Diffuse adenomyosis: comparison of endovaginal US and MR imaging with histopathologic correlation. *Radiology* 1996;199:151–158.
10. McCausland AM. Hysteroscopic myometrial biopsy: its use in diagnosing adenomyosis and its clinical application. *Am J Obstet Gynecol* 1996;174:1786–1794.
11. Loffer FD. Hysteroscopy with selective endometrial sampling compared with D&C for abnormal uterine bleeding: the value of a negative hysteroscopic view. *Obstet Gynecol* 1989;73:16–20.
12. Lindheim SR, Morales AJ. Comparison of sonohysterography and hysteroscopy: lessons learned and avoiding pitfalls. *J Am Assoc Gynecol Laparosc* 2002;9:223–231.
13. Bradley LD, Widrich T. State-of-the-art flexible hysteroscopy for office gynecologic evaluation. *J Am Assoc Gynecol Laparosc* 1995;2:263–267.
14. Wamsteker K, Emanuel MH, de Kruif JH. Transcervical hysteroscopic resection of submucous fibroids for abnormal uterine bleeding: results regarding the degree of intramural extension. *Obstet Gynecol* 1993;82:736–740.

5

IMAGING OF LEIOMYOMATA, THE UTERUS, AND THE PELVIS

REENA C. JHA
SANDRA J. ALLISON
SUSAN M. ASCHER

INTRODUCTION

Imaging is an essential tool in the evaluation, treatment, and postprocedural management of patients undergoing embolization. History and physical examination have limitations, and a number of conditions can mimic the symptoms associated with fibroids. Adnexal masses can mimic serosal fibroids. Similarly, adenomyosis, endometrial or cervical polyps, and endometrial hyperplasia or cancer can mimic the bleeding patterns associated with fibroids. For this reason, the diagnosis of fibroids must be confirmed with preoperative imaging, either ultrasound or magnetic resonance imaging (MRI). Just as important, imaging studies are an essential tool in assessing outcome, detecting recurrence, and diagnosing and managing complications. This chapter introduces the imaging methods that are essential to those practicing in this field.

ULTRASOUND IMAGING

Ultrasound is the primary modality used for imaging both the gravid and nongravid uterus. Transabdominal scans can be augmented by transvaginal and translabial scans, as well as sonohysterography. When more imaging is necessary after an inconclusive scan, MRI may clarify findings and direct management.

Technique

Generally, transabdominal scanning is performed first. The patient optimally has a full bladder to use as an acoustic window. In addition, the full bladder displaces gas-filled loops of bowel superiorly. A curvilinear probe of low to medium frequency (3.5B5 MHz) is routinely used. In the setting of massively enlarged uteri due to large leiomyomata, extended field-of-view imaging may prove useful, especially as a tool for surgical planning and consultation.

Transvaginal scanning can provide more detailed information about the endometrium. The higher frequencies insonated by transvaginal probes (5–7 MHz) provide improved spatial resolution. The ability to detect small leiomyomas is increased; however, their precise location with respect to the uterine cavity is uncertain at times (1). Improvement in spatial resolution is offset by limitations on probe position, given its intravaginal location.

Sonohysterography

This relatively new technique provides improved depiction of the uterine cavity over transvaginal scanning. A speculum examination is performed to evaluate orientation of cervix, followed by introduction of a 5- to 7-French catheter into the cervical external os. Under direct ultrasound visualization with an endocervical catheter in place, the uterine cavity is distended with 10 to 15 mL of saline. The saline-endometrial interface allows excellent depiction of endometrial and submucosal myometrial pathology (2). The procedure is tolerated well, requires no anesthesia, and has no reported complications (3,4).

Sonohysterography is typically performed for abnormal bleeding and is best done at the beginning of the cycle after menstruation when the endometrial lining is at its thinnest. This facilitates differentiation of an echogenic polyp from normal endometrial thickening during the secretory phase. With respect to leiomyomas, however, the best detection is during the secretory phase when endometrium is at its thickest and contrast between this and the hypoechoic leiomyoma is greatest (2).

Sonohysterography is more sensitive than transvaginal sonography and hysterosalpingography for detecting the presence and number of submucosal leiomyomata (5). Sonohysterography can provide additional information over transvaginal sonography alone, resulting in a decrease in the number of indeterminate diagnoses made on transvaginal sonography (6). Diagnostic confidence and interobserver agreement is considerably improved in the diagnosis of uterine abnormalities, especially in the diagnosis and classification of submucosal leiomyomata and its differentiation from endometrial polyps. Therefore, sonohysterography plays a role in preoperative assessment of women with leiomyomata (4). The percentage of leiomyoma projecting into the endometrial cavity is accurately depicted, thus directing management between hysteroscopy or myomectomy. Additional findings at sonohysterography may direct patient management toward either biopsy (blind or guided) or dilation and curettage (Fig. 5-1).

Application of Color Doppler

Color Doppler sonography can reveal the relative vascularity of uterine lesions (7). Color Doppler sonography/sonohysterography may be helpful in distinguishing an endometrial polyp with a single feeding vessel from an intracavitary submucosal leiomyoma, which usually has several vessels arising from the inner myometrium (8). In addition, color Doppler sonography (CDS) can be used to assess leiomyoma and uterine vascularity and flow patterns. Varied degrees of vascularity may be seen. Typically, leiomyomata have marked peripheral blood flow with decreased central flow or an avascular core (Fig. 5-2) (9). Information regarding leiomyoma vascularity obtained on CDS may be useful in determining which patients are best suited for uterine artery embolization (UAE) therapy (10). Specifically, Fleischer et al. (11) suggested that hypervascular leiomyomata as visualized by three-dimensional color Doppler imaging tended to decrease more in size than did isovascular or hypovascular leiomyomata after UAE. They demonstrated that utilizing three-dimensional color Doppler sonography to depict leiomyoma vascularity improved

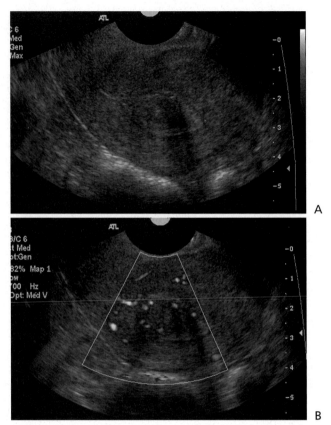

FIGURE 5-2. A: Patient presented with abnormal uterine bleeding. Sagittal gray-scale sonogram through the uterus demonstrates a mass projecting into the endometrial canal. Although the hypoechoic appearance favors an intracavitary leiomyoma, polyps are more common and may have this appearance. **B:** Doppler sonography demonstrates peripheral blood flow to the mass with relatively little central flow characteristic of leiomyoma. A single feeding vessel, characteristic of polyps, was not identified.

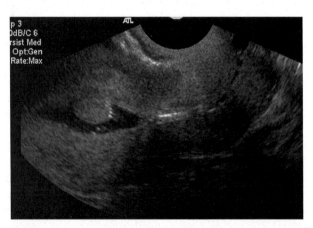

FIGURE 5-1. Sonohysterogram performed in patient with history of spotting. Preprocedural transvaginal sonogram demonstrated thickening of the endometrial complex. The image above demonstrates distention of the uterine cavity with saline. Note the echogenic catheter in the lower uterine segment. Mass projecting into the uterine cavity represents polyp causing apparent thickening of the endometrium on the previous scan.

the delineation of size, location, and extent of myometrial involvement. Aside from leiomyoma vascularity, CDS can depict collateral flow not depicted on uterine artery arteriography. A study by McLucas et al. (12) showed that peak systolic velocity has a relationship with the size of myomata and uterus before embolization. Higher peak systolic velocity values were associated with the number of vials of polyvinyl alcohol (PVA) particles used in embolization, as well as particle load used to embolize 1 L of uterine tissue. Therefore, preembolization Doppler studies may predict the patient's chance for failure (12). To date, sonographic contrast agents have not been used in the evaluation of leiomyomata or the post-UAE uterus.

Spectrum of Imaging Findings of Leiomyomas

Leiomyomas, also referred to as *fibroids* or *fibromyomas*, are the most common pelvic tumors. They are composed of bundles of smooth muscle that are interleaved. Sonographi-

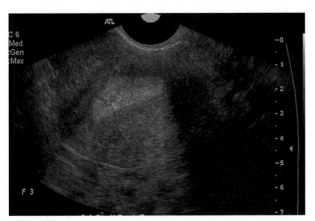

FIGURE 5-3. Intramural leiomyoma with uniform low echogenicity and poor sound through transmission typical of a leiomyoma primarily composed of smooth muscle.

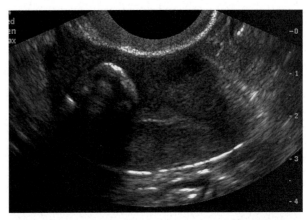

FIGURE 5-5. Transverse image of the uterine body demonstrating a degenerated myoma with coarse calcifications and associated posterior acoustic shadowing.

cally, leiomyomas may appear hyperechoic or hypoechoic, homogeneous or heterogeneous. The sonographic appearance of leiomyomata is largely dependent on its composition, i.e., relative amount of smooth muscle and areas of necrosis and/or degeneration (13). When the muscular component predominates, the leiomyoma appears as a hypoechoic solid mass with poor sound through transmission (Fig. 5-3). As a leiomyoma undergoes fibrous degeneration, echogenicity increases because of the presence of tiny cystic areas. These tiny cysts allow improved through transmission (Fig. 5-4). As degeneration progresses, cystic or hemorrhagic necrosis results in an anechoic mass with far acoustic enhancement. Calcifications, usually seen in older patients, present as echogenic foci with shadowing (Fig. 5-5).

Shadowing and acoustic attenuation is a defining sonographic characteristic of leiomyomata. It is a common misconception that attenuation from echogenic foci seen with myomas is always related to calcification within the myoma.

Radiations of sharp discrete shadowing that do not arise from demonstrable calcification are common in leiomyomata and are thought to be related to transition zones between fibrous tissue and smooth muscle (Fig. 5-6) (13).

Leiomyomata are also classified by location as submucosal, intramural, or subserosal (Fig. 5-7). Intramural is the most common location. Submucosal leiomyomata may be reliably distinguished from polyps by sonohysterography. Whereas polyps are isoechoic to endometrium and have preservation of the endometrial-myometrial interface, leiomyomata are broad based, hypoechoic, and well defined. There may be associated shadowing. Submucosal leiomyomata have an overlying layer of echogenic endometrium with related distortion of the endometrial-myometrial interface (Fig. 5-8) (14). Leiomyomata in other locations may become symptomatic if large enough, causing pressure effects on adjacent organs or ligaments. Subserosal leiomyomas may undergo torsion and necrosis. Leiomyomata

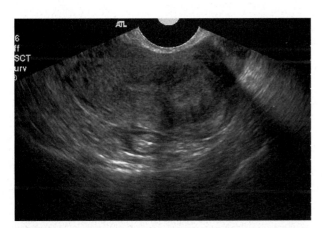

FIGURE 5-4. Transverse image of the uterus near the fundus depicting a leiomyoma with relatively increased echogenicity. The enhanced sound through transmission is related to tiny cystic areas of degeneration.

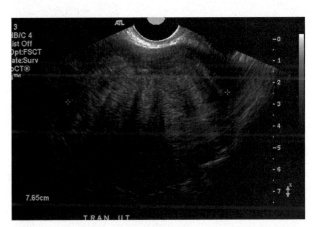

FIGURE 5-6. Transverse sonogram of the uterus with a large posterior leiomyoma demonstrates sharp radiating shadows without identifiable calcification. These shadows are thought to be related to interfaces between fibrous tissue and smooth muscle.

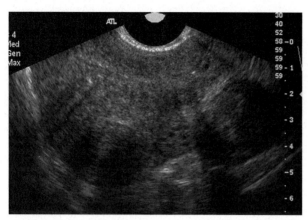

FIGURE 5-7. Sagittal image of the uterus demonstrates at least two hypoechoic masses projecting from the uterus posteriorly representing subserosal leiomyomata. Note the echogenic myoma with relatively enhanced sound through transmission.

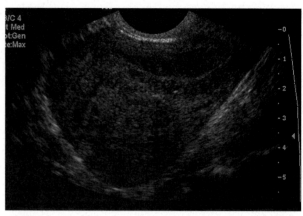

FIGURE 5-9. Enlargement of the uterus with anterior displacement of the endometrial complex without discrete mass. Follow-up magnetic resonance imaging demonstrated multiple anterior and posterior leiomyomata.

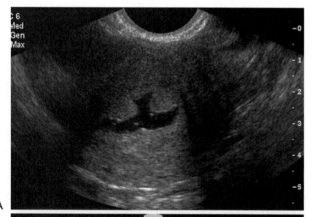

A

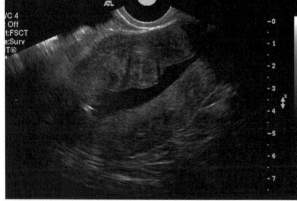

B

FIGURE 5-8. A: Sagittal image obtained during sonohysterography demonstrates two echogenic masses projecting into the uterine cavity in this patient with abnormal uterine bleeding. Note that the masses are isoechoic to the endometrium and there is preservation of the endomyometrial junction, which is typical for endometrial polyps. **B:** Sagittal image obtained in a different patient demonstrates two masses projecting into the uterine cavity. In this case, the masses are isoechoic to the myometrium, well defined, and broad based. Intact endometrium is seen overlying the masses. These findings are typical of leiomyomas.

located in the broad ligament may be challenging diagnostically and simulate ovarian or adnexal masses.

Leiomyomata may appear as single or multiple masses. Alternatively, they may present as part of a lobular enlarged uterus. In some cases the sole clue to the presence of leiomyomata is an irregularly enlarged uterus with distortion or obscuration of the endometrial stripe (Fig. 5-9) (15).

Sonographic Appearance Postembolization

Following UAE, leiomyomata appear to decrease in echogenicity and in general become hypoechoic. This is the expected finding given that devascularization followed by necrosis occurs. About 3 months after embolization, one should expect little if any flow on color Doppler sonography (Fig. 5-10) (9).

Tranquart et al. (16) demonstrated an absence of intraleiomyoma vessels as early as 3 months postembolization and persistence of perifibroid vessels. Uterine vascularization appears unchanged with sonography after embolization.

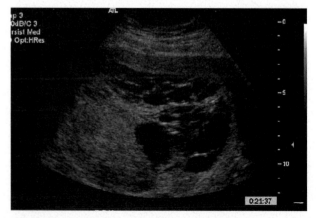

FIGURE 5-10. Transverse sonogram of the uterus after uterine artery embolization demonstrating multiple anechoic spaces within previously seen leiomyoma representing areas of necrosis.

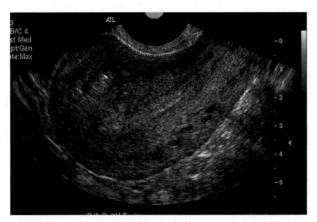

FIGURE 5-11. Adenomyosis. Sagittal sonogram of the uterus in a patient complaining of cyclical pelvic pain. The anteroposterior dimension of the uterus is abnormally large. The anterior myometrium is heterogeneous without a discrete mass. Echogenic area appears to extend from endometrium representing ectopic endometrial tissue. Note myometrial cyst. Follow-up magnetic resonance imaging demonstrated adenomyosis.

Adenomyosis

The sonographic signs of adenomyosis require the higher-frequency endovaginal transducers for detection. In addition, the signs are more reliably identified during real-time scanning and not on static images (17). In approximately 75% of patients, adenomyosis appears as areas of hypo-echogenicity or heterogeneity of the myometrium that may be focal or diffuse (18,19). The echogenic areas represent heterotopic endometrial tissue, whereas the hypoechoic regions represent smooth muscle. The relative amounts of each tissue type present determines the sonographic appearance. In approximately 50% of patients, small myometrial cysts are seen representing dilated cystic glands of hemorrhagic foci. Ectopic endometrial tissue may also appear as echogenic nodules or linear striations extending from the endometrium. This may cause poor definition of the endomyometrial junction. When attempting to distinguish adenomyosis from leiomyomata, the lack of contour abnormality or mass effect, elliptical shape, and ill-defined margins favor adenomyosis (Fig. 5-11) (5). Color Doppler sonography may demonstrate randomly scattered vessels or intratumoral signals and aid in accurately distinguishing adenomyosis from leiomyomata, which have peripheral scattered vessels or outer feeding vessels (20).

MAGNETIC RESONANCE IMAGING OF LEIOMYOMATA, THE UTERUS, AND THE PELVIS

MRI is an excellent method of visualizing the uterus. MRI is currently the most accurate imaging technique for the detection and localization of leiomyomata (21–24). MRI

has multiplanar capability and is able to accurately localize and measure lesions and thus overcome the limitations of ultrasound (25).

The imaging goals for patients selected as candidates for UAE are two-fold: to accurately assess for the presence, number, size, location, and character of leiomyomata; and to exclude concomitant pathology, particularly adenomyosis, which may be associated with clinical symptoms closely mimicking leiomyoma disease. For these reasons, MRI is the preferred modality to image potential UAE patients.

Magnetic Resonance Imaging of the Female Pelvis: Technique

Imaging is best performed with a high field strength magnet (>1 T) and a phased-array torso coil to maximize the signal-to-noise ratio. Patients fast for a minimum of 4 hours prior to the study. We do not routinely use antiperistaltics. The patients are asked to void prior to the examination.

The imaging technique for imaging the female pelvis is often diagnosis driven. The selection of size of field of view, slice thickness, and matrix depends on patient size, size of the uterus, and required resolution, respectively. T1-weighted sequences, either with gradient-echo or spin-echo technique, are used to assess the adnexa and to detect any bright signal that may be seen in hemorrhage or other proteinaceous material. Fat saturation is useful to increase the conspicuousness of bright signal intensity from proteinaceous material. The T2-weighted sequences acquired with turbo (fast) spin-echo sequences are ideal for defining the zonal anatomy of the uterus (Fig. 5-12) and are

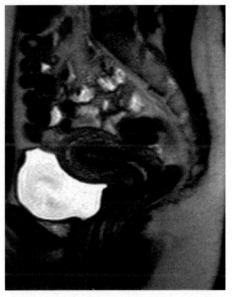

FIGURE 5-12. Normal uterus. On this T2-weighted sagittal image, the zonal anatomy of the uterus is well defined, with the endometrium bright in signal and outlined by the dark signal intensity of the junctional zone, which is continuous with the fibromuscular stroma of the cervix. The outer myometrium is intermediate in signal.

the most useful sequences for detecting leiomyomata. They are also vital in defining the junctional zone, which represents the innermost layer of the myometrium and is contiguous with the fibromuscular stroma of the cervix. Imaging the uterus in long and short axes allows for accurate localization of leiomyomata and the endometrial lining, as well as assessment of possible areas of adenomyosis. Use of thin-section, high-resolution, T2-weighted MRI sequences allows for better detection of adenomyosis as well as endometrial pathology. The T2-weighted images are also useful in detecting hydroureter or urinary compression, which may be a leiomyoma-related complication.

The typical appearance of leiomyomata at MRI has been well established (23,24). A typical leiomyoma demonstrates low signal intensity relative to myometrium on T2-weighted images and intermediate signal intensity on T1-weighted images and therefore is difficult to detect as discrete lesions on T1-weighted images (Fig. 5-13). A lobulated appearance of the uterus on a T1-weighted sequence is suggestive of this diagnosis, but T2-weighted images are vital in confirming this diagnosis and assessing concomitant uterine pathology. Nondegenerated leiomyomata are typically well-defined lesions of homogeneous low signal compared with adjacent normal myometrium on T2-weighted images. The low signal intensity on T2-weighted sequences is attributed to hyalinization (26,27). The presence of necrosis, and degeneration produces altered signal. Generally, MRI cannot accurately differentiate among hyaline, myxoid, or cystic degeneration (26). Red degeneration may show high signal on T1-weighted images

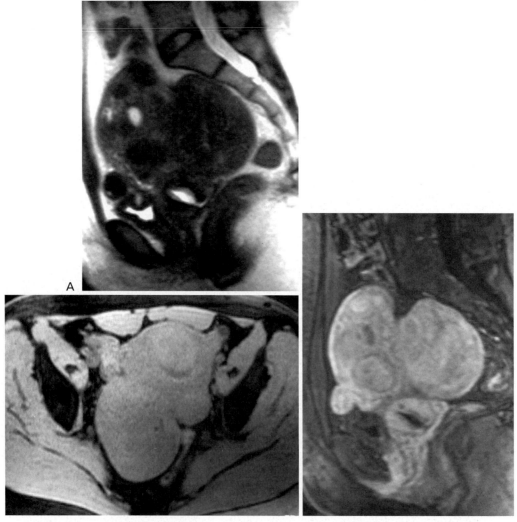

FIGURE 5-13. Typical magnetic resonance imaging examination of uterus before uterine artery embolization. **A:** T2-weighted sagittal image shows well-defined lesions of dark signal intensity that are typical for uterine leiomyomata, seen in subserosal and intramural locations. **B:** T1-weighted axial fat-saturated image shows a lobulated uterus, with a pedunculated subserosal mass representing a leiomyoma. The signal intensity of the leiomyomata are homogeneous with myometrium. **C:** T1-weighted sagittal gadolinium-enhanced image shows enhancement of the leiomyomata, with most lesions demonstrating signal slightly less than the myometrium.

and variable signal on T2-weighted images, which represent blood products (28). Classification of the subtypes of leiomyomata by MRI has been described, with fair accuracy rates in differentiating among subtypes; the highest accuracy is seen for hemorrhagic leiomyomata, with a sensitivity of 100% and specificity of 86% (29). Some leiomyomata have a high signal intensity rim on T2-weighted images, which represents a pseudocapsule of dilated lymphatic vessels, dilated veins, or edema (30). This rim may show enhancement on postgadolinium images. Leiomyomata may calcify, which is usually amorphous and coarse on plain radiography and may be seen on gradient-echo images as regions of signal loss due to susceptibility artifact.

Enhancement of the uterus with intravenous contrast is generally not necessary for making a diagnosis of a leiomyoma. Hricak et al. (31) have described MRI in the evaluation of benign uterine masses including leiomyomata. They determined that a combination of T1-weighted, proton-density, and T2-weighted images was able to detect leiomyomata in 92% of cases and characterize leiomyomata in 92% of cases (31). Most often, leiomyomata enhance heterogeneously less than the surrounding myometrium and remain well marginated. However, the addition of gadolinium enhancement did not improve detection or characterization. Gadolinium enhancement has been used to characterize leiomyomata that demonstrate high signal intensity on T2-weighted images. Cellular leiomyomata, which are composed of compact smooth muscle and little collagen, can have relatively higher signal on T2-weighted

images and demonstrate increased signal with gadolinium enhancement (Fig. 5-14) (32). Other investigators found undegenerated leiomyomata enhanced after gadolinium infusion, whereas those with hyaline degeneration did not (33).

The requirement for gadolinium enhancement in the UAE patient population has yet to be completely defined. We have found the ability to demonstrate lack of significant enhancement helpful as a method of assessing completeness of infarction (34). Use of gadolinium also may allow for the detection of ovarian artery supply, which may affect the success of UAE (Fig. 5-15). Furthermore, use of contrast can be helpful in localizing a pedunculated adnexal lesion as myometrial in origin.

We image all UAE candidates with MRI prior to treatment. Based on the findings, the patients may undergo UAE. Detection of concomitant or alternate pathology in a patient presenting with symptoms attributed to leiomyomata is a vital component in triaging these patients. Several reports have shown that MRI is highly accurate in the diagnosis of adenomyosis, with a high sensitivity and specificity of 86% to 100% and overall accuracy of 85% to 90.5% (24,31,35). MRI is also helpful in the detection of endometriomas. With the use of fat-suppressed T1-weighted sequences, accuracy rates are up to 96%, with sensitivity of 90% and specificity of 98% (36–39). Endometrial implants are more problematic, with a reported accuracy rate of 77% (40,41).

Based on our experience, relative contraindications to UAE include patients with a dominant pedunculated

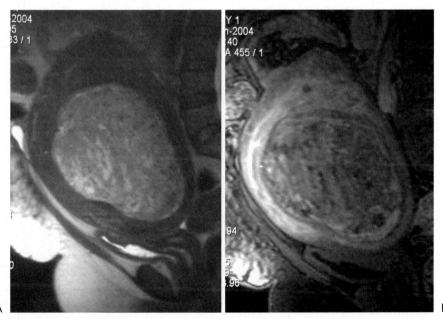

FIGURE 5-14. Cellular leiomyoma. **A:** T2-weighted sagittal image of the uterus shows heterogeneous well-defined mass with high signal intensity compared with the myometrium, which may be seen with a cellular leiomyoma or with degeneration of a leiomyoma. **B:** T1-weighted sagittal gadolinium-enhanced image shows enhancement of the leiomyoma.

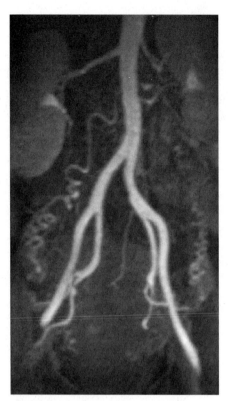

FIGURE 5-15. Enlarged ovarian artery collaterals in a patient before uterine artery embolization. T1-weighted gadolinium-enhanced magnetic resonance angiography of the pelvic vasculature shows bilateral tortuous arteries arising from the abdominal aorta at the level of the kidneys and extending into the pelvis, proving collaterals to the leiomyomatous uterus.

subserosal leiomyoma including a broad ligament leiomyoma (which may theoretically separate from the uterus post-UAE, and infarct in the peritoneal cavity) and cervical leiomyomata (which often have parasitized blood supply). A patient with overwhelming endometriosis and minimal leiomyoma burden may be a relative contraindication to UAE, whereas detecting changes of adenomyosis concomitant to leiomyomata may be useful in understanding patient symptoms prior to and subsequent to UAE. Patients with findings suggestive of extensive hemorrhagic degeneration prior to UAE, with high signal intensity on T1-weighted images (Fig. 5-16), may have a relative contraindication (34,42). We are currently not excluding patients with concomitant adenomyosis. A normal MRI of the uterus, or features suggestive of pelvic malignancy, is an absolute contraindication for UAE.

Adenomyosis

The diagnosis of adenomyosis by MRI is made by demonstrating abnormality of the junctional zone larger than 12 mm (35). Infiltration of endometrial glands into the inner myometrium leads to reactive thickening of the muscular layers, resulting in an enlarged junctional zone

(Fig. 5-17). Ancillary features include tiny foci of bright signal on T2-weighted images representing ectopic endometrium, cystic changes, or blood products, whereas bright signals on T1-weighted images represent the proteinaceous content of blood products. Irregularity of the junctional zone may be seen, and occasionally linear striations may be identified that represent invaginated endometrial glands. Adenomyosis may be focal or diffuse. When focal it is referred to as an *adenomyoma*. This may simulate a leiomyoma. The differentiating features between these lesions, aside from the criteria used to diagnose adenomyosis described previously, are that an adenomyoma must abut the

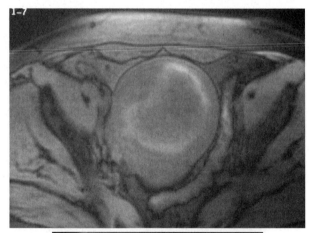

A

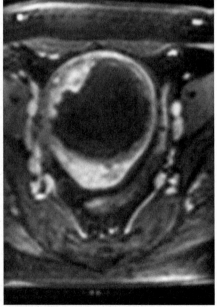

B

FIGURE 5-16. Degeneration of a leiomyoma in a patient before uterine artery embolization. **A:** T1-weighted axial fat-saturated image shows a lesion with high signal, particularly at the periphery. **B:** T1-weighted axial fat-saturated gadolinium-enhanced image shows only a minor area of enhancement along the margin. Some studies suggest poor response of lesions with these pre-UAE features.

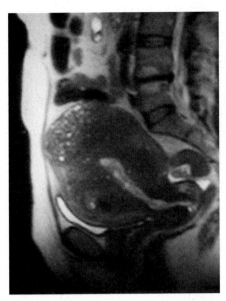

FIGURE 5-17. Florid adenomyosis in a patient with a presenting diagnosis of uterine leiomyomata. T2-weighted sagittal image shows marked thickening of the junctional zone, with numerous tiny foci of bright signal intensity seen scattered throughout the abnormal junctional zone.

junctional zone, have relatively poorly defined margins, and have little mass effect given its size, whereas a leiomyoma can be in any location of the uterus, have well-defined margins, and have mass effect of the adjacent tissues (43). Difficulties arise when the uterus contains diffuse small leiomyomata that are intramural and scattered throughout the junctional zone, making characterization of the junctional zone difficult. Transient uterine contractions may occasionally simulate adenomyosis, so care should be taken to ensure that the junctional zone thickening is fixed on image sequences obtained at separate time intervals (44). Gadolinium enhancement may occasionally be helpful because leiomyomata often demonstrate a well-defined margin, whereas adenomyosis tends to have a much more poorly defined heterogeneous pattern of enhancement.

Post Uterine Artery Embolization Imaging of Leiomyomata

The initial investigators who performed UAE used ultrasonography to evaluate the uterus before and after UAE (45,46). Given the limitations of sonography, many interventionalists are now using MRI in the evaluation of the UAE patient. Investigators have reported changes in volume of leiomyomata and the uterus, as well as alterations in signal characteristics. A significant decrease in the size of the uterus and leiomyomata has been described by various investigators (34,47,48). Post-UAE leiomyomata also show signal changes consistent with hemorrhagic infarction, with

increased signal on T1-weighted images (Fig. 5-18). Treated leiomyomata typically show more homogenous dark signal on T2-weighted images (24). Diminished vascularity is typically seen in leiomyomata treated with UAE (24,48-50).

Following UAE, region of interest analysis shows that the vascularity of the leiomyomata is significantly diminished, but the myometrial perfusion is maintained (34). Use of gadolinium allows assessment of degree of infarction, as only 60% of leiomyomata seen 3 months after UAE develop high signal intensity on T1-weighted images, suggesting red degeneration induced from embolization (34). Furthermore, investigators have suggested that the degree of infarction immediately after UAE based on gadolinium-enhanced MRI may be predictive of subsequent leiomyoma volume reduction (51).

MRI may be valuable in predicting the success of the procedure. Mizukami et al. (52) reported 15 patients imaged with MR pre-UAE and at 3, 6, and 12 months post-UAE. They suggest that leiomyomata with low signal on T2-weighted images pre-UAE have a poor response compared with those with intermediate or high signal. Burn et al. (42) reported poor response in patients with leiomyomata of high signal on T1-weighted images prior to embolization, whereas high signal intensity on T2-weighted images was predictive of a good response. We have also reported that high signal intensity on T1-weghted images is predictive of a poor response (34). These may represent leiomyomata that have already undergone hemorrhagic degeneration prior to embolization. Among other variables that may predict success, we have found that submucosal location has a high correlation with size reduction and that hypervascularity of a leiomyoma prior to UAE is strongly correlated with a decrease in leiomyoma perfusion post-UAE (34).

UAE as a treatment of adenomyosis with coexisting leiomyomata has shown mixed results in the few studies to date. Some investigators have shown initial clinical improvement with eventual failure (53), whereas others have shown an improvement in symptoms and a decrease in junctional zone thickness and, in some patients, devascularization of regions of adenomyosis (54). Assessment of the efficacy of UAE in the treatment of adenomyosis is limited by the coexistence of leiomyomata in these study groups. Adenomyosis is further discussed in Chapter 10.

Imaging Complications of Uterine Artery Embolization

Leiomyoma/Uterine Necrosis

Immediately following UAE, leiomyomata may undergo tissue necrosis, as is commonly seen after any embolization procedure, with dark foci seen on MRI repre-

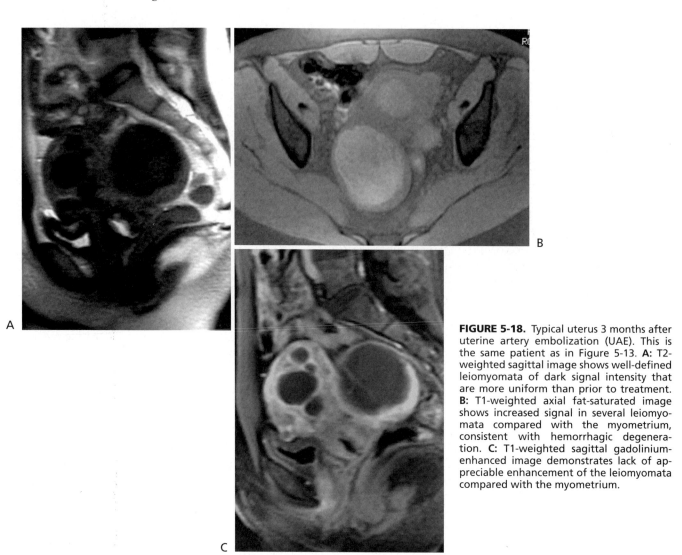

FIGURE 5-18. Typical uterus 3 months after uterine artery embolization (UAE). This is the same patient as in Figure 5-13. **A:** T2-weighted sagittal image shows well-defined leiomyomata of dark signal intensity that are more uniform than prior to treatment. **B:** T1-weighted axial fat-saturated image shows increased signal in several leiomyomata compared with the myometrium, consistent with hemorrhagic degeneration. **C:** T1-weighted sagittal gadolinium-enhanced image demonstrates lack of appreciable enhancement of the leiomyomata compared with the myometrium.

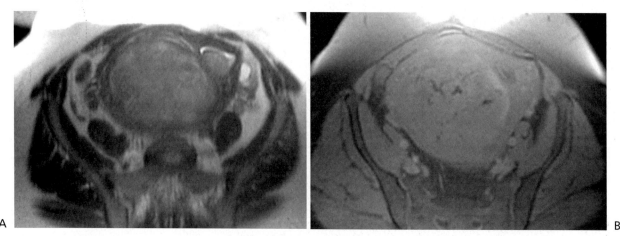

FIGURE 5-19. Leiomyoma necrosis 1 week after uterine artery embolization. **A:** T2-weighted axial image of the uterus shows a large leiomyoma with intermediate signal intensity. **B:** T1-weighted axial fat-saturated image shows small serpentine dark signal scattered throughout the leiomyoma. These represent foci of gas, which are typical in the postembolization period, and should not be confused with infection. This is not seen on 3-month post-UAE images.

senting susceptibility artifact from gas within the leiomyoma (Fig. 5-19). This may be mistaken for infection (55,56). Most often, routine follow-up is performed 3 to 6 months after the procedure, at which time the gas is no longer seen.

When UAE was first introduced, there was concern regarding the effects of the procedure on myometrial integrity. Several publications have reported maintenance of perfusion to the uterine wall. In the presence of persisting pain after UAE, myometrial injury may be suspected and MRI is indicated. Imaging of uterine necrosis is not well described, but the absence of enhancement of the uterine wall would be consistent with this diagnosis.

Vaginal Expulsion of Leiomyomata

Following UAE, the most common side effect of treatment reported by Walker and Pelage (57) in a series of 400 women treated with UAE was vaginal discharge, which occurred in 13% of patients. Frank vaginal expulsion of leiomyomata is unusual, and when seen it is most often in the setting of an initial submucosal leiomyomata and is reported to occur with an incidence of 0.5% to 12.5% (58-64). In most cases there is gradual sloughing of tissue, but occasionally there may be transcervical expulsion of a mass of tissue, with associated pelvic cramping, bleeding, fever, and leukocytosis. MRI may show the necrotic tissue displaced into the endometrial/endocervical canal (Fig. 5-20).

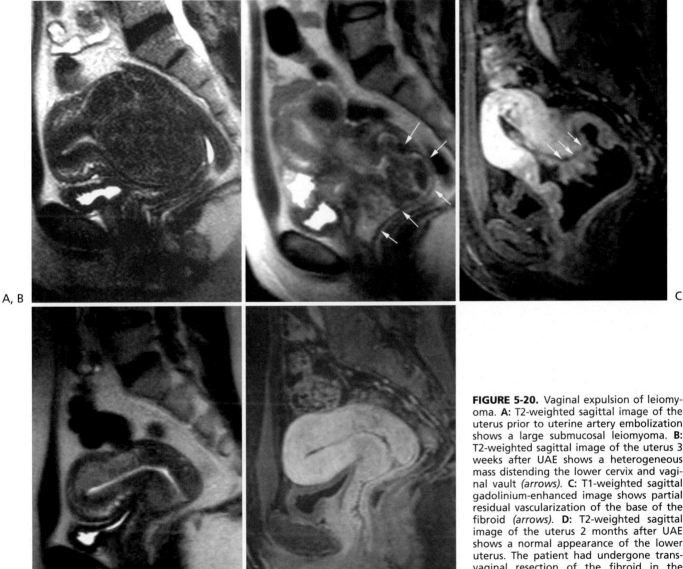

FIGURE 5-20. Vaginal expulsion of leiomyoma. **A:** T2-weighted sagittal image of the uterus prior to uterine artery embolization shows a large submucosal leiomyoma. **B:** T2-weighted sagittal image of the uterus 3 weeks after UAE shows a heterogeneous mass distending the lower cervix and vaginal vault *(arrows).* **C:** T1-weighted sagittal gadolinium-enhanced image shows partial residual vascularization of the base of the fibroid *(arrows).* **D:** T2-weighted sagittal image of the uterus 2 months after UAE shows a normal appearance of the lower uterus. The patient had undergone transvaginal resection of the fibroid in the interval, with control of symptoms. **E:** T1-weighted sagittal gadolinium-enhanced image reveals normal enhancement.

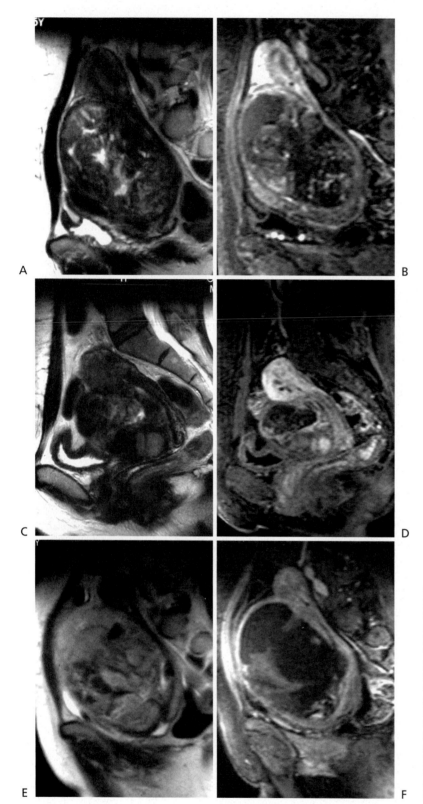

FIGURE 5-21. Leiomyosarcoma treated with uterine artery embolization. Pre-UAE: **A:** T2-weighted sagittal image shows a large heterogeneous mass suggestive of a leiomyoma that appears to be confined to the uterus. **B:** T1-weighted sagittal gadolinium-enhanced image shows heterogeneous enhancement of the lesion. Two months after UAE: **C:** T2-weighted sagittal image shows a significant decrease in size of the mass leiomyoma that appears to be confined to the uterus. **D:** T1-weighted sagittal gadolinium-enhanced image shows predominant devascularization with regions of heterogeneous enhancement. One year after UAE: **E:** T2-weighted sagittal image shows rapid regrowth of the large heterogeneous mass. **F:** T1-weighted sagittal gadolinium-enhanced image shows heterogeneous enhancement of the lesion with areas of revascularization.

Regrowth

Recurrence of leiomyomata may be seen after UAE (65). The usual appearance of an infarcted leiomyoma is complete absence of vascularity. If the fibroid is not completely avascular on initial postprocedural imaging, the residual viable tissue may regrow. On follow-up examinations, there is typically enlargement of the viable portions of the fibroid, even as the infarcted portions continue to recede. This concept is demonstrated in Chapter 10.

The mechanism for regrowth is poorly understood. The recruitment of alternate blood supply from the ovarian or vesicovaginal arteries may be one explanation (66). The collaterals may become of increasing importance when the major feeding uterine arterial flow undergoes blockade (Fig. 5-15). Over time, the viable fibroid tissue will recruit normal myometrial vessels to support the regrowth. Because these tumors are hormonally responsive, regrowth may also be related to the pathogenesis of the leiomyomata themselves.

Leiomyosarcoma

Malignant degeneration of a uterine leiomyoma is an uncommon event, with a reported incidence of 0.21% to 0.4% (67) in women undergoing surgery for a presumptive diagnosis of leiomyomata. The clinical symptoms are often nonspecific and simulate typical leiomyoma disease. Rapid growth of a leiomyoma has been suggested as worrisome, but in a review of 26 studies from 1962 to 1993, Parker et al. (68) reported that only 2.6% of patients with sarcoma had a history of rapid growth. The imaging features are also nonspecific and can be similar to those of a degenerating leiomyoma and difficult to diagnose unless obvious invasion is present. There have been reports of failure after UAE as a result of an underlying leiomyosarcoma (69,70). Although the diagnosis is usually made at the time of pathologic examination, the presence of regrowth of a heterogeneous hypervascular lesion after UAE should raise clinical suspicion and warrant more definitive therapy (Fig. 5-21).

CONCLUSION

UAE is emerging as a viable treatment option for women with symptomatic leiomyomata. Both ultrasound and MRI have valuable roles in the evaluation of these patients. The strength of ultrasound lies in the assessment of the endometrial cavity, particularly when sonohysterography is used. MRI plays a key role in the accurate assessment of the size and location of leiomyomata, as well as the evaluation of changes in leiomyoma and myometrial vascularity. With additional study, ultrasound and even MRI may also be useful in assessing alteration in the morphology of the ovaries and correlating these changes with hormonal changes before and after UAE. In the longer run, the most significant role of imaging will be in detecting recurrence of fibroids. MRI has a clear advantage in assessing whether the leiomyomata regrow and revascularize. If we were able to predict which patients may have regrowth based on imaging features, there would be a significant added value from MRI.

REFERENCES

1. Mayer DP, Shipilov V. Ultrasonography and magnetic resonance imaging of uterine fibroids. *Obstet Gynecol Clin North Am* 1995;22:667–725.
2. Sohaey R, Woodward P. Sonohysterography: technique, endometrial findings, and clinical applications. *Semin Ultrasound CT MR* 1999;20:250–258.
3. Jorizzo JR, Riccio GJ, Chen Y, et al. Sonohysterography: The next step in the evaluation of the abnormal endometrium. *Radiographics* 1999;19:S17–S30.
4. Bernard JP, Rizk E, Camatte S, et al. Saline contrast sonohysterography in the preoperative assessment of benign intrauterine disorders. *Ultrasound Obstet Gynecol* 2001;17:145–149.
5. Lev-Toaff AS, Toaff ME, Liu JB, et al. Value of sonohysterography in the diagnosis and management of abnormal uterine bleeding. *Radiology* 1996;201:179–184.
6. Becker E Jr, Lev-Toaff AS, Kaufman EP, et al. The added value of transvaginal sonohysterography over transvaginal sonography alone in women with known or suspected leiomyoma. *J Ultrasound Med* 2002;21:237–247.
7. Fleischer AC, Shappel HW, Parker LP, et al. Doppler sonography of endometrial masses. *J Ultrasound Med* 2002;21:861–865.
8. Fleischer AC, Shappell HW. Color Doppler sonohysterography of endometrial polyps and submucosal fibroids. *J Ultrasound Med* 2003;22:601–604.
9. Weintraub JL, Romano WJ, Kirsch MJ, et al. Uterine artery embolization, sonographic imaging findings. *J Ultrasound Med* 2002;21:633–637.
10. Muniz CJ, Fleischer AC, Donnelly EF, et al. Three-dimensional color Doppler sonography and uterine artery arteriography of fibroids: assessment of changes in vascularity before and after embolization. *J Ultrasound Med* 2002;21:129–133.
11. Fleischer AC, Donnelly EF, Campbell MG, et al. Three-dimensional color Doppler sonography before and after fibroid embolization. *J Ultrasound Med* 2000;19:701–705.
12. McLucas B, Perrella R, Goodwin S, et al. Role of uterine artery Doppler flow in fibroid embolization. *J Ultrasound Med* 2002;21:113–120.
13. Kliewer MA, Hertzberg, BS, George PY. Acoustic shadowing from uterine leiomyomas: sonographic-pathologic correlation. *Radiology* 1995;196:99–102.
14. Davis PC, O'Neill MJ, Yoder IC, et al. Sonohysterographic findings of endometrial and subendometrial conditions. *Radiographics* 2002;22:803–816.
15. Gross BH, Silver TM, Jaffee MH. Sonographic features of uterine leiomyomas: analysis of 41 proven cases. *J Ultrasound Med* 1983;2:401–406.
16. Tranquart F, Brunereau L, Cottier JP, et al. Prospective sonographic assessment of uterine artery embolization for the treatment of fibroids. *Ultrasound Obstet Gynecol* 2002;19:81–87.

17. Reinhold C, Tafazoli F, Mehio A, et al. Uterine adenomyosis: endovaginal US and MR imaging features with histopathologic correlation. *Radiographics* 1999;19:S147–S160.

18. Reinhold C, Atri M, Mehio A, et al. Diffuse uterine adenomyosis: morphologic criteria and diagnostic accuracy of endovaginal sonography. *Radiology* 1995;197:609–614.

19. Fedele L, Bianchi S, Dorta M, et al. Transvaginal ultrasonography in the diagnosis of diffuse adenomyosis. *Fertil Steril* 1992;58:94–97.

20. Chiang CH, Chang MY, Hsu JJ, et al. Tumor vascular pattern and blood flow impedance in the differential diagnosis of leiomyoma and adenomyosis by color Doppler sonography. *J Assist Reprod Genet* 1999;16:268–275.

21. Weinreb JC, Barkoff ND, Megibow A, et al. The value of MR imaging in distinguishing leiomyomas from other solid pelvic masses when sonography is indeterminate. *AJR Am J Roentgenol* 1990;154:295–299.

22. Zawin M, McCarthy S, Scoutt LM, et al. High-field MRI and US evaluation of the pelvis in women with leiomyomas. *Magn Reson Imaging* 1990;8:371–376.

23. Hricak H, Tscholakoff D, Heinrichs L, et al. Uterine leiomyomas: correlation of MR, histopathologic findings and symptoms. *Radiology* 1986;158:385–391.

24. Togashi K, Ozasa H, Konish I, et al. Enlarged uterus: differentiation between adenomyosis and leiomyoma with MR imaging. *Radiology* 1989;171:531–534.

25. Broekmans FJ, Heitbrink MA, Hompes PGA, et al. Quantitative MRI of uterine leiomyomas during triptorelin treatment: reproducibility of volume assessment and predictability of treatment response. *Magn Reson Imaging* 1996;14:1127–1135.

26. Oguchi O, Mori A, Kobayashi Y, et al. Prediction of histopathologic features and proliferative activity of uterine leiomyoma by magnetic resonance imaging prior to GnRH analogue therapy: correlation between T2-weighted images and the effect of GnRH analogue. *J Obstet Gynaecol* 1995;21:107–117.

27. Ooto H, Nambu Y, Nonogaki H, et al. Treatment with LH-RH analog, buserelin, for uterine leiomyoma: assessment with MR imaging. *Endometriosis Kenkyukai Kaishi* 1989;10:245–249.

28. Kawakami S, Togashi K, Konishi I, et al. Red degeneration of uterine leiomyoma: MR appearance. *J Comput Assist Tomogr* 1994;18:925–928.

29. Schwartz LB, Zawin M, Carcangiu ML, et al. Does pelvis magnetic resonance imaging differentiate among the histologic subtypes of uterine leiomyomata? *Fertil Steril* 1998;70:580–587.

30. Mittl RL, Yeh I-T, Kressel HY. High signal intensity rim surrounding uterine leiomyomas on MR images: pathological correlation. *Radiology* 1991;180:81–83.

31. Hricak H, Finck S, Honda G, et al. MR imaging in the evaluation of benign uterine masses. *AJR Am J Roentgenol* 1992;158:1043–1050.

32. Yamashita Y, Torashima M, Takahashi M, et al. Hyperintense uterine leiomyomas at T2-weighted MR imaging: differentiation with dynamic enhanced MR imaging and clinical implications. *Radiology* 1993;189:721–725.

33. Okizuka H, Sugimura K, Takemori M, et al. MR detection of degenerating uterine leiomyomas. *J Comput Assist Tomogr* 1993;17:760–776.

34. Jha RC, Ascher SM, Imaoka I, et al. Symptomatic fibroleiomyomata: MR imaging of the uterus before and after uterine arterial embolization. *Radiology* 2000;217:228–235.

35. Reinhold C, McCarthy S, Bret PM, et al. Diffuse adenomyosis: comparison of endovaginal US an MR imaging with histopathological correlation. *Radiology* 1996;199:151–158.

36. Olive DL, Schwartz LB. Endometriosis. *N Engl J Med* 1993;328:1759–1769.

37. Togashi K, Nishimura K, Kimura I, et al. Endometrial cysts: diagnosis with MR imaging. *Radiology* 1991;180:73–78.

38. Zawin M, McCarthy SM, Scoutt L, et al. Endometriosis: appearance and detection with MR imaging. *Radiology* 1989;171:693–696.

39. Arrive L, Hricak H, Martin MC. Pelvic endometriosis: MR imaging. *Radiology* 1989;171:687–692.

40. Bis KG, Vrachliotis TG, Agrawal R, et al. Pelvic endometriosis: MR imaging spectrum with laparoscopic correlation and diagnostic pitfalls. *Radiographics* 1997;17:639–655.

41. Takahashi K, Okada M, Ozaki T, et al. Diagnosis of pelvic endometriosis by magnetic resonance imaging using "fat-saturation" technique. *Fertil Steril* 1994;62:973–977.

42. Burn P, McCall JM, Chinn R, et al. Uterine fibroleiomyoma: MR imaging appearances before and after embolization of uterine arteries. *Radiology* 2000;214:729–734.

43. Ascher SM, Jha RC, Reinhold C. Benign myometrial conditions: leiomyomas and adenomyosis. *Top Magn Reson Imaging* 2003;14:281–304.

44. Masui T, Katayama M, Kobayashi S, et al. Psuedolesions related to uterine contraction: characterization with multiphase-multisection T2-weighted MR imaging. *Radiology* 2003;227:345–352.

45. Goodwin SC, Vedantham S, McLucas B, et al. Preliminary experience with uterine artery embolization for uterine fibroids. *J Vasc Interv Radiol* 1997;8:517–526.

46. Worthington-Kirsch RL, Popky GL, Hutchins FL. Uterine artery embolization for the management of leiomyomas: quality-of-life assessment and clinical response. *Radiology* 1998;208:625–629.

47. Bradley EA, Reidy JF, Forman RG, et al. Transcatheter uterine artery embolization to treat large uterine fibroids. *Br J Obstet Gynaecol* 1998;105:231–234.

48. Burn P, McCall JM, Chinn R, et al. Embolization of uterine fibroids. *Br J Radiol* 1999;72:159–161.

49. Brophy DP, Rabkin DJ, Kim D, et al. Selective preservation of myometrial rather than fibroid enhancement after bilateral uterine fibroid embolization: objective enhancement with contrast-enhanced magnetic resonance imaging. *Radiology* 1999;213[p]:133(abstr).

50. O'Neill MJ, Fan C, Kaufman JA, et al. MR imaging of fibroid, myometrial and endometrial volume and perfusion characteristics in women with symptomatic uterine fibroids: pre and post transcatheter embolization of the uterine arteries. *Radiology* 1999;213[p]:348(abstr).

51. Katsumori T, Nakajima K, Tokuhiro M. Gadolinium-enhanced MR imaging in the evaluation of uterine fibroids treated with uterine artery embolization. *AJR Am J Roentgenol* 2001;177:303–307.

52. Mizukami N, Yamashita Y, Matsukawa T, et al. The value of MR imaging in predicting the treatment effect of arterial embolization therapy for uterine leiomyomas. *Radiology* 1999;213[p]:347(abstr).

53. McLucas B, Adler L, Perrella R. Uterine fibroid embolization: nonsurgical treatment for symptomatic fibroids. *J Am Coll Surg* 2001;192:95–105.

54. Jha RC, Takahama J, Imaoka I, et al. Adenomyosis: MRI of the uterus treated with uterine artery embolization. *AJR Am J Roentgenol* 2003;181:851–856.

55. Vott S, Bonilla SM, Goodwin SC, et al. CT findings after uterine artery embolization. *J Comput Assist Tomogr* 2000;24:846–848.

56. Godfred CD, Zbella EA. Uterine necrosis after uterine artery embolization for leiomyoma. *Obstet Gynecol* 2001;98 [5 Pt 2]:950–952.

57. Walker WJ, Pelage JP. Uterine artery embolization for symptomatic fibroids: clinical results in 400 women with imaging follow up. *BJOG* 2002;109:1262–1272.

58. Berkowitz RP, Hutchins FL Jr, Worthington-Kirsch RL. Vaginal expulsion of submucosal fibroids after uterine artery embolization. A report of three cases. *J Reprod Med* 1999;44:373–376.

59. Huang LY, Cheng YF, Huang CC, et al. Incomplete vaginal expulsion of pyoadenomyoma with sepsis and focal bladder necrosis after uterine artery embolization for symptomatic adenomyosis: case report. *Hum Reprod* 2003;18:167–171.

60. Kroencke TJ, Gauruder-Burmester A, Enzweiler CN, et al. Disintegration and stepwise expulsion of a large uterine leiomyoma with restoration of the uterine architecture after successful uterine fibroid embolization: case report. *Hum Reprod* 2003;18:863–865.

61. Laverge F, D'Angelo A, Davies NJ, et al. Spontaneous expulsion of three large fibroids after uterine artery embolization. *Fertil Steril* 2003;80:450–452.

62. Murgo S, Simon P, Golzarian J. Embolization of uterine fibroids. *Rev Med Brux* 2002;23:435–442.

63. Panageas E, Kier R, McCauley TR, et al. Submucosal uterine leiomyomas: diagnosis of prolapse into the cervix and vagina based on MR imaging. *AJR Am J Roentgenol* 1992;159:555–558.

64. Pollard RR, Goldberg JM. Prolapsed cervical myoma after uterine artery embolization. A case report. *J Reprod Med* 2001;46:499–500.

65. Marret H, Alonso AM, Cottier JP, et al. Leiomyoma recurrence after uterine artery embolization. *J Vasc Interv Radiol* 2003;14:1395–1399.

66. Nikolic B, Spies JB, Abbara S, et al. Ovarian artery supply of uterine fibroids as a cause of treatment failure after uterine artery embolization: a case report. *J Vasc Interv Radiol* 1999;10:1167–1170.

67. Dover RW, Ferrier AJ, Torode HW. Sarcomas and the conservative management of uterine fibroids: a cause for concern? *Aust N Z J Obstet Gynaecol* 2000;40:308–312.

68. Parker WH, Fu YS, Berek JS. Uterine sarcoma in patients operated on for presumed leiomyoma and rapidly growing leiomyoma. *Obstet Gynecol* 1994;83:414–418.

69. Common AA, Mocarski EJM, Kolin A, et al. Therapeutic failure of uterine fibroid embolization caused by underlying leiomyosarcoma. *J Vasc Interv Radiol* 2001;12:1449–1452.

70. Joyce A, Hessami S, Heller D. Leiomyosarcoma after uterine artery embolization. A case report. *J Reprod Med* 2001;46:278–280.

6

SURGICAL THERAPIES FOR UTERINE LEIOMYOMATA

JEFFREY Y. LIN

INTRODUCTION

Surgical therapies for women with uterine leiomyomata and significant symptoms are the oldest and most utilized treatment options. Although both abdominal hysterectomy and myomectomy were successfully performed in the mid-nineteenth century in Europe and the United States, it was not until the twentieth century that hysterectomy became the definitive treatment for leiomyomata. Hysterectomy combines surety of symptom relief with low morbidity, low mortality, and minimal risk of fibroid recurrence. Beginning in the 1960s, myomectomy arose as a popular alternative to hysterectomy for women who desired uterine conservation. Given the current trend to delay childbearing in more industrialized nations, conservative options continue to grow more important. With the recent trend of greater patient involvement in medical decision making, development of new nonsurgical and surgical alternatives has accelerated. Nevertheless, all new modalities need to be critically compared to hysterectomy and myomectomy.

TRADITIONAL HYSTERECTOMY

Currently, about 600,000 hysterectomies are performed annually in the United States, with an overall annual cost of about $5 billion (USD). About one third of hysterectomies performed list leiomyomata as a diagnosis on discharge from the hospital (1).

Hysterectomy has many commendable attributes as a therapy for women with uterine leiomyomata. Over the 160-year history of hysterectomy as treatment for leiomyomata, there has been a gradual evolution of approaches and techniques. Most of the evolution has been with the intent to reduce morbidity, because the efficacy of hysterectomy in alleviating uterine bleeding, pelvic compressive symptoms, dysmenorrhea, pelvic pain, and dyspareunia associated with leiomyomata is well established. Hysterectomy can also correct ureteral obstruction secondary to leiomyomata and

establish certainty regarding the absence of uterine cancer. Concern regarding the possibility of adnexal disease can be conveniently addressed at the time of hysterectomy, especially when an abdominal or laparoscopic surgical approach is performed.

Perioperative mortality after hysterectomy appears to be about 12 per 10,000 procedures overall; hysterectomies performed for leiomyomata carry an even lower risk (2). Significant morbidity associated with hysterectomy is about 9% and may include urinary tract infection, thromboembolic complications, sepsis or pelvic abscess, intestinal or urologic injury, intestinal obstruction, hemorrhage, nerve injury, and anesthetic risks (3). Childbearing ability is lost in women of reproductive age after hysterectomy, but with assisted reproduction, ovum retrieval with subsequent *in vitro* fertilization and embryo transfer to a surrogate woman is possible.

Psychological, emotional, and spiritual issues may accompany hysterectomy. The uterus is important in the reproductive process and for many women has strong symbolic importance. The spiritual impact of hysterectomy on a woman may be influenced by cultural issues, history of reproductive losses, and infertility issues. The physical aspects of sexuality in women who have undergone recent hysterectomy are reasonably well studied and are apparently minimal (4). Frequently, symptoms that may contribute to sexual dysfunction, such as dyspareunia and pelvic pain, may be alleviated by hysterectomy, thus leading to improved sexual satisfaction (4,5). However, one should be cautious in attributing no effect of hysterectomy on sexuality, because there is considerable individual variation to the spiritual and physiologic interplay of sexuality. The effect of hysterectomy on sexuality must also be separated from the effect of hypoestrogenism and decreased androgen levels if concomitant bilateral salpingo-oophorectomy is performed at the time of hysterectomy. Changes in hormonal milieu that mark the end of reproductive life have a significant effect on gender identity, mood, libido, and vaginal function.

The technical aspects of traditional total hysterectomy can be quite varied, but the general principles are well established. Total hysterectomy by traditional techniques may be performed transabdominally or transvaginally. The transabdominal route typically uses a vertical midline or transverse lower abdominal incision. The transverse incision may involve division of the rectus abdominis muscle or separation of the muscle from its insertion on the pubic symphysis. The choice of incision depends on the size and mobility of myomatous uterus, the presence of adhesions, and the possibility of needing access to the upper abdomen. Division and ligation of the round and uteroovarian ligaments are accomplished, usually with suture ligation or occasionally with surgical staples. Subsequently, the ascending portion of the uterine artery and vein and the lower medial cardinal ligament are divided in a similar fashion. The bladder must be dissected and separated from the anterior endopelvic fascia, which covers the lower uterine segment, anterior cervix, and upper vagina. In most cases, full ureteral dissection and development of the rectovaginal septum are not necessary. The cervix is removed and the vaginal apex sutured closed or the edges of the mucosa oversewn. The abdomen is then closed. Typical operating time is approximately 45 minutes to several hours, and hospitalization lasts 2 to 4 days. In uncomplicated cases, a woman may satisfactorily recover and return to work in 4 to 6 weeks. Anesthetic appropriate for abdominal hysterectomy includes epidural, spinal, or general anesthetic. Medicare reimbursement for abdominal hysterectomy in 2003 was approximately $988 USD (15.22 relative value units [RVU]).

Transvaginal or simply vaginal hysterectomy entails removal of the uterus through the vagina. In women with uterine leiomyomata, the size and degree of mobility of the uterus, the dimensions of the pelvic outlet and midpelvis, and the presence of any periuterine adhesions determine the feasibility of safe transvaginal removal of the uterus. Vaginal hysterectomy has been shown to be very feasible in women without uterovaginal prolapse as well (6). Greater exposure can be obtained with creation of a Schuchardt incision or mediolateral episiotomy.

The vaginal mucosa is first incised, a colpotomy is made either posteriorly or anteriorly, and the base of the cardinal and uterosacral ligaments is divided and ligated. At this point, a large fibroid uterus can be reduced in size by removing the cervix and central portion of the corpus, bisecting the corpus, or by morcellation (7). Morcellation should be avoided if an intact uterus is needed for careful histopathologic examination. In a woman with adequate pelvic anatomy who has a uterus with some degree of descensus, a fibroid uterus of up to 18 weeks' gestational size can potentially be removed by this technique. This is followed by exteriorization of the uterus through the vagina, with subsequent ligation of the uteroovarian and round ligaments. The ovaries and fallopian tubes can be removed through the vagina as well, particularly in parous women.

Inspection of the upper pelvis and abdomen is extremely limited with the vaginal approach. The peritoneum is often closed, and the vaginal mucosa is closed as well with absorbable suture. Operative blood loss is similar to abdominal hysterectomy, and operating times may be shorter in well-selected candidates. Postoperative hospitalization is generally 1 to 3 days, bowel function returns rapidly, and patients return to work in 3 to 4 weeks (6–8). In women who are good candidates for vaginal hysterectomy, one should also consider the need for concomitant repair of pelvic floor defects such as vaginal apex prolapse, cystourethrocele, rectocele, and paravaginal defects, as well as bilateral salpingo-oophorectomy.

Supracervical or subtotal hysterectomy for uterine leiomyomata has become increasingly popular over the last 12 years. Although this can only be performed through the transabdominal route, a laparoscopic approach is also feasible in many cases. The approach is similar to total abdominal hysterectomy with amputation of the uterine corpus at the junction of the cervix. The cervical stump is then oversewn with heavy absorbable suture. The operating time is shorter, and the risk for vesical or ureteral injuries is somewhat lower than with total hysterectomy. The physiologic advantages of supracervical hysterectomy are controversial. Proponents of supracervical hysterectomy have suggested that preservation of the cervix and much of the base of the cardinal ligament may reduce the risk of vaginal apex prolapse, improve bladder and sexual function, and have reduced risk for perioperative infection. Theoretically, by preserving the cervix, the genital hiatus in the levator ani muscles is not enlarged and the parasympathetic nerve supply from the sacrum is less disrupted. A number of randomized clinical trials have attempted to address these issues (9). With short-term follow-up, there have been no demonstrable differences in voiding function, sexual satisfaction, or complication rates when supracervical hysterectomy is compared to total hysterectomy. Of note, some women who have undergone supracervical hysterectomy have light postoperative cyclic bleeding that is bothersome. No substantive comparative data exist for pelvic floor defects in women who have undergone supracervical or total hysterectomy. Women who retain the cervix still are recommended to have annual cervical cytology for cervical cancer screening, and women who have a history of cervical dysplasia probably should be discouraged from having a supracervical hysterectomy. Treatment of cervical stump carcinoma by radical trachelectomy and lymphadenectomy is technically difficult and radiotherapy more problematic as a consequence of the loss of the uterine corpus for separation of the small intestine from brachytherapy sources. Reimbursement for supracervical hysterectomy and total hysterectomy is generally equivalent.

A variation of vaginal hysterectomy was introduced in 1990 and was described as laparoscopically assisted vaginal hysterectomy (10). In this operation, the laparoscope and laparoscopic instruments are inserted into the abdomen, with subsequent division of the round and uteroovarian or infundibulopelvic ligaments. If any peri-uterine or periadnexal adhesions are noted, they may also be divided. The remainder of the hysterectomy is completed transvaginally with removal of the uterus and potentially the adnexa through the vagina. This is generally performed with three laparoscopic entry sites. One study suggested that women with fibroids that are up to 8 to 10 cm in diameter and weigh less than 450 g may be reasonable candidates for laparoscopically assisted vaginal hysterectomy (11). Although this approach was initially thought to be able to convert women with an indication for abdominal hysterectomy to this less invasive opera-tion, subsequent studies demonstrated potential increased cost secondary to the increased operating room time and heavy reliance on expensive disposable laparoscopic instruments (12,13). Additional studies also suggested that many laparoscopically assisted vaginal hysterectomies and salpingo-oophorectomies could be performed strictly through a transvaginal route by an experienced gynecologic surgeon (14).

Laparoscopic hysterectomy has been performed with increasing regularity since 1992 (15,16). Most are supracer-vical, but more recently there is a trend to perform total laparoscopic hysterectomy. The laparoscopic approach allows for full visualization of abdominal and even retroperitoneal structures and allows for extensive adhesion lysis if necessary. Typically, four laparoscopic ports are placed in the lower abdomen, and the conduct of the operation is very similar to abdominal hysterectomy. Ligation and division of the ligaments are most often accomplished using bipolar electrocautery or the harmonic scalpel and less often with an endoscopic stapler, sutures, or ligating clips. Retrieval of the detached fibroid uterus can be accomplished with an endoscopic morcellating device, which reduces the uterus to strips of tissue that can be removed through the laparoscopic ports. Alternatively, the detached uterus can be removed transvaginally prior to closure of the vaginal cuff. Morcellation of the uterus may carry a small risk of producing iatrogenic endometriosis (17). Although rates of operative injuries to the urinary tract during laparoscopic hysterectomy (1.4%) were initially higher than those incurred with traditional abdominal hysterectomy, this can be significantly reduced with greater surgical experience (18). For typical gynecologic surgeons, laparoscopic hysterectomy may offer a better recovery than abdominal hysterectomy but with about a two-fold increased risk for complications (19). Although very large fibroid uteri have been removed by the laparoscopic approach, more typically uteri with fibroids less than 8 cm in diameter or up to 16 weeks' gestational size are appropriate candidates (20). Very large and particularly broad fibroid uteri and the presence of significant adhesions may inordinately increase the risk of laparoscopic surgery

and may make the traditional approach by laparotomy more attractive. Although definitive trials have not been con-ducted, laparoscopic hysterectomy may offer quicker recovery, less postoperative pain, and less adhesion forma-tion than abdominal hysterectomy (11). One disadvantage of laparoscopic surgery is that CO_2 insufflation of the abdomen generally precludes the use of conduction anesthesia. There is also the risk of specific trocar-related complications such as enteric and vascular injury, as well as a risk for hypercarbia from CO_2 insufflation or CO_2 embolization. Electrosurgical injuries may occur; these may be direct injuries or the result of coupled or capacitive electrical discharge. Some patients may find the small scars from laparoscopic trocars in the midabdomen less aesthetic than a very low and small transverse abdominal incision.

The choice of the approach for hysterectomy should be based on the medical indications for the hysterectomy, the particular expertise of the gynecologic surgeon, and the desires of the patient. An example of this principle is if a woman has, in addition to symptoms from fibroids, another component of pelvic pain such as chronic appendicitis, peritoneal endometriosis, or an adnexal mass or needs ureteral assessment for hydroureter, then an abdominal approach by laparotomy or laparoscopy should be utilized. Ovarian masses can be partially visualized from a primary transvaginal approach but generally cannot be removed atraumatically through the vagina. In North America, the necessary surgical skills for removing a bulky fibroid uterus vaginally safely vary among surgeons. One should always remember that the primary benefits of vaginal and laparoscopic approaches are ease of patient recovery and decreased patient discomfort. Increased efficacy of the procedure and increased operative safety are generally not attributable to less invasive approaches. Although recovery times for less invasive surgery are shorter, cost savings with laparoscopic approaches may be offset by longer operating room times and equipment charges. In deciding between laparotomy and laparoscopy, a very bulky uterus, severe fibrotic adhesions, or a very vascular tumor may point away from the laparoscopic approach. The choice of supracervical versus total hysterectomy may often be left to the patient, provided there is no underlying history of cervical disease or significant risk factors for cervical cancer.

MYOMECTOMY

Myomectomy is well recognized as a valid alternative to hysterectomy for women with significant symptoms from uterine leiomyomata who wish to preserve the potential for childbearing. Conservation of the uterus for other reasons may be acceptable, provided that the patient is fully informed regarding the additional risks associated with myomectomy. Knowledge of the patient's childbearing desires, her prior reproductive history, and her likelihood for successful conception are essential for surgical counseling. As a general rule, myomectomy affords conservation of the uterus for childbearing and, in some patients, improved gender identity as a benefit. Contrary to many patients' expectations, myomectomy by laparoscopy or laparotomy is not a lesser procedure compared to hysterectomy performed by the same approach. Negative perioperative aspects of myomectomy relative to hysterectomy include increased mean surgical blood loss and possibly increased adhesion formation leading to increased risk for intestinal obstruction (21). Febrile morbidity is common after myomectomy, but the risk of significant pelvic infection is less than that of hysterectomy (22). Although there is a paucity of good data, alleviation of menorrhagia and pelvic pressure symptoms after myomectomy has been reported to be about 81% (23). Importantly, alleviation of fibroid symptoms by hysterectomy is certain and permanent, whereas the results achieved by myomectomy may be incomplete and temporary. Although it is hard to accurately assess given differences in preoperative fibroid distribution, duration to menopause, and symptom severity, the likelihood of significant fibroid regrowth after myomectomy is about 15% to 25% (23,24). Compared with uterine artery embolization, one study suggested that the need for repeated treatment of fibroid symptoms was higher in embolization patients than in myomectomy patients during the immediate 3-year post-treatment period (25). There is also the remote possibility of not diagnosing a uterine sarcoma or endometrial cancer if the uterus is conserved. The durations of hospitalization and postoperative recovery are very similar between myomectomy and hysterectomy. Medicare reimbursement to the surgeon for myomectomy in 2003 was approximately $942 USD (14.58 RVU).

Women who undergo myomectomy need to have preoperative counseling regarding the risk of uterine rupture and placentation problems with subsequent pregnancies (26). Although the exact criteria for delivery of a term pregnancy by elective cesarean section in a woman who has undergone a myomectomy may be undefined, most experts recommend cesarean section for women in which the myomectomy was very extensive and necessitated the repair of a transmural defect. Although uterine rupture during pregnancy in women who have undergone myomectomy is rare and the exact frequency is unknown, it may result in intrapartum fetal demise and maternal hemorrhage. Older studies looking at uterine rupture after prior cesarean section and myomectomy suggest a 0.1% risk of rupture for myomectomy (27). Ideally, in those women at increased risk for rupture, the elective cesarean section should be scheduled at term before labor is anticipated. Testing the integrity of the uterine wall prior to pregnancy by hysterogram is of uncertain benefit. There is a theoretical risk associated with myomectomy and the subsequent development of placenta accreta (28).

The impact of fibroids on fertility and recurrent pregnancy loss is unpredictable; therefore, the benefit of myomectomy in women with fibroids and infertility or pregnancy loss is unclear. Whereas some women with fibroids who have reproductive problems may benefit from myomectomy, all other potential causes for infertility and pregnancy loss already should have been evaluated given the morbidity associated with myomectomy. The possibility of periadnexal adhesions and endometrial synechiae with even endometrial cavity obliteration postmyomectomy needs to be included in the preoperative discussion. Although extreme peritubal adhesions associated with myomectomy may be circumvented with egg retrieval for *in vitro* fertilization, endometrial cavity obliteration (Asherman syndrome) is difficult to manage successfully. Although the rate of successful pregnancy after myomectomy is difficult to measure because of many confounding variables, in one report it was as high as 44% in the 2-year period following myomectomy (29). There appear to be no data supporting routine myomectomy for the purpose of improving reproductive outcome in women with even large fibroids who have minimal symptoms (26). Although this procedure may be attractive in women with enormous fibroids, one must consider the state of the uterus after an extensive myomectomy.

Myomectomy can be performed through a variety of transabdominal incisions, through a primary laparoscopic approach, and rarely through the vagina (via colpotomy). The goal is complete extirpation of all fibroids, although one may consider the impact of individual fibroid removal on tubal function. Preoperative imaging of fibroids by ultrasound, MRI, hysterosonogram, or hysterosalpingogram may be helpful but is not necessary. After adequate visualization of the fibroids, a minimal number of sagittally oriented incisions are made through the uterine serosa and through the outer myometrium to the surface of the fibroid. The choice of cutting instruments is not clearly critical to a good outcome, but operative speed is important in reducing blood loss (30). Injection of vasopressin into the uterine incision sites has been shown to decrease blood loss as well (31). The use of tourniquets or vascular clamps to temporarily occlude the uterine arterial blood supply has not been shown to be helpful (30). Fibroids located in the broad ligament adjacent to the uterine artery and ureter, fibroids in the cervix, and posterior wall fibroids tend to be more difficult to resect. Layered repair with absorbable suture of the myometrial defect is hemostatic and improves the structural integrity of the uterine wall. Good hemostasis may reduce the risk for adhesions, and use of adhesion-reducing materials such as methylcellulose or hyaluronate/methylcellulose sheets covering the uterine incisions has been demonstrated to reduce adhesion formation (32). Rarely is hysterectomy required after the fibroids have been removed (<1%), although this contingency should be discussed with the patient preoperatively (22).

Laparoscopic myomectomy seems to be a highly comparable operation to abdominal myomectomy with regard to efficacy. Several series have reported reasonable pregnancy outcomes after laparoscopic myomectomy, suggesting preservation of fertility and a low risk of uterine rupture (14,33–36). One study suggested superior hemostasis with use of the harmonic scalpel versus the monopolar cautery (37). Operative blood loss with laparoscopic myomectomy is comparable to that with abdominal myomectomy (36,38). A few small studies suggest that rates of conception after laparoscopic myomectomy may be equal to or better than the rates after abdominal myomectomy (36,39). Closure of the uterine defect with laparoscopic suturing appears important to achieving a low risk of uterine rupture. With laparoscopic myomectomy, removal of fibroids from the abdomen is accomplished with a morcellating device or through a colpotomy.

A subsequent myomectomy or hysterectomy tends to be technically more difficult, primarily because of periuterine adhesions. The myometrium tends to be fibrotic, and the fibroids are more difficult to excise. These typically are performed by laparotomy. In women undergoing a repeat myomectomy, not only are the rates of blood transfusion and conversion to hysterectomy slightly higher, but the rate of subsequent live birth (8.6%) is quite low in older women with greater numbers of fibroids having the least chance for successful pregnancy (31). Women who undergo subsequent myomectomies are obviously older than women who undergo primary myomectomy.

The choice of myomectomy by laparotomy or laparoscopy is largely based on the training and judgment of the surgeon. Many of the issues associated with abdominal hysterectomy and laparoscopic hysterectomy are the same as with myomectomy. One should take into account the additional time required to perform extensive laparoscopic suturing after removing many or very large fibroids (>9–10 cm), remembering that additional time may incur increased blood loss (40). There has been some question regarding the increased likelihood of fibroid recurrence after laparoscopic myomectomy, but the existing data are inadequate. Removal of a fibroid that is pedunculated and in a posterior location can be accomplished transvaginally with creation of a colpotomy in the space of Douglas, but visualization and the ability to repair a significant myometrial defect are limited.

HYSTEROSCOPIC SURGERY

Hysteroscopic surgery may offer symptom relief and uterine conservation in a subset of women with uterine leiomyomata. Hysteroscopic procedures are of generally short duration, are performed in an ambulatory surgery setting, and need only a brief period of recovery. Most surgeons utilize 1.5% glycine or 3% sorbitol distention media and a monopolar electrocautery loop for resection. Only certain women with menorrhagia and submucosal fibroids and associated dysmenorrhea are candidates. The size of the fibroid uterus is an important factor, as risk of complications seems to rise with uteri greater than 12 weeks' gestational size. In women with submucous fibroids and recurrent pregnancy loss without other etiologies, hysteroscopic resection of the intracavitary portion of the fibroid may also be beneficial. Most studies demonstrate a reduction in bleeding symptoms of about 85% (41,42). Additionally, fibroid resection may be accompanied by endometrial resection or ablation. Interestingly, the success rate is lower in patients with fibroids and menorrhagia than in those with dysfunctional uterine bleeding (43). Obviously, in cases where the endometrium is also ablated, fertility is not a priority. Recently, a technique for removing submucous fibroids completely has been described (44). It is unclear whether this is superior to typical hysteroscopic resection.

MYOLYSIS

Myolysis is a surgical technique that has the intention of destroying fibroids. Electrocautery, cryosurgical, and laser destruction of fibroids and their immediate blood supply has been reported with laparoscopic, hysteroscopic, and image-guided approaches (45). In the late 1980s, laparoscopic myolysis with the neodymium:yttrium aluminum garnet (Nd:YAG) laser was performed but was limited by availability of the laser (46,47). Subsequent use of a bipolar electrocautery needle was also used with good reduction of fibroid size (48). Concern developed regarding the risks for uterointestinal adhesions and subsequent uterine rupture during pregnancy after myolysis (49,50). Cryomyolysis can be performed laparoscopically or via hysteroscope, depending on the location of the fibroids (51,52). Image-guided techniques using laser or cryotherapy may be superior to surgical approaches (53,54). Magnetic resonance imaging may detect small incremental increases or decreases in targeted tissue temperature, allowing for very precise treatment. Focused high-intensity ultrasound therapy has also been tested (55). To date no randomized clinical trials have been performed comparing these modalities with myomectomy or uterine artery embolization.

UTERINE ARTERY LIGATION

Laparoscopic uterine artery occlusion or ligation is a relatively new procedure that was probably developed as a result of the success of uterine artery embolization. Successful bilateral laparoscopic ligation or coagulation of the most proximal portion of the uterine artery has been reported, with a 76% reduction in dominant fibroid diameter and an 80% to 90% improvement in pain and bleeding in treated patients (56,57). Posttreatment pregnancies have been reported, but the first trimester loss rate seems high, suggesting that this procedure should be reserved for women with fibroids who are not interested in childbearing (58). Limited data exist comparing surgical artery ligation with uterine artery embolization (59,60). Hospitalization for the procedure is typically 24 hours or less, and recovery time is about 2 weeks.

USE OF PREOPERATIVE MEDICATIONS PRIOR TO SURGERY FOR LEIOMYOMATA

Medical treatment of women with fibroids prior to planned surgical intervention has been proposed. Therapies have included androgens, gonadotropin-releasing hormone (GnRH) analogues, and selective estrogen receptor modulators. These therapies may act directly on the endometrium to reduce bleeding as well as fibroid volume temporarily. Certainly, temporary volume reduction can make vaginal, laparoscopically assisted, and laparoscopic hysterectomy more attractive in women with large, broad uterine leiomyomata (61). If amenorrhea is induced with GnRH analogues and surgery is delayed for 3 months in women with fibroids, menorrhagia, and anemia, preoperative hemoglobin levels can be improved, reducing the risk for transfusion.

In women planning to undergo myomectomy, induction of amenorrhea with correction of preoperative anemia may be of value. However, operative blood loss, operating time, and extent of uterine surgery seem to be unchanged with the use of preoperative GnRH therapy (62). There also has been some suggestion that the rate of recurrent leiomyomata is higher in women who had been treated with preoperative GnRH therapy prior to myomectomy (61–63). Adverse effects may occur with GnRH analogues as well; therefore, in the absence of anemia, premyomectomy treatment is not warranted.

Prior to hysteroscopic surgery, pretreatment with a GnRH analogue for 1 month may be of some benefit (42).

CONCLUSIONS

Surgical therapies have the longest history of use in the management of women with symptoms attributable to uterine fibroids. Hysterectomy and myomectomy are the primary surgical treatment options and are evolving to less invasive techniques, which include the laparoscopic approach. Clinical decision making has often been based on personal physician experience and case series of various therapies that have significant biases with respect to fibroid size and distribution. Better-designed studies and even some randomized trials have been conducted comparing traditional surgical approaches with newer, less invasive surgical

options and uterine artery embolization. These studies have attempted to critically compare rates of symptom relief and complications, duration of symptom relief, total economic costs, and patient satisfaction, but they have been hampered by small sample size and a dependence on economic modeling rather than real data (9,25,59,64). Primarily because of the extensive variations in fibroid size and distribution, the inherent subjectivity in patients' perception and tolerance of symptoms, and the individual variations in surgeons' technique, randomized clinical trials will be necessary to determine the superiority of a modality for a given subset of women with fibroids.

REFERENCES

1. Lepine LA, Hillis SD, Marchbanks PA, et al. Hysterectomy surveillance—United States, 1980–1993. *MMWR CDC Surveill Summ* 1997;46:1–15.
2. Wingo PA, Huezo CM, Rubin GL, et al. The mortality risk associated with hysterectomy. *Am J Obstet Gynecol* 1985;152: 803–808.
3. Weaver F, Hynes D, Goldberg JM, et al. Hysterectomy in Veterans Affairs Medical Centers. *Obstet Gynecol* 2001;97: 880–884.
4. Roovers JP, van der Bom JG, van der Vaart CH, et al. Hysterectomy and sexual wellbeing: prospective observational study of vaginal hysterectomy, subtotal abdominal hysterectomy, and total abdominal hysterectomy. *BMJ* 2003;327:774–778.
5. Zobbe V, Gimbel H, Andersen BM, et al. Sexuality after total vs. subtotal hysterectomy. *Acta Obstet Gynecol Scand* 2004;83: 191–196.
6. Miskry T, Magos A. Randomized, prospective, double-blind comparison of abdominal and vaginal hysterectomy in women without uterovaginal prolapse. *Acta Obstet Gynecol Scand* 2003;82:351–358.
7. Benassi L, Rossi T, Kaihura CT, et al. Abdominal or vaginal hysterectomy for enlarged uteri: a randomized clinical trial. *Am J Obstet Gynecol* 2002;187:1561–1565.
8. Taylor SM, Romero AA, Kammerer-Doak DN, et al. Abdominal hysterectomy for the enlarged myomatous uterus compared with vaginal hysterectomy with morcellation. *Am J Obstet Gynecol* 2003;189:1579–1582, discussion 1582–1583.
9. Lumsden MA. Embolization versus myomectomy versus hysterectomy: which is best, when? *Hum Reprod* 2002;17:253–259.
10. Kovac SR, Cruikshank SH, Retto HF. Laparoscopy-assisted vaginal hysterectomy. *J Gynecol Surg* 1990;6:185–193.
11. Hwang JL, Seow KM, Tsai YL, et al. Comparative study of vaginal, laparoscopically assisted vaginal and abdominal hysterectomies for uterine myoma larger than 6 cm in diameter or uterus weighing at least 450 g: a prospective randomized study. *Acta Obstet Gynecol Scand* 2002;81:1132–1138.
12. Summitt RL Jr, Stovall TG, Steege JF, et al. A multicenter randomized comparison of laparoscopically assisted vaginal hysterectomy and abdominal hysterectomy in abdominal hysterectomy candidates. *Obstet Gynecol* 1998;92:321–326.
13. Campbell ES, Xiao H, Smith MK. Types of hysterectomy. Comparison of characteristics, hospital costs, utilization and outcomes. *J Reprod Med* 2003;48:943–949.
14. Darai E, Soriano D, Kimata P, et al. Vaginal hysterectomy for enlarged uteri, with or without laparoscopic assistance: randomized study. *Obstet Gynecol* 2001;97:712–716.

15. Liu CY. Laparoscopic hysterectomy. A review of 72 cases. *J Reprod Med* 1992;37:351–4.

16. Jones RA. Laparoscopic hysterectomy: a series of 100 cases. *Med J Aust* 1993;159:447–449.

17. Sepilian V, Della Badia C. Iatrogenic endometriosis caused by uterine morcellation during a supracervical hysterectomy. *Obstet Gynecol* 2003;102:1125–1127.

18. Wattiez A, Soriano D, Cohen SB, et al. The learning curve of total laparoscopic hysterectomy: comparative analysis of 1647 cases. *J Am Assoc Gynecol Laparosc* 2002;9:339–345.

19. Garry R, Fountain J, Mason S, et al. The eVALuate study: two parallel randomised trials, one comparing laparoscopic with abdominal hysterectomy, the other comparing laparoscopic with vaginal hysterectomy. *BMJ* 2004;328:129.

20. O'Shea RT, Cook JR, Seman EI. Total laparoscopic hysterectomy: a new option for removal of the large myomatous uterus. *Aust N Z J Obstet Gynaecol* 2002;42:282–284.

21. Stricker B, Blanco J, Fox HE. The gynecologic contribution to intestinal obstruction in females. *J Am Coll Surg* 1994;178:617–620.

22. LaMorte AI, Lalwani S, Diamond MP. Morbidity associated with abdominal myomectomy. *Obstet Gynecol* 1993;82:897–900.

23. Buttram VC Jr, Reiter RC. Uterine leiomyomata: etiology, symptomatology, and management. *Fertil Steril* 1981;36:433–445.

24. Acien P, Quereda F. Abdominal myomectomy: results of a simple operative technique. *Fertil Steril* 1996;65:41–51.

25. Broder MS, Goodwin S, Chen G, et al. Comparison of long-term outcomes of myomectomy and uterine artery embolization. *Obstet Gynecol* 2002;100:864–868.

26. ACOG practice bulletin. Surgical alternatives to hysterectomy in the management of leiomyomas. Number 16, May 2000 (replaces educational bulletin number 192, May 1994). *Int J Gynaecol Obstet* 2001;73:285–293.

27. Garnet JD. Uterine rupture during pregnancy. An analysis of 133 patients. *Obstet Gynecol* 1964;23:898–905.

28. Quakernack K, Bordt J, Nienhaus H. [Placenta percreta and rupture of the uterus (author's transl)]. *Geburtshilfe Frauenheilkd* 1980;40:520–523.

29. Fauconnier A, Dubuisson JB, Ancel PY, et al. Prognostic factors of reproductive outcome after myomectomy in infertile patients. *Hum Reprod* 2000;15:1751–1757.

30. Ginsburg ES, Benson CB, Garfield JM, et al. The effect of operative technique and uterine size on blood loss during myomectomy: a prospective randomized study. *Fertil Steril* 1993;60:956–962.

31. Frederick J, Fletcher H, Simeon D, et al. Intramyometrial vasopressin as a haemostatic agent during myomectomy. *Br J Obstet Gynaecol* 1994;101:435–437.

32. Pellicano M, Bramante S, Cirillo D, et al. Effectiveness of autocrosslinked hyaluronic acid gel after laparoscopic myomectomy in infertile patients: a prospective, randomized, controlled study. *Fertil Steril* 2003;80:441–444.

33. Landi S, Fiaccavento A, Zaccoletti R, et al. Pregnancy outcomes and deliveries after laparoscopic myomectomy. *J Am Assoc Gynecol Laparosc* 2003;10:177–181.

34. Malzoni M, Rotond M, Perone C, et al. Fertility after laparoscopic myomectomy of large uterine myomas: operative technique and preliminary results. *Eur J Gynaecol Oncol* 2003;24:79–82.

35. Stringer NH, Strassner HT, Lawson L, et al. Pregnancy outcomes after laparoscopic myomectomy with ultrasonic energy and laparoscopic suturing of the endometrial cavity. *J Am Assoc Gynecol Laparosc* 2001;8:129–136.

36. Seracchioli R, Rossi S, Govoni F, et al. Fertility and obstetric outcome after laparoscopic myomectomy of large myomata: a randomized comparison with abdominal myomectomy. *Hum Reprod* 2000;15:2663–2668.

37. Ou CS, Harper A, Liu YH, et al. Laparoscopic myomectomy technique. Use of colpotomy and the harmonic scalpel. *J Reprod Med* 2002;47:849–853.

38. Silva BA, Falcone T, Bradley L, et al. Case-control study of laparoscopic versus abdominal myomectomy. *J Laparoendosc Adv Surg Tech A* 2000;10:191–197.

39. Campo S, Campo V, Gambadauro P. Reproductive outcome before and after laparoscopic or abdominal myomectomy for subserous or intramural myomas. *Eur J Obstet Gynecol Reprod Biol* 2003;110:215–219.

40. Takeuchi H, Kuwatsuru R. The indications, surgical techniques, and limitations of laparoscopic myomectomy. *JSLS* 2003;7:89–95.

41. Munoz JL, Jimenez JS, Hernandez C, et al. Hysteroscopic myomectomy: our experience and review. *JSLS* 2003;7:39–48.

42. Gemer O, Kapustian V, Kroll D, et al. Perioperative factors for predicting successful hysteroscopic endometrial ablation. *J Reprod Med* 2003;48:677–680.

43. Yin CS, Wei RY, Chao TC, et al. Hysteroscopic endometrial ablation without endometrial preparation. *Int J Gynaecol Obstet* 1998;62:167–172.

44. Litta P, Vasile C, Merlin F, et al. A new technique of hysteroscopic myomectomy with enucleation in toto. *J Am Assoc Gynecol Laparosc* 2003;10:263–270.

45. Goldfarb HA. Bipolar laparoscopic needles for myoma coagulation. *J Am Assoc Gynecol Laparosc* 1995;2:175–179.

46. Goldfarb HA. Myoma coagulation (myolysis). *Obstet Gynecol Clin North Am* 2000;27:421–430.

47. Nisolle M, Smets M, Malvaux V, et al. Laparoscopic myolysis with the Nd:YAG laser. *J Gynecol Surg* 1993;9:95–99.

48. Donnez J, Squifflet J, Polet R, et al. Laparoscopic myolysis. *Hum Reprod Update* 2000;6:609–613.

49. Arcangeli S, Pasquarette MM. Gravid uterine rupture after myolysis. *Obstet Gynecol* 1997;89:857.

50. Vilos GA, Daly LJ, Tse BM. Pregnancy outcome after laparoscopic electromyolysis. *J Am Assoc Gynecol Laparosc* 1998;5:289–292.

51. Rupp CC, Nagel TC, Swanlund DJ, et al. Cryothermic and hyperthermic treatments of human leiomyomata and adjacent myometrium and their implications for laparoscopic surgery. *J Am Assoc Gynecol Laparosc* 2003;10:90–98.

52. Olive DL, Rutherford T, Zreik T, et al. Cryomyolysis in the conservative treatment of uterine fibroids. *J Am Assoc Gynecol Laparosc* 1996;3:S36.

53. Cowan BD, Sewell PE, Howard JC, et al. Interventional magnetic resonance imaging cryotherapy of uterine fibroid tumors: preliminary observation. *Am J Obstet Gynecol* 2002;186:1183–1187.

54. Hindley JT, Law PA, Hickey M, et al. Clinical outcomes following percutaneous magnetic resonance image guided laser ablation of symptomatic uterine fibroids. *Hum Reprod* 2002;17:2737–2741.

55. Stewart EA, Gedroyc WM, Tempany CM, et al. Focused ultrasound treatment of uterine fibroid tumors: safety and feasibility of a noninvasive thermoablative technique. *Am J Obstet Gynecol* 2003;189:48–54.

56. Liu WM, Ng HT, Wu YC, et al. Laparoscopic bipolar coagulation of uterine vessels: a new method for treating symptomatic fibroids. *Fertil Steril* 2001;75:417–422.

57. Lichtinger M, Hallson L, Calvo P, et al. Laparoscopic uterine artery occlusion for symptomatic leiomyomas. *J Am Assoc Gynecol Laparosc* 2002;9:191–198.

58. Chen YJ, Wang PH, Yuan CC, et al. Pregnancy following treatment of symptomatic myomas with laparoscopic bipolar coagulation of uterine vessels. *Hum Reprod* 2003;18:1077–1081.

59. Hald K, Langebrekke A, Klow NE, et al. Laparoscopic occlusion of uterine vessels for the treatment of symptomatic fibroids: initial experience and comparison to uterine artery embolization. *Am J Obstet Gynecol* 2004;190:37–43.

60. Park KH, Kim JY, Shin JS, et al. Treatment outcomes of uterine artery embolization and laparoscopic uterine artery ligation for uterine myoma. *Yonsei Med J* 2003;44:694–702.

61. Lethaby A, Vollenhoven B, Sowter M. Pre-operative GnRH analogue therapy before hysterectomy or myomectomy for uterine fibroids. *Cochrane Database Syst Rev* 2001:CD000547.

62. Vercellini P, Trespidi L, Zaina B, et al. Gonadotropin-releasing hormone agonist treatment before abdominal myomectomy: a controlled trial. *Fertil Steril* 2003;79:1390–1395.

63. Sharma M, Buck L, Mastrogamvrakis G, et al. Cost effectiveness of pre-operative gonadotrophin releasing analogues for women with uterine fibroids undergoing hysterectomy or myomectomy. *BJOG* 2003;110:712, author reply 712–713.

64. Al-Fozan H, Dufort J, Kaplow M, et al. Cost analysis of myomectomy, hysterectomy, and uterine artery embolization. *Am J Obstet Gynecol* 2002;187:1401–1404.

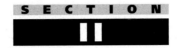

SECTION
II

THE UTERINE EMBOLIZATION PROCEDURE FOR FIBROIDS

7

PATIENT SELECTION AND PREPARATION FOR UTERINE ARTERY EMBOLIZATION

DAVID M. HOVSEPIAN

INTRODUCTION

Central to the successful outcome of any procedure is the appropriate selection of patients. Nowhere is this more important than in the treatment of symptomatic leiomyomata by uterine artery embolization (UAE). Because the symptoms associated with myomata are not specific, it is important to assess them in the context of the presenting clinical problems. Deciding who is an appropriate candidate involves careful evaluation of the myomata—specifically their size, location, and attributes. Imaging plays a particularly vital role to preprocedural planning for UAE because it allows assessment of the myomata and of concurrent conditions that may imitate or exacerbate the symptom complex.

By offering the service of UAE, interventional radiologists (IRs) may find themselves playing a central role in patient evaluation, often at the initial point of consultation. In some cases, evaluation reveals clear contraindications to UAE or surgery. Triaging patients to the most appropriate care is vital to any UAE program. As will become apparent, patient preference strongly influences the choice of treatment. This chapter investigates the role of the IR in screening potential UAE patients, determining whether or when intervention is necessary, and choosing the best treatment option.

THE EVOLVING ROLE OF INTERVENTIONALISTS IN PATIENT CARE

The practice of uterine embolization for treatment of myomata has developed unlike any other in interventional radiology. Its development has been largely driven by patients seeking a less invasive alternative to hysterectomy, which was often the only choice given them until recently. This change in attitude among patients has dovetailed with the development of the Internet, which has dramatically

improved the opportunities of patients to explore the options available to them.

The Internet has revolutionized the practice of medicine in general, both by giving patients easier access to doctors and by allowing doctors to provide information that reaches patients outside of their immediate practice. Rising patient interest in gathering more medical information about UAE has coincided perfectly with an easy means of obtaining it. Many women have amassed a great deal of information about myoma treatments, including UAE, before ever scheduling an appointment with a doctor.

However, for those IR physicians who provide UAE services, the Information Age brings with it additional responsibilities. Many times the interventionalist is the first physician a patient encounters when she finally seeks treatment for myomata. It is essential that the IR perform a thorough assessment of symptoms, including prior gynecologic history, concurrent medical conditions, and relevant physical findings. The interventionalist must be knowledgeable of the clinical presentation of myomata with respect to other common gynecologic conditions in the differential diagnosis. With the additional advantage of imaging training, the IR must be able to establish with reasonable certainty whether symptoms are attributable to myomata or to some other underlying cause.

Many IRs continue to see their role primarily as consultant. They are understandably nervous to take self-referrals and the added responsibility that comes with being a primary care physician. Even those interventionalists who provide primary evaluations would agree that patients' interests are best served by having a thorough gynecologic evaluation to supplement their own consultation. Most IRs are not skilled in performing a bimanual pelvic examination, nor do they possess more than a basic knowledge of leiomyoma physiology or natural history. They do not have the breadth of knowledge or experience with gynecologic diseases that gynecologists have, so it seems that a collaborative approach to patient evaluation and management would serve only to enhance the care that IRs can provide.

PREPROCEDURAL EVALUATION

The preprocedural evaluation should include a detailed history of both gynecologic and general medical conditions. A gynecologic history includes the following information: the chief complaint and a description of any pelvic symptoms (e.g., pain or pressure; urinary frequency; constipation; flank, back, or leg pain), menstrual history, reproductive history, and whether menopausal symptoms are present. The menstrual history should document the duration of the menstrual cycle, the number of heavy days, the presence or absence of intermenstrual bleeding, the frequency of sanitary wear change (pads, tampons, or both) on heavy days, and the presence (or absence) of clot passage, flooding, or anemia.

The general medical history should include all other medical conditions, prior surgeries, allergies, medication use, and a review of symptoms. It is often during this portion of the history that one uncovers issues that can impact directly on postprocedural management or recovery, such as a sensitivity to narcotics or an intolerance of nonsteroidal antiinflammatory medications, both of which are mainstays of post-UAE pain management. Also, by examining the presenting symptoms in the context of a patient's overall medical history, an accurate diagnosis can be assured with greater confidence.

DECIDING WHO NEEDS TREATMENT

The decision to treat should be based solely on symptoms. Of the approximately 5.5 million women with symptomatic myomata in the United States, approximately 85% will have symptoms in one of the following two categories, with a significant overlap group (1). The first category is menstrual disturbance, which includes heavy menses (menorrhagia), extreme menstrual cramps (dysmenorrhea), or intermenstrual bleeding (metrorrhagia). A nearly equal percentage will develop a sensation of pressure, pain, or compression upon adjacent organs by the enlarged uterus and especially by myomata that protrude from the exterior surface (Fig. 7-1).

UAE appears equally effective in treating both classes of symptoms. Most women who undergo UAE experience sufficient symptomatic relief such that they do not seek additional treatment. No statistically significant correlation between symptom relief and any characteristic demographic or anatomic feature has been identified (2). One subset of patients, however, may be an exception to this rule. Occasionally, when urinary frequency is the sole complaint, there may be no symptomatic relief, which has also been

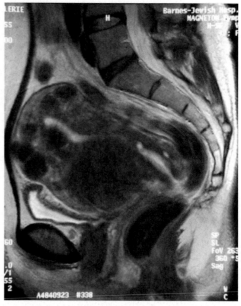

FIGURE 7-1. Bladder compression. Sagittal T2-weighted magnetic resonance image reveals an enlarged uterus with multiple low-signal-intensity myomata. The uterus occupies the entire pelvis. It compresses the urinary bladder, which cannot fill to its normal capacity, leading to urinary frequency.

noted after hysterectomy in this same setting (3). When urinary frequency is but one of a number of other myoma-related problems, it is often one of the first to show noticeable improvement after successful embolization. This apparent discrepancy may reflect the fact that isolated urinary symptoms are more likely a result of primary bladder pathology than myomata, which tend to cause a combination of symptoms.

Back pain is another commonly associated complaint. Many times an enlarged uterus will press upon the sacrum and cause nerve root irritation. Because lumbar disc disease is so prevalent, a sagittal MRI scan that includes the lumbar spine is often a helpful tool for determining if disc disease is contributing to the symptoms. If the uterus fails to make contact with any posterior structures, a careful look at the discs and neural foramina is suggested. The uterus can refer pain to the lower spine in the absence of direct compression of spinal structures; however, it is distinguishable by usually occurring cyclically before or during the menstrual cycle. If a patient has daily back pain or back pain that is worse on rising in the morning or with certain positions, then a primary spinal cause should be considered.

Given the presenting symptoms, it then becomes important to determine if the symptoms can be explained by the leiomyomata. Most commonly, after a gynecologic examination has revealed an enlarged or nodular uterus, an ultrasound scan is requested. Although this is adequate for confirming the presence of myomata, it offers little information to support the likelihood of myomata causing the symptoms at hand, except perhaps in the situation in

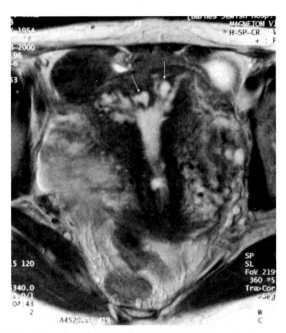

FIGURE 7-2. Adenomyosis. Axial T2-weighted magnetic resonance image showing a solitary pedunculated submucosal myoma that is unlikely to be interfering with menses. The normal junctional zone architecture is lost. There are numerous high-signal foci throughout the anterior myometrium *(arrows)*, which is characteristic of this disease. These foci represent endometrial glandular elements that have invaded the myometrium.

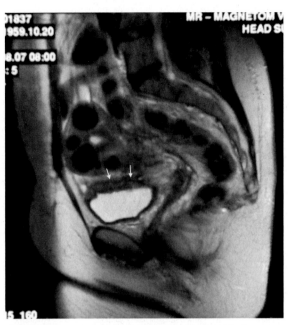

FIGURE 7-3. Endometriosis. Sagittal T2-weighted magnetic resonance scan demonstrates thickening of the dome of the urinary bladder with some high-signal foci within *(arrows)*. Urinary symptoms cycled with menses. The uterus, located directly superior, may contain a small submucosal myoma but otherwise is unremarkable.

which a sonohysterogram for bleeding demonstrates submucosal myoma(ta). MRI, on the other hand, can provide details of size, location, and viability. Conditions that produce similar symptoms, such as adenomyosis (Fig. 7-2) and endometriosis (Fig. 7-3), can be reliably detected and diagnosed. Pelvic MRI has been shown to alter treatment planning prior to UAE in 15% of patients (4).

Correlating leiomyomata location to the presenting symptoms is relatively straightforward. For instance, intermenstrual bleeding is not typical of most leiomyomata. It is usually a result of other pathologic processes, such as endometrial hyperplasia, polyps, or carcinoma. MRI or sonohysterography may help establish an alternative diagnosis, but an endometrial biopsy is still advisable in this case before proceeding with UAE.

Purely submucosal myomata are relatively uncommon, but they can cause severe vaginal bleeding that can be surprisingly disproportionate to their size. Vaginal bleeding can also result from large intramural lesions that encroach upon the endometrial cavity (Fig. 7-4). The mechanism by which bleeding occurs is not entirely clear. One theory has been that myomata that cause hemorrhage must extend into the endometrial cavity and thin the endometrium to the point of ulceration. However, because the majority of myomata remain largely intramural and do not have an exposed surface, this theory has been largely discredited.

One interesting theory holds that myoma-related menorrhagia results from obstruction of the venous plexus of the endometrium or the radial or arcuate veins into which they drain and that it can be caused by myomata in any location (5). Alternatively, it has been suggested that leiomyomata may disrupt the normal contractile function of the uterus, which predisposes to uncontrolled bleeding, or that the increase in endometrial surface area somehow plays a role in heavy bleeding.

Subserosal and small intramural leiomyomata are unlikely to interfere with menstrual flow or cause infertility. Large subserosal myomata or multiple intramural myomata that enlarge the uterus can result in pelvic pain, pressure, and mass effect on adjacent organs (Fig. 7-5). The presence of multiple leiomyomata is not uncommon. In our practice, nearly three quarters of patients have five or more myomata. Often one or more of these may be hypovascular or avascular, but even if the dominant myoma is in the process of degenerating, UAE will often impact enough on the remaining myomata that symptoms are alleviated. Calcified myomata (Fig. 7-6) are often incidental findings on abdominal radiographs. Areas of calcification, if large and coalescent, may also be seen by MRI as areas of signal void. There can be viable areas contained within them, so embolization may still have a beneficial effect despite their otherwise indolent appearance (Fig. 7-7).

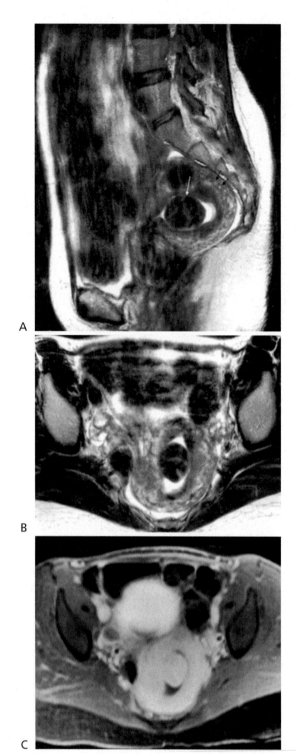

FIGURE 7-4. Pedunculated submucosal myoma. **A:** Sagittal T2-weighted magnetic resonance scan reveals a retroverted uterus that contains a large submucosal myoma *(arrow)* with no definite point of attachment, as well as an intramural myoma. There is asymmetrical junctional zone thickening superiorly and some high-signal-intensity foci in the adjacent myometrium that support the additional diagnosis of adenomyosis *(black arrows).* **B:** Axial T2-weighted magnetic resonance scan confirms the pedunculated nature of the myoma and suggests that it is attached along the right margin. **C:** After gadolinium contrast administration, both the uterus and myoma significantly enhance.

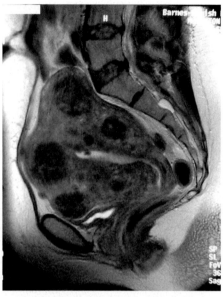

FIGURE 7-5. Multiple leiomyomata. Sagittal T2-weight magnetic resonance image. Numerous intramural myomata distort the normal outer contours of the uterus and press upon the urinary bladder, sacrum, and colon. As a result, there were complaints of urinary frequency, back pain, and constipation, all of which improved after UAE. The patient also had menstrual symptoms, perhaps due to the presence of small submucosal myomata, which also resolved.

It is important to determine whether the myomata are viable. If only ultrasound is available, viability can be assessed using Doppler (6), but contrast-enhanced imaging, either CT or MRI, gives a clearer indication of tumor vascularity (7–10). MRI is often the preferred of the two modalities because it provides superior tissue characterization and enhancement detail. The pattern of enhancement on MRI can often be quite bizarre, and viable areas interspersed with patches of necrosis should nevertheless respond to UAE.

Despite efforts to develop guidelines that provide clear-cut indications for UAE, widening awareness of the procedure has resulted in an increasing number of asymptomatic women asking if they are candidates. Their intention is either to prevent further growth of currently asymptomatic lesions or to hopefully decrease their abdominal girth. In support of the first group, there is evidence that volume reduction for larger uteri is less and occurs in proportion to the initial uterine volume (8). For patients whose main problem is a protuberant abdomen, it is important to remember a basic tenet of geometry—namely, a reduction in uterine volume of 50% roughly corresponds to a diameter reduction of only 20%. Although the myomata tend to soften as they infarct, which often reduces or even eliminates symptoms with minimal shrinkage, there may be little or no effect on the patient's waistline.

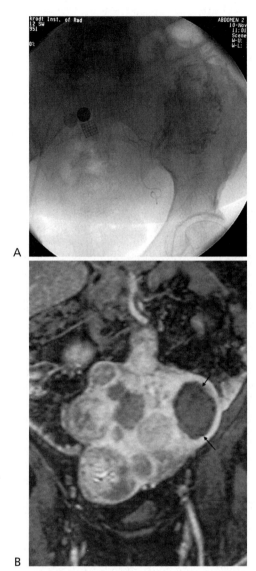

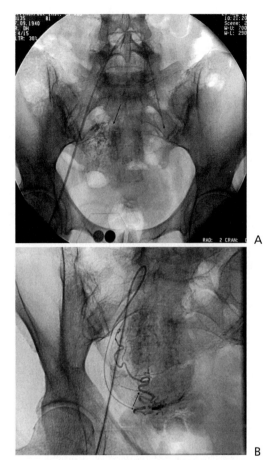

FIGURE 7-6. Calcified nonviable myoma. **A:** Radiograph taken during UAE demonstrates a large, calcified myoma in the left pelvis. A 3-French microcatheter has been placed in the left uterine artery. A radiation dosimetry badge overlies the sacrum. **B:** Coronal volumetric interpolated breathhold examination (VIBE) magnetic resonance image after gadolinium contrast administration shows areas of signal void peripherally, corresponding to the calcifications, and no significant enhancement of this nonviable myoma *(arrows).*

FIGURE 7-7. Calcified viable myoma. **A:** Radiograph of the pelvis taken during UAE demonstrates a calcified myoma in the right pelvis *(arrow).* A 4-French catheter has been advanced over the aortic bifurcation prior to access of the left uterine artery. A dosimetry badge overlies the right superior pubic ramus. **B:** During embolization, contrast agent injected into the right uterine artery reveals a large vessel feeding this myoma *(arrow),* which is still largely viable. Symptoms improved after UAE.

DETERMINING WHO IS A CANDIDATE FOR UTERINE ARTERY EMBOLIZATION

One group of patients particularly suited to UAE for treatment of symptomatic myomata are those who have not responded to conventional treatments. Indeed, the first report that brought UAE to the attention of physicians and patients in the United States included only those patients who had experienced prior treatment failures or recurrences (11). Repeat surgery after myomectomy is technically

challenging because of adhesion formation and may not be feasible, depending on the location of the myomata. UAE is ideally suited in this setting because it requires only that the uterine arteries be patent.

Preoperative MRI can demonstrate important anatomic features of the arterial supply that may impact treatment planning (Figs. 7-8 and 7-9). MRI also provides information about the viability of the leiomyomata and the likelihood that embolization will be effective. For instance, a myoma that has high signal intensity on T1-weighted images and shows no sign of enhancement after gadolinium administration is likely to have undergone "red" or hemorrhagic degeneration, and UAE is unlikely to improve on what is occurring naturally.

Deciding who is an appropriate candidate for UAE is probably better approached by determining the opposite, that is, whether UAE is contraindicated. The first important consideration is uterine or myoma size. There is no definite upper limit to the size of a uterus that will likely benefit

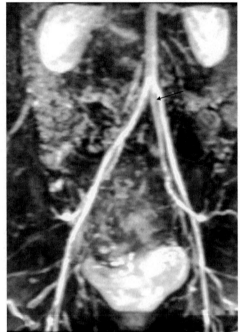

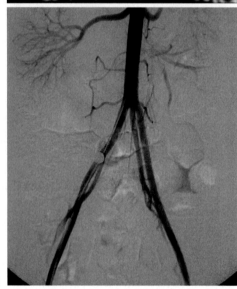

FIGURE 7-8. Variant anatomy. **A:** Coronal view from a magnetic resonance angiogram reveals that the origin of the left internal iliac artery arises from the aortic bifurcation *(arrow)*. **B.** Preliminary pelvic angiogram taken during the UAE procedure confirms the accuracy of the anatomy as depicted by magnetic resonance imaging.

symptoms satisfactorily (1). Undoubtedly, failure to acceptably reduce mass effect was a significant factor.

Pedunculated leiomyomata are a unique subset. When they develop on the surface of the uterus and are attached by a narrow stalk (Fig. 7-10), the point of attachment may disintegrate after UAE, and the myoma may become free to roll about the abdominal cavity. This situation may require surgery because of peritoneal irritation. The current convention among many IRs is that if the base of attachment is less than 50% of the diameter of the myoma, myomectomy is preferable if it can be done safely.

Similarly, a pedunculated submucosal fibroid or an intramural myoma that intrudes sufficiently into the endometrial cavity may slough after embolization (1,12–16). Although this may ultimately relieve symptoms and produce the desired outcome, the process of expulsion can often be quite painful and require hospitalization. In most instances, the cervix is capable of dilating and allowing expulsion of the myoma without any additional manipulation.

Occasionally, passage is arrested in the cervical canal, exposing devitalized tissue to contamination by vaginal flora. Infectious complications may develop and rapidly escalate if they are not caught early. Patients with pedunculated submucous myomata must be counseled regarding the expected symptoms of myoma expulsion and be told whom to contact if they suspect that such an eventuality is occurring. Arrested passage is usually readily remediable by the gynecologist, who can perform a speculum examination and extraction with the patient under conscious sedation and analgesia. Typically, such intervention is warranted if the myoma has not passed spontaneously within a 48- to 72-hour period of observation.

Preoperative imaging may be helpful for determining whether or not the location of the myoma poses any specific risks, such as those described previously, but occasionally a concern is raised that ultrasound and MRI may be insufficient to exclude the possibility of leiomyosarcoma. Ultrasound or MRI may not distinguish leiomyomata from their malignant counterparts. Additionally, MRI can sometimes be confusing because of the varied and bizarre appearance taken on by benign leiomyomata both before and after gadolinium contrast administration.

The time course of growth and the rapidity of symptom development may provide clues to the possibility of malignancy because a leiomyoma is unlikely to outpace the benchmark of a normal pregnancy. Fortunately, leiomyosarcomata are rare. In one series in which 198 women were operated on for rapidly enlarging myomata, none of the lesions were found to be sarcomata (17). In that same series, only one of 1,332 patients with presumed benign myomata was found to have a sarcoma (0.075%). A sarcoma that is embolized may or may not succumb to embolization. Recurrences or technical failures should be carefully reviewed before they are dismissed as merely insufficiently treated benign myomata.

from UAE, but the patient's expectations must be realistic. It has been shown that for every 100 cc of uterine volume increase there is a 2% decrease in the overall amount of shrinkage after UAE (8). For this reason, many IRs suggest that for a uterus greater than 20 cm in its longest dimension, which corresponds roughly to a 20-week-size pregnancy, the amount of shrinkage may be unsatisfactory. In one series, 4.5% of woman ultimately underwent hysterectomy for definitive treatment after UAE failed to resolve their

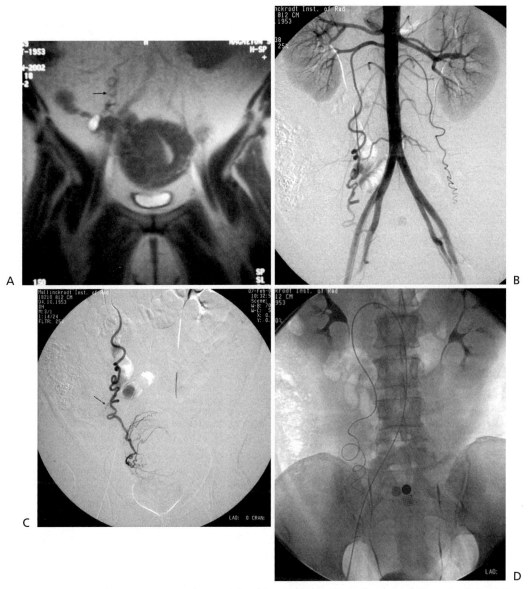

FIGURE 7-9. Ovarian artery contribution. **A:** Coronal T1-weighted image shows the corkscrew appearance of the right ovarian artery, whose black outline is readily discernible against the high-signal intraperitoneal adipose tissue *(arrow)*. **B:** Anteroposterior arteriogram taken at the outset of a uterine artery embolization procedure demonstrates both ovarian arteries without the need for selective catheterization, indicating their possible contribution to the uterine circulation. The right ovarian artery arises from the lower of two right renal arteries, and its course exactly matches the magnetic resonance scan. **C:** Selective catheterization was performed with a 3-French microcatheter. The triangular shape of the ovarian blush can be seen laterally in the midportion of the artery *(arrow)*. The dilated ovarian artery continues on to supply the entire right side of the uterus. **D:** Radiograph of the microcatheter, which was advanced beyond the ovary prior to delivery of the embolic agent. Contrast is visible in both renal collecting systems, and there is no evidence of hydronephrosis. A dosimetry badge overlies the sacrum.

UTERINE ARTERY EMBOLIZATION IN PATIENTS WITH CONCURRENT GYNECOLOGIC CONDITIONS

Some patients may have coexistent conditions that impact on the likelihood of a successful outcome or even predispose them to complications. The two most common of these conditions are endometriosis and adenomyosis, and their possible influence on the case must be discussed in detail prior to embarking on UAE. Treatments for these entities are quite different, and failure to discover these conditions may account for reported failures of UAE (18).

Adenomyosis is characterized by an enlarged, tender uterus, with symptoms of dysmenorrhea and menorrhagia (19). Adenomyosis is a difficult diagnosis to make clinically. MRI clearly depicts the junctional zone of the uterus and is sensitive to diffuse or focal thickening of the endometrium, which is the hallmark of adenomyosis. MRI may also demonstrate high-signal glandular foci within the myometrium on T2-weighted images, which further

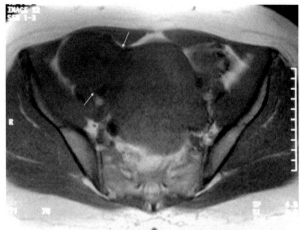

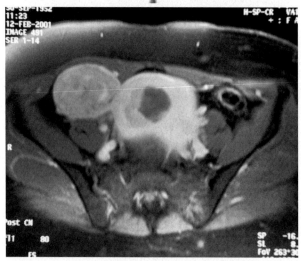

FIGURE 7-10. Pedunculated subserosal myoma. **A:** Axial T1-weighted magnetic resonance image shows a large myoma arising from the right side of the uterus. Its base of attachment appears broad *(arrows)*. **B:** Image taken at the same level after gadolinium contrast administration now demonstrates a narrow connection that measures 50% or less of the diameter of the myoma.

supports the diagnosis. Adenomyosis appears concurrently with leiomyomata in approximately 10% to 20% of patients (20).

The only definitive treatment for adenomyosis is hysterectomy. Early reports of UAE for treatment of adenomyosis show promise that embolization may be effective in controlling the associated symptoms (21,22). These preliminary data suggest that the outcome of embolization for treatment of myomata is not affected by the presence of mild to moderate adenomyosis. There also appears to be control of symptoms in patients with dominant or pure adenomyosis, at least in the short term. However, there are no long-term studies confirming its overall effectiveness. Adenomyosis does require a healthy vascular substrate that may be inhibited by UAE (23,24), but little is known about the ability of the adenomyosis process to recover or rekindle after em-

bolotherapy. Infarcting myomata, on the other hand, have been shown to undergo a well-described unrecoverable progression to disintegration and replacement by hyaline, which is an inert, acellular material (25).

Endometriosis is a condition that can cause abnormal menstruation accompanied by cramps and pain, which can be severe (26,27). It is characterized by ectopic endometrial tissue implants within the pelvic cavity. MRI features of these methemoglobin-rich foci are characteristic (28) and serve to distinguish endometriosis from other disease processes. Laparoscopy with laser ablation and/or restrictive surgery can be curative. Embolotherapy has no role in the treatment of endometriosis (29,30).

Prior infection or surgery may alter the normal ability of the tissues to recover after UAE and predispose to abscess formation, uterine necrosis, or inflammatory changes that affect adjacent organs. For instance, bowel perforation has been observed in cases of uterine necrosis in which intestines have become adherent to inflamed areas and eventually broken down (12,31,32).

Prior surgery may alter the collateral arterial blood supply to the uterus and inhibit successful reperfusion after embolization. Bowel loops that become adherent to the uterus after surgery may become a collateral source of blood supply to myomata with which they come in contact. This situation may preclude embolization if vital organs are supplied by the same circulation.

Women with a history of poor wound healing may be at greater risk for complications, but there is no convention on how to characterize this heterogeneous group and provide guidelines for UAE. Germane to any angiographic procedure are the health of the kidneys, the history of a contrast allergy, and any bleeding diathesis. Because most of these issues can be addressed and ameliorated, they fall into the category of relative contraindications.

One final consideration is that of concurrent hormonal therapy, specifically the use of the gonadotropin releasing hormone agonist, leuprolide acetate (Lupron). Although this standard treatment for shrinking myomata may alleviate myoma-related symptoms while the patient is taking the medication, hypoestrogenism is not recommended for longer than 6 months (33), and symptoms tend to recur when the patient no longer takes the drug and the myomata rebound to their pretreatment size (34).

As the myomata shrink, the uterine arteries shrink correspondingly, perhaps as a direct result of supply and demand (35). Therefore, some investigators request that Lupron therapy be discontinued up to 3 months prior to UAE to allow the arteries to resume their normal size and physiologic response to embolotherapy. It is possible that this is unnecessary and may even lead to reduced overall shrinkage of myomata, because the amount of tissue that must be treated will be greater after the Lupron effect dissipates and the myomata regrow. Moreover, for women for whom Lupron was prescribed for treatment of menorrhagia, 3 months of no therapy may not be acceptable.

CONTRAINDICATIONS TO UTERINE EMBOLIZATION

There are few contraindications to UAE, and many contraindications are only relative. Clearly, a viable intrauterine pregnancy is an absolute contraindication to UAE, as is active infection of the uterus and/or adnexa. Chronic endometritis, on the other hand, may only be a relative contraindication, because protective antibiotic coverage during and after UAE may be adequate to suppress any serious infectious complications and allow full recovery. Suspected pelvic malignancy is a contraindication to UAE unless embolization is used in a palliative or adjunctive role.

CHOOSING THE BEST TREATMENT OPTION

A main concern regarding selection of appropriate candidates for UAE is the issue of fertility. Although this may seem an issue more appropriate to the list of contraindications mentioned previously, this single issue is often at the heart of deciding which treatment option is best for a given patient.

From a fertility standpoint, patients fall into three main categories: those actively seeking to get pregnant, those interested in preserving fertility, and those for whom future childbearing is not a consideration. To address women in this last category, there are no barriers to UAE. However, there is an important age-related issue for these women, who are often in their mid-forties—specifically, that a small percentage of women 45 years old or older may develop amenorrhea after UAE (36).

For a woman who wishes to keep her option of fertility open, discussion must include all of the issues involved, particularly her current age and its impact on her fertility. Because successful pregnancies with no obvious side effects have been reported (37,38), it is apparent that for any given woman, carrying a pregnancy to term is certainly possible. However, whether there are any negative impacts of UAE on either the uterus or ovaries that will interfere with the ability to conceive is entirely unknown.

The issue of fertility is one that most significantly affects the group of women who are actively seeking to get pregnant. If there are one or two dominant myomata causing an anatomic deformity of the uterine cavity and/or occupying enough of the cavity so that normal placentation is unlikely to occur, a myomectomy is the treatment of choice. If there are so many myomata that myomectomy is no longer feasible (Fig. 7-11), then UAE may be the best alternative because medical treatment (chemically induced menopause) and hysterectomy are clearly counter to the intent.

For some women, the desire to avoid surgery altogether is the prime motivation for seeking uterine-sparing alternatives, such as UAE. Whether it is from concerns about complications of surgery, a prior bad experience, or a wish to maintain one's body organs (or specifically gender

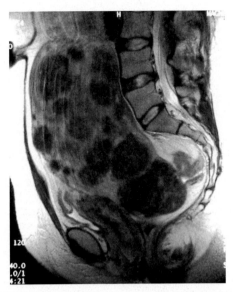

FIGURE 7-11. Myriad leiomyomata. Sagittal T2-weighted magnetic resonance scan shows an enlarged uterus at the level of the umbilicus. There are innumerable myomata within it, precluding myomectomy.

identity), the patient's wishes clearly enter into the equation.

For many women, hysterectomy is an appropriate choice. Many are concerned about leaving devitalized myomata tissue that could become infected. Some want to have these tumors removed from their body and wish not to have the chance of recurrence in the future or entertain a risk of cancerous development. Others want their waistline to decrease for personal or professional reasons. It should be noted, however, that women older than the age of 45 are frequently counseled by their gynecologists to undergo bilateral salpingo-oophorectomy, in addition to removal of the uterus, because of the malignant potential of the endometrium, cervix, and ovaries. As of this date, there is no evidence that leaving those organs intact predisposes to a higher than expected rate of untreatable malignancy, but surgical intervention may be warranted if ultrasound or MRI raises concern about any of the pelvic organs.

The more difficult group to address is those women who are currently asymptomatic but feel that the myomata are growing and wish to address them before significant problems arise. It is a logic that is hard to argue against, but one must keep in mind that serious complications can arise following UAE, and one must constantly weigh the risks, however small, with the perceived benefit. Currently, there are no data to support the use of UAE as a prophylactic measure.

CONCLUSION

When patients are properly screened and counseled, UAE has been shown to be a safe and effective means of managing myoma-related symptoms. As experience with this procedure grows, it is clear that patient selection is perhaps the most important step to ensuring a good outcome. By learning to evaluate a patient's clinical situation in the context of the imaging findings, only then can one provide the proper guidance in deciding among the choice of therapies.

REFERENCES

1. Spies JB, Ascher SA, Roth AR, et al. Uterine artery embolization for leiomyomata. *Obstet Gynecol* 2001;98:29–34.
2. Spies JB, Roth AR, Jha RC, et al. Leiomyomata treated with uterine artery embolization: factors associated with successful symptom and imaging outcome. *Radiology* 2002;222:45–52.
3. Lipman JC, Smith SJ, Spies JB, et al. IV. Uterine fibroid embolization: follow-up. *Tech Vasc Interv Radiol* 2002;5:44–55.
4. Omary RA, Vasireddy S, Chrisman HB, et al. The effect of pelvic MR imaging on the diagnosis and treatment of women with presumed symptomatic uterine fibroids. *J Vasc Interv Radiol* 2002;13:1149–1153.
5. Buttram VC Jr, Reiter RC. Uterine leiomyomata: etiology, symptomatology, and management. *Fertil Steril* 1981;36:433–445.
6. Ryu RK, Chrisman HB, Omary RA, et al. The vascular impact of uterine artery embolization: prospective sonographic assessment of ovarian arterial circulation. *J Vasc Interv Radiol* 2001;12:1071–1074.
7. Burn PR, McCall JM, Chinn RJ, et al. Uterine fibroleiomyoma: MR imaging appearances before and after embolization of uterine arteries. *Radiology* 2000;214:729–734.
8. Jha RC, Ascher SM, Imaoka I, et al. Symptomatic fibroleiomyomata: MR imaging of the uterus before and after uterine arterial embolization. *Radiology* 2000;217:228–235.
9. Katsumori T, Nakajima K, Tokuhiro M. Gadolinium-enhanced MR imaging in the evaluation of uterine fibroids treated with uterine artery embolization. *AJR Am J Roentgenol* 2001;177:303–307.
10. Yamashita Y, Torashima M, Takahashi M, et al. Hyperintense uterine leiomyoma at T2-weighted MR imaging: differentiation with dynamic enhanced MR imaging and clinical implications. *Radiology* 1993;189:721–725.
11. Goodwin SC, Vedantham S, McLucas B, et al. Preliminary experience with uterine artery embolization for uterine fibroids. *J Vasc Interv Radiol* 1997;8:517–526.
12. Ravina J, Ciraru-Vigneron N, Aymard A, et al. Uterine artery embolisation for fibroid disease: results of a 6 year study. *Min Invas Ther Allied Technol* 1999;8:441–447.
13. Pelage JP, Le Dref O, Soyer P, et al. Fibroid-related menorrhagia: treatment with superselective embolization of the uterine arteries and midterm follow-up. *Radiology* 2000;215:428–431.
14. McLucas B, Adler L, Perrella R. Uterine fibroid embolization: nonsurgical treatment for symptomatic fibroids. *J Am Coll Surg* 2001;192:95–105.
15. Andersen PE, Lund N, Justesen P, et al. Uterine artery embolization of symptomatic uterine fibroids. Initial success and short-term results. *Acta Radiol* 2001;42:234–238.
16. Katsumori T, Nakajima K, Mihara T, et al. Uterine artery embolization using gelatin sponge particles alone for symptomatic uterine fibroids: midterm results. *AJR Am J Roentgenol* 2002;178:135–139.
17. Parker WH, Fu YS, Berek JS. Uterine sarcoma in patients operated on for presumed leiomyoma and rapidly growing leiomyoma. *Obstet Gynecol* 1994;83:414–418.
18. Smith SJ, Sewall LE, Handelsman A. A clinical failure of uterine fibroid embolization due to adenomyosis. *J Vasc Interv Radiol* 1999;10:1171–1174.
19. Azziz R. Adenomyosis: current perspectives. *Obstet Gynecol Clin North Am* 1989;16:221–235.
20. Vavilis D, Agorastos T, Tzafetas J, et al. Adenomyosis at hysterectomy: prevalence and relationship to operative findings and reproductive and menstrual factors. *Clin Exp Obstet Gynecol* 1997;24:36–38.
21. Ahn C, Lee WH, Sunwoo TW, et al. Uterine artery embolization for the treatment of symptomatic adenomyosis of the uterus. *J Vasc Interv Radiol* 2000;11:191.
22. Siskin GP, Tublin ME, Stainken BF, et al. Uterine artery embolization for the treatment of adenomyosis: clinical response and evaluation with MR imaging. *AJR Am J Roentgenol* 2001;177:297–302.
23. Schindl M, Birner P, Obermair A, et al. Increased microvessel density in adenomyosis uteri. *Fertil Steril* 2001;75:131–135.
24. Kobayashi TK, Ueda M, Nishino T, et al. Cellular changes following uterine artery embolization for the treatment of adenomyosis. *Cytopathology* 2001;12:270–272.
25. Siskin GP, Eaton LA Jr, Stainken BF, et al. Pathologic findings in a uterine leiomyoma after bilateral uterine artery embolization. *J Vasc Interv Radiol* 1999;10:891–894.
26. Mahmood TA, Templeton AA, Thomson L, et al. Menstrual symptoms in women with pelvic endometriosis. *Br J Obstet Gynaecol* 1991;98:558–563.
27. Fedele L, Bianchi S, Bocciolone L, et al. Pain symptoms associated with endometriosis. *Obstet Gynecol* 1992;79:767–769.
28. Bis KG, Vrachliotis TG, Agrawal R, et al. Pelvic endometriosis: MR imaging spectrum with laparoscopic correlation and diagnostic pitfalls. *Radiographics* 1997;17:639–655.
29. Davis GD. Management of endometriosis and its associated adhesions with the CO_2 laser laparoscope. *Obstet Gynecol* 1986;68:422–425.
30. Sutton CJ, Jones KD. Laser laparoscopy for endometriosis and endometriotic cysts. *Surg Endosc* 2002;16:1513–1517.
31. Godfrey CD, Zbella EA. Uterine necrosis after uterine artery embolization for leiomyoma. *Obstet Gynecol* 2001;98:950–952.
32. Pirard C, Squifflet J, Gilles A, et al. Uterine necrosis and sepsis after vascular embolization and surgical ligation in a patient with postpartum hemorrhage. *Fertil Steril* 2002;78:412–413.
33. Friedman AJ, Daly M, Juneau-Norcross M, et al. Long-term medical therapy for leiomyomata uteri: a prospective, randomized study of leuprolide acetate depot plus either oestrogen-progestin or progestin "add-back" for 2 years. *Hum Reprod* 1994;9:1618–1625.
34. Friedman AJ, Harrison-Atlas D, Barbieri RL, et al. A randomized, placebo-controlled, double-blind study evaluating the efficacy of leuprolide acetate depot in the treatment of uterine leiomyomata. *Fertil Steril* 1989;51:251–256.
35. Coddington CC, Brzyski R, Hansen KA, et al. Short term treatment with leuprolide acetate is a successful adjunct to surgical therapy of leiomyomas of the uterus. *Surg Gynecol Obstet* 1992;175:57–63.
36. Chrisman HB, Saker MB, Ryu RK, et al. The impact of uterine fibroid embolization on resumption of menses and ovarian function. *J Vasc Interv Radiol* 2000;11:699–703.
37. Ciraru-Vigneron N, Ravina J, Aymard A, et al. Pregnancy after embolisation of uterine myomata. *Min Invas Ther Allied Technol* 1999;8:407–410.
38. McLucas B, Goodwin S, Adler L, et al. Pregnancy following uterine fibroid embolization. *Int J Gynaecol Obstet* 2001;74:1–7.

8

PERIPROCEDURAL PATIENT MANAGEMENT

JOSEPH BONN
JAMES B. SPIES

Uterine artery embolization (UAE) for treatment of symptomatic leiomyomata poses unique challenges to the interventional radiologist. UAE is typically performed as an elective procedure on relatively healthy, middle-aged women, and the procedure is not painful. However, it sets in motion a host of postoperative symptoms, including pelvic pain and nausea, anorexia, low-grade fever, and fatigue, known as the *postembolization syndrome,* which represent the primary clinical challenge in managing these patients.

To optimally care for the patient intraoperatively and during postembolization recovery, the interventional radiologist should be familiar with a wide range of anxiolytics, analgesics, and antiemetics and should be prepared to prescribe them for use in the immediate perioperative period and for the several days at home after hospital discharge. In particular, the interventional radiologist should gain experience with the use of patient-controlled analgesia (PCA) pumps and nonsteroidal antiinflammatory drugs (NSAIDs), which together form the basis of post-procedural pain management.

The clinical skill that the interventionalist needs for managing these patients is unlike that previously necessary in this field, but it can serve as a basis for the care we provide patients undergoing similar procedures that result in pain, nausea, and other constitutional symptoms. It represents a new level of clinical expertise for practitioners and solidifies our role in patient care. In this chapter, we provide the reader with a review of the recovery after uterine embolization and a detailed discussion of the medications and treatment strategies in common use for its management. With this knowledge, most interventionalists should feel comfortable with the ancillary issues associated with the care of these patients.

DEVELOPING A CARE PLAN FOR UTERINE ARTERY EMBOLIZATION PATIENTS

UAE can be an extremely tolerable procedure when the technique is optimal and when there is a well-defined protocol for the care of these patients after embolization. It is important that each member of the UAE team understand the procedure and its postprocedural course. This includes any nurses, nurse practitioners, or physician assistants who may care for these patients. It is best that a standard approach to postprocedural management be developed, with written standard orders, physician contact protocol, and written discharge instructions. If possible, one nursing unit should be designated as the preferred postprocedural site of care. This allows one group of nurses to become skilled in assessing and managing these patients, and this will significantly enhance the consistency of care.

There are a variety of different approaches to the care of these patients, and we focus on one successful approach in use at Jefferson Medical College, Philadelphia, Pennsylvania, with suggestions for alternative medications and procedures in use elsewhere. It is important for each interventionalist to develop his or her own approach and, as experienced is gained, to modify it to enhance its effectiveness.

PREOPERATIVE AND INTRAOPERATIVE MEDICAL MANAGEMENT

The patient's introduction into the pharmacology of UAE begins during the initial consultation, at which time the specifics of the procedure are explained, and the operator's medical management protocol is described. The discussion includes the level of mental awareness the patient should expect during the procedure (with adjustments made for each patient's anticipated tolerance level), the timing, duration, and severity of postprocedural pain, and the other elements of the postembolization syndrome, including fever, fatigue, nausea, and anorexia. For each topic discussed, the corresponding medications that will be administered should be described to the patient, and all of the patient's questions about the drugs should be answered.

On the day of the procedure, in preparation for conscious sedation, the patient is instructed not to have anything to eat or drink after midnight the night before, except for any prescribed medications that may be taken with a sip of water that morning. At Jefferson, while the patient is being admitted, a nurse or clinical coordinator palpates and localizes the femoral pulse that will be used for access and places 1 inch of EMLA anesthetic cream (lidocaine 2.5%, prilocaine 2.5% cream) on the skin over the pulse. In the approximately 45 minutes until the initial needle access into the femoral artery, while the patient is being brought to the procedure room and the groin is being prepped and draped, this topical anesthetic will remove most of the initial sting that occurs during the subcutaneous administration of local anesthetic, a sting that many patients focus on and remember surprisingly well. Another approach is for the patient to be sedated prior to the injection of local anesthesia, thus alleviating any discomfort that might occur.

It is our practice to give the patient a 10-mg oral dose of metoclopramide (Reglan) with a sip of water. Metoclopramide is a dopamine antagonist that increases upper gastrointestinal motility and relaxes the pyloric sphincter and duodenal bulb, resulting in a shorter gastric emptying time and an antiemetic effect against postembolization nausea. At Georgetown University School of Medicine, Washington, D.C., routinely the patient is given 4 mg of intravenous ondansetron (Zofran) immediately before the procedure, and an additional dose is given 6 hours later. This medication is safe, has few side effects, and appears to prevent significant nausea in many patients. The nausea associated with the procedure may be related to the narcotics used after the procedure or to the ischemic pain from the procedure. Regardless of the cause, the nausea can be a substantial management problem, and prevention measures are clearly helpful. The use of antiemetics is discussed in detail later.

PROPHYLACTIC ANTIBIOTICS

From the earliest publications on UAE for treatment of fibroids, there have been reports of infection occurring in the first days after uterine embolization (1,2). There also have been rare reports of sepsis in the first month after embolization (3).

To prevent infectious complications, some use 1 g of intravenous cefazolin or 1 g of vancomycin if the patient is allergic to penicillin (4–6). Some operators treat with additional doses of oral antibiotics such as levofloxacin (Levaquin) for up to 5 days after the procedure, with the same goal of reducing contamination of the ischemic uterus with skin flora transported through the catheter or via the embolic agent (5). It has not yet been established whether prophylactic antibiotics reduce the incidence of infection, and the Georgetown group has reported the occurrence of *Clostridium difficile* after UAE related to antibiotic use. For this reason, routine antibiotics are no longer used there and have not been used since 2002. Given the lack of evidence supporting their use, prophylactic antibiotics should be used judiciously, and the duration of use should be limited.

ADDITIONAL PATIENT CARE CONSIDERATIONS

Secure intravenous access is essential during and after UAE while the patient is hospitalized. Such access allows administration of medications and fluids but also can be used for resuscitation if needed. A bladder catheter is placed by some operators to prevent obscuration of the uterine arteries during the embolization as the bladder fills with contrast and to ease the patient's difficulty in urinating after UAE, a difficulty incurred by the postoperative pain, which worsens as the bladder distends. Other operators weigh the small but real risk of cystitis associated with bladder catheters and favor using this aid as needed, rather than empirically.

UAE is like many other interventional procedures in that the procedure can be performed reliably under intravenous conscious sedation, with anxiolytics and sedatives to calm the patient who is awake enough to sense the activity in the room, analgesics to dull or remove any procedural pain (in this case caused by the early effects of uterine ischemia), and antiemetics for nausea. The topic will not be elaborated here, but the importance of vital sign monitoring, including pulse oximetry, and of utilizing nurses or anesthetists with substantial training and experience in sedation and patient resuscitation cannot be overemphasized.

CONSCIOUS SEDATION DURING UTERINE ARTERY EMBOLIZATION

The most commonly used anxiolytic and sedative for interventional procedures performed under conscious sedation is midazolam (Versed), a short-acting benzodiazepine central nervous system depressant that can be administered either intravenously or intramuscularly. Sedation is achieved within 3 to 5 minutes after intravenous injection, and the time of onset is affected by the total dose administered and by the concurrent administration of narcotics. Midazolam has the additional property of being an amnestic, so patients do not recall details of the procedure, particularly the painful portions. An additional benefit is that, during UAE, the patient can be maintained on a light level of sedation because the early segments of the procedure are relatively pain free. This allows the patient to assist in the procedure by keeping still (especially during road mapping) and holding her breath as needed during angiographic filming.

Oversedation effects of midazolam can be reversed by flumazenil (Romazicon), a specific benzodiazepine receptor antagonist that reverses benzodiazepine-induced effects but not the effects of other medications used in conscious sedation (specifically barbiturates, anesthetics, and opioids). Because the sedative effects of concomitant analgesics persist during flumazenil treatment and the sedation from midazolam may outlast the transient flumazenil effect, patients should be monitored for resedation and respiratory depression once the flumazenil wears off. Given the relatively light sedation required for most patients undergoing UAE, it is unlikely that flumazenil will be called on for sedation reversal, but the operator should understand its use in the rare instances when it may be necessary.

A variety of narcotics can be used for analgesia during interventional procedures, although fentanyl (Sublimaze) is commonly used as an adjunct to midazolam for sedation as well as for its analgesic effects. In particular, it has the beneficial properties of rapid onset and short duration. These characteristics provide the nurse or anesthesiologist with greater security, knowing that a patient's pain can be overcome quickly but that the narcotic effect will not be so prolonged as to raise concerns about cumulative overdosing. Fentanyl usually is given in increments of 50 μg intravenously and is titrated, along with midazolam, to reach the desired sedative effect. Although fentanyl is safe when used judiciously, it is important for the interventionalist and nurse to be familiar with the opioid antagonist naloxone, which is administered as an intravenous push dose of 0.4 to 2 mg at 2- to 3-minute intervals, titrated to the patient's response up to a maximum of 10 mg.

An additional pharmacologic supplement occasionally used for conscious sedation during interventional procedures is droperidol (Inapsine), a butyrophenone derivative that produces dopaminergic and α-adrenergic receptor blockade resulting in sedation and, more importantly, antiemesis. When droperidol is given in small doses, the incidence of postoperative nausea and vomiting is reduced. When it is given with narcotics, droperidol can be more effective as an adjunctive sedative without the significant anxiolytic or amnestic effects of a benzodiazepine such as midazolam.

RECOVERY AFTER UTERINE EMBOLIZATION

Prior to discussing patient postprocedural management, it is important to review the recovery that typically occurs after embolization. Although we have gained considerable anecdotal experience over the years by observing the recovery of patients after this procedure, it is only in the last 12 months that data from clinical studies have become available and provided sufficient detail to be useful for understanding the typical recovery after UAE.

The first study to present substantive data on recovery was the Ontario Uterine Fibroid Embolization Trial (7), published in October 2003. This was a cohort of 555 patients treated between November 1998 and November 2000, and as such it reflects the embolization technique in common use at that time. Each patient was embolized with polyvinyl alcohol particles, some of which included supplemental embolic materials. The embolization endpoint in this group was complete stasis (standing column of contrast) in the uterine artery. This endpoint represents a more extensive occlusion than is typically used currently, and thus the details of recovery may not reflect current practice. However, at a minimum, it provides details on patients who experience more than the typical pain currently seen.

Of the patients in the Ontario study, 30% had pain during the procedure, and 92% had pain after the procedure. All patients were surveyed by telephone 2 weeks after the procedure and reported their peak level of pain on a scale from 1 to 10 (1 = minimal pain, 10 = worst imaginable pain). The mean pain score was 7.0 (SD 2.47), with 58% of patients reporting peak pain between 7.0 and 10.0, which is clearly significant pain. When asked to rate their pain using descriptors, 35% said that their pain was very uncomfortable, and 22% said it was unbearable. Ten percent said their postprocedural pain management was ineffective. The mean length of hospital stay (LOS) was 1.3 nights (range 0–11 nights), with 13% having a 2-night LOS and 5% having a 3-night LOS. Pain was the reason for extended stay in 93% of cases. The authors noted that there were a few cases in which organizational or operational difficulties caused delays in receiving analgesic. While in the hospital, 13% of patients expressed dissatisfaction with care related to information gaps, conflicts, and other issues. Most of the patients dissatisfied with their care were among those with the most severe pain. Appropriate pain control monitoring and management were cited as common problems, and 24% of patients said their interventionalist did not visit them in the hospital after the procedure.

After discharge, almost all patients reported abdominal cramping pain. The mean duration of prescription analgesic use was 6.8 days, and only 2% of patients were still taking analgesics after 2 weeks. Nine percent reported that pain control was inadequate with the prescribed oral analgesics. Other symptoms experienced included vaginal discharge

(21%), spotting (22%), and bleeding (32%), with 3% reporting vaginal passage of tissue. Fever was reported by 29% and dysuria by 2%. One third experienced hot flashes, and 8% had mood swings. Puncture site pain and/or difficulty walking were reported by 8%. Ten percent of patients returned to emergency rooms after UAE, and 3% were readmitted. During the first month after embolization, eight women underwent hysterectomy, for a rate of 1.5%. The mean time to return to work was 13.1 days, with 81% returning to work within 2 weeks. Patients with high levels of pain after the procedure were more likely to have a prolonged hospitalization, return to the hospital, be readmitted, and report dissatisfaction with their care, thus underscoring the key role of postprocedural patient management in ensuring a tolerable experience for patients.

A more recent study has been completed that details the recovery after embolization in a group of patients treated in 2002 and 2003 (8). The data set was derived from 100 patients undergoing uterine embolization randomized to either tris-acryl gelatin microspheres or polyvinyl alcohol particles in a study designed to assess differences in recovery from the procedure and the effectiveness of embolics for UAE (9). The key difference between the study by Bruno et al. and that of the Ontario group was the endpoint of embolization. Whether using microspheres or polyvinyl alcohol particles, the degree of uterine artery occlusion in current practice is much less extensive, with residual flow (although minimal) still present. The other difference is the use of better defined and more proactive pain management protocols after embolization. In this study, the peak visual analog scale (VAS) score (rating of pain on a 0 to 10 cm scale, analogous to the scale used in the Ontario Study) was 3.03, and for the first week it was 4.89. The study also summed morphine use (mean 47 mg in hospital), outpatient Percocet use (mean of 11 tablets), and Motrin use (mean of 18 tablets). Additional details of the recovery are given in Tables 8-1 and 8-2. From Table 8-2, the course

of recovery is noted to be relatively mild, with only 11% of patients experiencing pain with a score greater than 7 in hospital, and only 19% experiencing that level of pain at any time during the first week after treatment. The greatest degree of pain was within the first 3 days after treatment. During the first week, 33% developed a temperature of 37.5°C to 38.5°C, and only 2% had fever greater than 38.5°C. Sixty-two percent of patients returned to normal activities within 2 weeks, and an additional 24% within 15 to 21 days. Ninety-four percent of patients missed fewer than 10 days of work.

POSTPROCEDURAL MANAGEMENT

Based on the previous summary, the patient undergoing UAE should be prepared for pelvic pain and the symptoms of postembolization syndrome. In particular, the marked pelvic pain and the nausea associated with UAE recovery will be the patient's greatest concern and should be the focus of the interventional radiologist's attention in the immediate postoperative period.

The ischemic pain after embolization usually peaks within a few hours and starts to recede by 6 hours after the procedure. By the morning after the procedure, most patients have relatively mild or no pain. With the transition to oral analgesics and the progression of inflammation of the newly infarcted fibroids, there is usually a resurgence of pain for 2 to 3 days after discharge, which usually begins to recede by 48 to 72 hours after embolization. This pain is most commonly described as menstrual-type cramps, although the cramps can become severe if regular medication regimens are not followed.

Postembolization syndrome generally encompasses symptoms of low-grade fever, anorexia, and fatigue typical of any patient undergoing embolization. These symptoms should be expected to begin 1 or 2 days after the procedure

TABLE 8.1 MEAN VALUES OF BASELINE CHARACTERISTICS, SHORT-TERM OUTCOMES, AND THREE-MONTH OUTCOMES

Short-Term Outcome Measures	N	Mean	SE	95% CI
Maximum VAS score in hospital	99	3.03	0.26	2.50, 3.55
Maximum VAS score first week	92	4.89	0.26	4.38, 5.40
Maximum temperature (C°) in hospital	91	37.14	0.05	37.05, 37.24
Maximum temperature (C°) first week	93	37.44	0.05	37.35, 37.53
Number of PCA doses attempted	96	70.58	6.72	57.24, 83.93
Number of PCA doses given	97	28.14	1.62	25.60, 32.03
Total PCA dose (normalized to morphine mg)	98	46.69	3.48	39.78, 53.59
Total Zofran dose (mg)	98	3.43	0.36	2.71, 4.15
Total Phenergan dose (mg)	98	12.33	1.41	9.53, 15.13
Total Percocet dose (number of tablets)	92	10.68	1.19	8.32, 13.05
Total Motrin dose (number of tablets)	91	17.89	0.58	16.75, 19.03

PCA, patient-controlled analgesia; VAS, visual analog scale.
Adapted from Bruno J, Allison S, McCullough M, et al. Recovery after uterine artery embolization for leiomyomas: a detailed analysis of its duration and severity. *J Vasc Interv Radiol* 2004 *(in press)*.

TABLE 8.2 MEAN VALUES OF FIRST-WEEK OUTCOMES BY DAY

	N	Mean	SE	95% CI	VAS Score <4 (n)	VAS Score 4–7 (n)	VAS Score >7 (n)
Maximum VAS Score							
In-hospital score	99	3.03	0.26	2.50, 3.55	67	21	11
Day 2	93	4.33	0.26	3.81, 4.84	52	38	15
Day 3	93	3.44	0.23	2.98, 3.91	56	33	4
Day 4	93	2.37	0.20	1.97, 2.78	73	17	3
Day 5	93	1.74	0.18	1.39, 2.10	80	10	3
Day 6	91	1.30	0.16	0.98, 1.63	86	3	2
Day 7	88	1.29	0.19	0.90, 1.67	84	2	2
Peak outpatient VAS score days 2–7	92	4.89	0.26	4.38, 5.40	31	42	19

	N	Mean	SE	95% CI	Temperature <37.5°C (n)	Temperature 37.5–38.5°C (n)	Temperature >38.5°C (n)
Maximum Temperature (°C)							
Day 1	85	36.95	0.05	36.86, 37.05	80	5	0
Day 2	92	37.10	0.05	37.01, 37.20	84	7	1
Day 3	92	37.10	0.06	36.97, 37.19	72	20	0
Day 4	93	36.94	0.05	36.84, 37.03	85	8	0
Day 5	93	36.92	0.05	36.83, 37.01	88	4	1
Day 6	88	36.85	0.05	36.76, 36.95	84	3	1
Day 7	83	36.80	0.05	36.71, 36.90	78	4	1
Maximum temperature week 1	85	37.44	0.05	37.35, 37.53	50	33	2

VAS, visual analog scale.
Adapted from Bruno J, Allison S, McCullough M, et al. Recovery after uterine artery embolization for leiomyomas: a detailed analysis of its duration and severity. *J Vasc Interv Radiol* 2004 *(in press)*.

and last for 3 to 4 days. Although these flulike symptoms are uncomfortable for some, they are usually self-limited and play a minor part early in the patient's recovery. As the pain recedes by day 3 or 4, the fatigue, anorexia, and malaise become the primary residual symptoms limiting patient activity.

As with many painful surgical procedures, anticipating the pain response should help the patient and nurse get a head start on delivering the analgesic medications that otherwise might not be as effective after the pain has peaked. With this in mind, the patient who is about to undergo UAE should be instructed on the use of the PCA pump during the preprocedural discussion or as she is being prepped and draped on the angiographic table. The PCA analgesia pump should be set up by the nursing staff and be ready for use during the procedure, if needed. Pain often begins as the embolization is being completed, and many patients will need immediate clinician-administered doses to control it.

PATIENT-CONTROLLED ANALGESIA

Several different analgesics can be administered in a PCA pump, including morphine and hydromorphone (Dilaudid), although for UAE some operators prefer the highly potent but very short-acting narcotic fentanyl. Some have advocated a PCA pump setting that delivers both a basal dose and a dose on demand. The basal dose is helpful in the first postoperative hours if the dozing patient who is still recovering from her procedural sedation neglects to activate the on-demand PCA dose delivery (10). The basal dose should not be so high as to overly sedate the patient, which may lead to prolonged periods during which the patient neglects to activate the on-demand dose until too late into the pain cycle. At Jefferson, patients are instructed that they may begin using the PCA pump during the procedure and do not have to wait until afterwards. The digital readout on the pump allows the nurse to follow the amount of additional analgesic the patient is self-dosing, so the nurse can adjust the patient's conscious sedation dosing accordingly.

Prior to developing a PCA dosing schedule, the interventionalist needs to consult with the pain management service in their own institution to ensure that the plan meets with hospital policy. For instance, in some hospitals, the patient is not allowed access to the PCA while receiving other sedation or narcotics, and some hospitals do not allow for continuous intravenous narcotics as a basal dose. Many centers have standard PCA protocols, and it is best to use these where possible because the nursing staff is familiar with them.

A typical PCA dosing schedule for fentanyl begins with a fentanyl concentration of 10 μg/mL. The basal PCA dose is usually set at 1 mL per hour, which is equal to 10 μg of fentanyl per hour delivered without activating the pump. The on-demand PCA feature delivers a dose of fentanyl, in the same concentration, at 1 mL no more frequently than every 6 minutes (the "lockout" period), which is equal to 10 μg per dose or a maximum of 100 μg per hour. For morphine, a typical schedule would include an initial clinician-administered bolus of 4 mg, with a demand dose range from 0.5 to 2 mg every 8 minutes. A PCA delivering Dilaudid may be set to administer a concentration of 0.2 mg/mL. The on-demand setting delivers a 1-mL dose with a 6-minute lockout period, for a maximum of 10 mL per hour, or 2 mg. A basal dose may be used, but some have found it helpful simply to supplement the on-demand analgesia with 1- to 2-mg bolus supplements.

All interventionalists should become very familiar with the clinical pharmacology of pain management, narcotics in general, and their own drug of choice in particular. A number of clinical pharmacology handbooks provide good reviews on the subject (11,12). As prescribing operators gain more experience with the PCA, its variables (e.g., analgesic concentration, basal dose rate, frequency of on-demand activation, and amount of analgesic per on-demand activation) can be adjusted to the needs and reactions of the patient. In addition, if a particular analgesic is found not to be effective or durable, a different analgesic can be substituted.

Others have reported taking a more comprehensive approach to PCA analgesia, having the patient start the pump before the procedure, tailoring the basal or continuous dose to the patient's body weight (adjusted for the morbidly obese), and allowing high on-demand doses (30 to 60 μg of fentanyl every 6 minutes) during the UAE. After the procedure, the continuous dose is reduced by 40%, and the PCA is maintained overnight before being converted to oral analgesia tailored to the patient's PCA usage (10).

Only a minority of investigators have used epidural anesthesia for more dense, continuous, local pain control. Most interventionalists adhere to the more traditional intravenous regimens because of the risks of the epidural procedure and the added time and expense. One such epidural anesthesia protocol for UAE has the catheters placed by anesthesiologists, who then administer continuous infusions of the long-acting anesthetic bupivacaine hydrochloride 0.125% and fentanyl citrate 5 μg/ml, which are titrated to the individual patient's pain levels, averaging 8 mL per hour of the mixture, or 40 μg of fentanyl per hour.

At Jefferson, in addition to a PCA-delivered narcotic, the patient is given the option of at least one supplemental oral analgesic, which usually is a version of oxycodone, most commonly Percocet when oxycodone is combined with acetaminophen and Percodan when it is combined with aspirin. Both acetaminophen and aspirin are antipyretics as well, which is helpful for treating the low-grade fever typical of the postembolization syndrome. The patient is reminded that she has control over her PCA dosing, but she must request the additional oral analgesics. This approach may not be allowed under pain management protocols at other institutions.

At Georgetown, once the PCA is started, additional clinician-administered doses of the PCA drug (usually morphine) are the standard means of controlling pain not managed with the standard doses. Usually the additional doses are given in 4-mg increments and are repeated every 5 to 10 minutes up to approximately 12 to 16 mg until there is relief. If there is no relief at that point, the patient may be a nonmetabolizer of morphine and thus not respond. Such a patient may get relief with an alternative medication such as fentanyl.

It is important that the nurses overseeing the patient's recovery instruct any companions, such as relatives or friends, that they are not to assist the patient and operate the PCA themselves because it is the patient's level of consciousness that helps provide the failsafe prevention of a narcotic overdose, which the companion might unknowingly override.

NONSTEROIDAL ANTIINFLAMMATORY DRUGS

Opioid analgesia alone may not provide adequate relief for the patient who is experiencing the intense ischemic pain from UAE, so it is important to recognize the role that inflammation plays in the initial response to injury from organ embolization. Thus, it is important to develop a regimen based on both nonsteroidal antiinflammatory drugs (NSAIDS) and narcotics. Many interventionalists rely on the potent, long-lasting NSAID ketorolac (Toradol) in synergistic combination with a narcotic to treat pelvic pain immediately after UAE. Ketorolac is a potent NSAID whose analgesic action is based on the inhibition of prostaglandin synthesis; thus, it has no sedative or anxiolytic properties. Its strength can be related to a known opioid in that the recommended intravenous dose of 30 mg provides analgesia comparable to 4 mg of intravenous morphine. However, ketorolac has the potential adverse effects of platelet inhibition and gastrointestinal bleeding from peptic ulcers. It should not be used for more than 5 days because of the increased risk of these complications. Ketorolac is available in intravenous or intramuscular parenteral form, with a recommended total daily dose of 120 mg (30 mg every 6 hours). We have experimented with giving the ketorolac in a split dose into each of the uterine arteries in the same manner as chemoembolization, that is, after the first several milliliters of embolic particles have occluded the majority of the uterine artery outflow. The unproven hypothesis is that ketorolac is retained in a more concentrated dose in the uterus where the maximum antiin-flammatory effect is needed and may be achieved in this manner.

Most practices keep the patient in the hospital overnight and convert the patient to oral medications the morning of the first postoperative day. Again, the mainstay of therapy after discharge is the programmed use of oral NSAIDS for several days. If ketorolac is being used, during the transition from the parenteral to the oral form, a standard recommendation is to begin with two tablets (20 mg) followed by one tablet (10 mg) every 4 to 6 hours, not to exceed 40 mg every 24 hours. Another choice, ibuprofen (Motrin), is usually given at the 600- or 800-mg dose level every 6 hours, with a total daily dose of no more than 4,000 mg. Other choices that have been used include naproxen (Naprosyn), naproxen sodium (Anaprox), and indomethacin tablets or suppositories (Indocin).

ANTIEMETICS

In the immediate post-UAE patient, it is sometimes difficult to distinguish nausea caused by narcotic analgesia from pain-related postembolization nausea. If the former is suspected either by the time of the nausea or by previous history, the narcotic analgesia may be switched or its dose reduced to test the theory and relieve the symptoms. Sometimes the nausea occurs with first ambulation or the first meal after embolization. In practice, it is difficult to distinguish nausea secondary to the procedure itself from medication-related nausea. In either case, antiemetics can help.

Antiemetics in common use include prochlorperazine (Compazine), promethazine (Phenergan), and ondansetron. These drugs have been shown to be effective in several postoperative clinical trials and are usually given parenterally in the immediate postoperative period. Prochlorperazine is administered as a single 10-mg intravenous or intramuscular dose, with the total parenteral dose not exceeding 40 mg per day. Promethazine is given 12.5 to 25 mg intravenously every 4 to 6 hours as needed. Ondansetron is administered most commonly as a single 4-mg intravenous or intramuscular dose, although 8-mg doses are sometimes used when the lower dose is ineffective. If one of these antiemetics is not effective in controlling postembolization nausea and vomiting in the UAE patient, another medication should be tried.

The postembolization nausea that may be marked in the immediate postoperative period typically recedes the night of the procedure or the next day. However, the patient should still have an antiemetic available for use at home if needed. Oral dosing for prochlorperazine (Compazine) is 10 mg every 4 to 6 hours, promethazine (Phenergan) 25 mg every 4 to 6 hours, and ondansetron (Zofran) 4 to 8 mg every 4 to 6 hours. Given the relatively minimal nausea most patients have after discharge, these drugs should be taken only on an as-needed basis. If the nausea is severe enough for the patient to require the drug, the patient may have trouble keeping an oral version down, so a more effective alternative may be the suppository version. One such effective antiemetic is prochlorperazine (Compazine), which is available as a 25-mg suppository.

POSTDISCHARGE CARE

As discussed previously, following discharge home, most patients will experience the pain, low-grade fever, nausea, anorexia, and fatigue of the postembolization syndrome for several days. Cramping pelvic pain and nausea will predominate for the first 24 to 48 hours. A protocol of a strong oral narcotic analgesic and a potent NSAID taken on a strict schedule should be adequate for most patients' postoperative pain, although it is important to consider substitutions, especially for the narcotic analgesic in patients who do not respond to the standard regimen. Patients are also advised to adhere to a scheduled dosing of the analgesic and the antiinflammatory agent because this proactive treatment provides greater pain relief than a reactive approach that waits for the pain to become significant before medication is taken. At Jefferson, the analgesic and antiinflammatory regimen includes oxycodone/acetaminophen (Percocet) in a 5-mg/325-mg dose given as one to two tablets every 3 hours, interlaced with ketorolac in a 10-mg tablet given every 6 hours (not to exceed 40 mg per day). The interlacing schedule is set for the first 24 to 48 hours, during the period of most severe pain, so that no more than 3 hours passes between analgesic medications. (An additional benefit of the Percocet mixture is the antipyretic properties of the acetaminophen ingredient.) As the more severe pain recedes, the time periods between doses can be lengthened, the number of Percocet tablets reduced per dose, or the Percocet discontinued in favor of the nonsedating and less potent ketorolac.

An alternative regimen is used at Georgetown. The patient is prescribed ibuprofen 800 mg every 6 hours for 4 days and then as needed thereafter. This is supplemented by one or two Percocet 5-mg/325-mg tablets every 3 to 4 hours as needed. If the patient does not tolerate Percocet, then another moderate-strength oral narcotic is substituted. The patient is also given Phenergan 25 mg orally every 4 to 6 hours as needed for nausea.

As with any prolonged analgesic regimen, constipation can easily develop from the narcotic's inhibition of intestinal motility, and if not prevented, it can be a source of considerable patient discomfort. Patients should be advised to maintain adequate hydration in the first week after the procedure, empirically start a stool softener either just before or after the procedure, and add a laxative if the stool softener is inadequate. As discussed previously, oral or rectal antiemetics should be available on an as-needed basis.

Patients return to activity after UAE at a rate that mirrors a variety of factors, which include the severity of the original symptoms, the size and location of the fibroids, and individual tolerances to illness, pain, and recovery. It is important to emphasize rest and hydration, maintenance of a schedule of analgesics and antiinflammatories, and a proactive stance toward constipation. Patients are advised not to immerse the femoral artery incision in water (bathing or swimming) for 5 days, although they may shower right away.

To reinforce the instructions outlined, the patient should be given written discharge instructions that explain the medications for pain and nausea, measures to take for prevention of constipation, diet and activity restrictions, answers to frequently asked questions, physician contact information for urgent and emergent problems, and follow-up visit guidelines. Even when instructions are given verbally at the time of discharge, there are often questions and confusion, and a written set of instructions will prevent many anxious phone calls.

PATIENT FOLLOW-UP

To ensure that a technically successful procedure results in a successful outcome, a regular follow-up protocol is important.

It is our practice to call our patients at home the day after discharge to inquire how they fared their first night and to reinforce their medication protocol. A follow-up office visit at 1 to 2 weeks usually reveals that their postembolization symptoms are markedly reduced or resolved and allows the interventionalist an opportunity to detect any lingering postembolization symptoms or early signs of endometritis, infectious or otherwise. A repeat imaging study at 3 months after UAE provides important comparative size information and ensures that the fibroids have been successfully treated. If this study is combined with a follow-up office visit, there is an opportunity to discuss mid-term progress, especially for patients with bulk symptoms whose fibroid shrinkage may just be reaching its maximum, and to ensure that the imaging results correlate with the clinical outcome.

In the immediate postprocedural period, the interventional radiologist must make his or her team available at all times for urgent or emergent calls from post-UAE patients. Increasing pelvic or abdominal pain, rather than the decreasing pain levels one would expect to see 1 or 2 weeks after UAE, may be an early sign of prolonged or recurrent postembolization syndrome. One must have a very low threshold for diagnosing and treating infectious endometritis in these patients, especially if they present with a fever. We will admit these patients, obtain blood, urine, and cervical cultures, and begin intravenous antibiotics empirically until the results of laboratory cultures are available,

while returning the patients to earlier levels of parenteral analgesics and NSAIDs for treatment of their symptoms. A review of 400 patients undergoing UAE detected endometritis in 0.5% of the postoperative group (13).

Other postoperative conditions that may require urgent or emergent responses include pain from an incompletely expelled submucosal fibroid or persistent vaginal discharge. The former, seen in 2.5% of patients in the same large review, may be diagnosed by pelvic examination or by imaging studies and often will require hysteroscopic or simple dilation and curettage (D&C) to complete the removal, usually with prompt pain relief (13). Vaginal discharge is usually a comfort and social concern; patients are reassured that the drainage is a normal result of fibroid ischemia in some patients and that it will resolve on its own within a few days or weeks. When the discharge has a foul odor, we culture the drainage, treat the patient with oral doxycycline 100 mg twice a day for 10 days, and switch to a different antibiotic as needed when organism sensitivities return. Rarely, these patients will require a simple D&C if the drainage does not improve. It is important that interventional radiologists see their UAE patients for these postoperative concerns, diagnose and treat them when possible, and develop referral lines with gynecologist colleagues for times when a different type of care is required.

CONCLUSION

The relatively straightforward medical management of the patient before and during UAE becomes a significant challenge in the postoperative period when the interventional radiologist becomes the primary clinician treating the many manifestations of the postembolization syndrome, especially pain and nausea. The regimens outlined and reviewed in this chapter represent the lengthy experience of a variety of interventional radiologists, although most of the information is not derived from prospective, randomized, controlled trials. Above and beyond individual medications, dosing schedules, and the operator's personal experience, a number of principles should govern the process of periprocedural management of the UAE patient. As described in a recent editorial on post-UAE recovery, the medication protocol should be well defined, and it should incorporate the training of all medical personnel involved in the patient's care (14). It should include details about all medications given before, during, and after the procedure, with special instructions for transitioning the patient to oral medications at home. The protocol should be consistent and predictable and based on well-founded principles, yet it should be flexible to accommodate the wide range of patient tolerances and requirements.

Ultimately, the interventional radiologist who is most knowledgeable of the medications used in the care of UAE patients and of the potential problems that a patient might experience will prove the one most likely to ensure a smooth recovery.

REFERENCES

1. Goodwin S, Vedantham S, McLucas B, et al. Preliminary experience with uterine artery embolization for uterine fibroids. *J Vasc Interv Radiol* 1997;8:517–526.
2. Ravina J, Herbreteau D, Ciraru-Vigneron N, et al. Arterial embolisation to treat uterine myomata. *Lancet* 1995;346:671–672.
3. Vashisht A, Studd J, Carey A, et al. Fatal septicaemia after fibroid embolisation. *Lancet* 1999;354:307–308.
4. Goodwin S, McLucas B, Lee M, et al. Uterine artery embolization for the treatment of uterine leiomyomata: midterm results. *J Vasc Interv Radiol* 1999;10:1159–1165.
5. Siskin G, Stainken B, Dowling K, et al. Outpatient uterine artery embolization for symptomatic uterine fibroids: experience in 49 patients. *J Vasc Interv Radiol* 2000;11:305–311.
6. Pron G, Bennett J, Common A, et al. Technical results and effects of operator experience on uterine artery embolization for fibroids: the Ontario Uterine Fibroid Embolization Trial. *J Vasc Interv Radiol* 2003;14:545–554.
7. Pron G, Mocarski E, Bennett J, et al. Tolerance, hospital stay, and recovery after uterine artery embolization for fibroids: the Ontario Uterine Fibroid Embolization Trial. *J Vasc Interv Radiol* 2003;14:1243–1250.
8. Bruno J, Allison S, McCullough M, et al. Recovery after uterine artery embolization for leiomyomas: a detailed analysis of its duration and severity. *J Vasc Interv Radiol* 2004 *(in press)*.
9. Spies J, Allison S, Sterbis K, et al. Polyvinyl alcohol particles and tris acryl gelatin microspheres for uterine artery embolization for leiomyomas: results of a randomized comparative study. *J Vasc Interv Radiol* 2004 *(in press)*.
10. Ryan J, Gainey M, Glasson J. Simplified pain-control protocol after uterine artery embolization [Letter]. *Radiology* 2000;224:610–613.
11. Wells BG, DiPiro JT, Schwinghammer TL, et al. *Clinical pharmacology.* Stamford, CT: Appleton Lange, 1998.
12. Anderson PO, Knoben JE, Troutman WG, eds. *Pharmacotherapy handbook,* 3rd ed. Stamford, CT: Appleton & Lange, 1999.
13. Spies J, Spector A, Roth A, et al. Complications after uterine artery embolization for leiomyomata. *Obstet Gynecol* 2002;100:873–880.
14. Spies J. Recovery after uterine artery embolization: understanding and managing short-term outcomes. *J Vasc Interv Radiol* 2003;4:1219–1222.

9

TECHNIQUE OF UTERINE ARTERY EMBOLIZATION AND CHOICE OF EMBOLICS

JEAN-PIERRE PELAGE
MICHEL WASSEF
PASCAL LACOMBE
ALEXANDRE LAURENT

INTRODUCTION

The method of uterine fibroid embolization has been extensively described in the literature (1–7). In essence, it involves the placement of a catheter into the uterine arteries and injecting embolization particles into the uterine arteries to obtain fibroid infarction and shrinkage. There are some differences in technique among centers—some catheterize the uterine arteries directly using 4- or 5-French catheters (3,5,8,9), whereas others use microcatheters (2,10,11). When considering the choice of an embolization agent, the physical properties of the agent (granulometric distribution, compressibility) and the method of delivery should be considered. Nonspherical polyvinyl alcohol (PVA) particles were the first embolization agents used for uterine fibroid embolization (1–5,9–11). Spherical embolization particles, such as tris-acryl microspheres, have been developed to address some of the disadvantages of nonspherical particles, such as the unpredictable level of arterial occlusion and the clumping associated with them (12–14). Recently, spherical PVA particles have been introduced (15,16). To date, there is no consensus opinion on the type and size of embolization materials to be used for uterine fibroid embolization. In addition, the appropriate technique of embolization (i.e., angiographic endpoint) with each of the available products is an ongoing debate.

USUAL TECHNIQUE OF CATHETERIZATION

Local anesthesia and intravenous sedation (combination of narcotics and benzodiazepines) are used because embolization is performed with the patient undergoing conscious sedation (2–5,11,17). Typically, the right groin is prepared for the procedure and draped in the usual sterile fashion. The common femoral artery is punctured, and a 4- or 5-French sheath is placed (2–5,7,11,17). A 0.032- or

0.035-inch angled hydrophilic guidewire is then used, and a 4- or 5-French visceral catheter (often cobra shaped) is placed over the wire and used to select the contralateral iliac system (2–5,8,17). The contralateral internal iliac artery is catheterized, and digital subtraction angiography is performed in order to identify the origin of the uterine artery and the presence of any variations (8). In most cases, the origin of the uterine artery is easily identified using the contralateral oblique projection (Fig. 9-1). The 4- or 5-French catheter is advanced into the anterior division of the internal iliac artery, and the uterine artery is selected using road-mapping technique (8). The tip of the catheter is placed into the transverse segment of the uterine artery, ideally distal to the origin of cervicovaginal branches, and

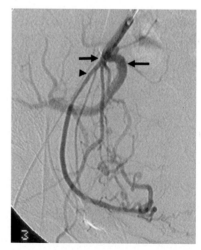

FIGURE 9-1. A 38-year-old woman with uterine fibroids. Digital subtraction angiogram of the right internal iliac artery in left anterior oblique projection (contralateral oblique) shows division into two main stems *(arrows)*. The uterine artery, which is the first branch from the anterior division, is easily identified *(arrowhead)*.

digital subtraction angiography is performed before emboli-zation (Fig. 9-2) (4,8,18). After embolization of the contralateral uterine artery, the initial visceral cobra-shaped catheter, a Levin 1 catheter, or a Simmons 2 catheter is used to select the ipsilateral internal iliac artery after forming a Waltman loop (5,6,8,10,19,20). The same procedure is then repeated to catheterize the uterine artery (5,6,8,10).

TWO-CATHETER TECHNIQUE

Some authors favor a bilateral, as opposed to the more usual unilateral, femoral approach with simultaneous embolization of both uterine arteries (4,21). Catheterization from the contralateral side using a cross-over technique is usually easier and therefore requires less fluoroscopy time, particularly for less-experienced radiologists (4,21). The Waltman loop is more prone to kinking when a unilateral approach is used (6,20). Once the two catheters are in place, simultaneous injection of both uterine arteries is performed before and after embolization (Fig. 9-3). This method gives greater flexibility of embolization, allowing switching back and forth between the two sides and ensuring a stable final endpoint. It also results in a lower radiation dose because both sides are embolized simultaneously. However, this technique is best completed with simultaneous embolization performed by two separate operators, and it may be associated with an increased risk of admittedly rare femoral artery puncture site complications (4,21,22).

DIFFICULT CATHETERIZATION OF THE UTERINE ARTERY

In most cases, a cobra-shaped catheter will easily hook over the aortic bifurcation and follow an angiographic wire into the hypogastric artery. For difficult catheterization of the contralateral uterine artery, a long sheath may be useful to stabilize the primary catheter. In the case of difficult catheterization of the ipsilateral uterine artery or when kinking of the catheter is observed after Waltman loop formation, puncture of the contralateral femoral artery is sometimes required (6,23). In most cases, identification of the origin of the uterine artery should be made using the contralateral oblique view (8,18). If the vessel origin is not demonstrated, then the ipsilateral oblique projection should be performed to best characterize the precise origin of the uterine artery (Fig. 9-4) (8,18). Failure of catheterization using a 4- or 5-French catheter is frequently observed when the uterine artery is tortuous or has a high origin from the hypogastric artery with an acute angulation from the anterior division of the hypogastric artery (17). A micro-catheter used with a flexible microwire is particularly useful in these circumstances (Figs. 9-4 and 9-5) (6). Similarly, for thin uterine arteries, direct catheterization from the

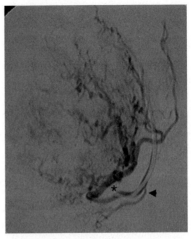

FIGURE 9-2. A 40-year-old woman with uterine fibroids. Digital subtraction angiogram shows characteristic course of the left uterine artery. The tip of the 4-French cobra-type catheter *(star)* is carefully placed distal to the cervicovaginal artery *(arrowhead).*

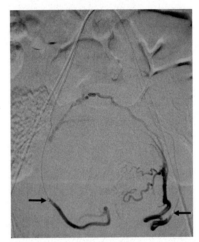

FIGURE 9-3. A 28-year-old woman with multiple uterine fibroids seeking fertility after treatment. Digital subtraction angiogram obtained after bilateral and simultaneous injection into the uterine arteries using microcatheters *(arrows).*

hypogastric artery using a microcatheter with the primary catheter positioned in the anterior division of the hypogastric artery should be performed (Fig. 9-5). In order to allow easy injection of the particles at the time of embolization, large-lumen (0.024 to 0.027 inch) microcatheters are particularly useful.

PITFALLS IN UTERINE ARTERY EMBOLIZATION

There are a variety of reasons for embolization failure, and these are discussed in detail in Chapter 10. However, a brief introduction in the context of a discussion on technique is provided here.

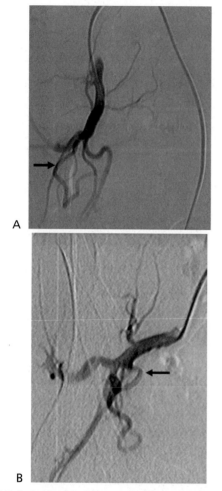

FIGURE 9-4. A 44-year-old woman with uterine fibroids. Digital subtraction angiogram of right internal iliac artery in left anterior oblique projection (contralateral) 30° oblique **(A)** and right anterior oblique projection (homolateral) 30° oblique **(B)**. The origin of the uterine artery (*arrow,* **A** and **B**) is well identified on homolateral oblique projection because of its upper origin. Note acute angulation of the origin of the uterine artery from the internal iliac artery.

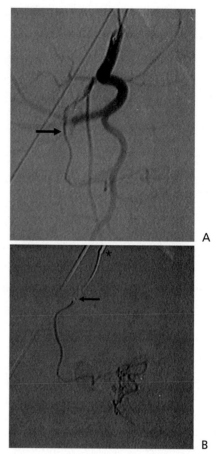

FIGURE 9-5. A 40-year-old woman with multiple uterine fibroids treated with subcutaneous injection of gonadotropin-releasing hormone agonists 2 weeks before arteriography. **A:** Digital subtraction angiogram of the right internal iliac artery in left anterior oblique projection shows a thin uterine artery *(arrow).* **B:** Selective catheterization of the uterine artery is performed using a microcatheter with the 4-French cobra-type catheter left into the anterior division of the internal iliac artery.

The goal of uterine fibroid embolization is complete ischemic infarction of all uterine fibroids. Failure of complete devascularization of the fibroids may affect long-term clinical response (Fig. 9-6) (23). Embolization of uterine fibroids is mainly based on a preferential flow to the fibroids; therefore, it is crucial to prevent spasm or flow restriction. Spasm may result in poor flow into the perifibroid plexus, which is the target of embolization, and may lead to insufficient delivery of embolic material (14,23). When spasm is encountered on one side, it is possible to embolize the other side or to leave the catheter in place for several minutes (21,23).

During embolization, it is difficult to determine whether stasis is related to a stable embolization endpoint or to catheter-induced spasm. Spasm or reduced arterial diameter leading to difficult catheterization seems to be more frequent in women recently treated with gonadotropin-releasing hormone agonists or after the use of intraarterial lidocaine (Fig. 9-5) (5,17,24). The most common cause of spasm is catheter related, where the relatively rigid catheter distorts the course of the tortuous uterine artery. Variable approaches have been used to prevent or treat spasm (23). Options include waiting until spasm resolves, catheterizing past the spasm with a hydrophilic wire, using a microcatheter, or treatment with vasodilators (Fig. 9-7) (5,23). Intraarterial injection of nitroglycerin is associated with an inconsistent effect and may be associated with vasovagal attacks and hypotension (5,11,17,23).

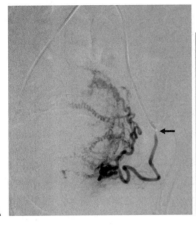

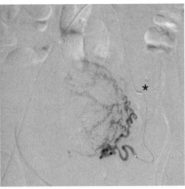

A   B

FIGURE 9-6. A 42-year-old woman with multiple uterine fibroids. **A:** Digital subtraction angiogram of selective injection into an enlarged left uterine artery shows spasm at the tip of the 4-French catheter *(arrow).* **B:** Superselective catheterization of the transverse segments of the uterine artery distal to the spasm is successfully performed using a microcatheter. Note that the 4-French catheter has been pulled out into the anterior division of the internal iliac artery *(star).*

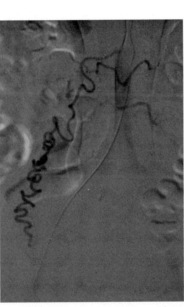

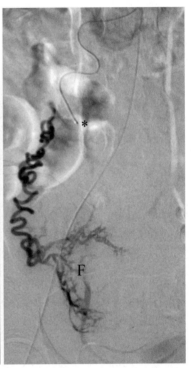

A, B   C

FIGURE 9-7. A 42-year-old woman with a large transmural fundal uterine fibroid. **A:** Flush aortogram shows two enlarged ovarian arteries originating below the renal arteries *(arrows).* **B:** Digital subtraction angiogram of selective injection into the right ovarian artery using a 5-French Mickaelsson-type catheter shows characteristic tortuous course of the vessel. **C:** Superselective catheterization and injection using a microcatheter *(star)* confirm that the fibroid *(F)* is supplied by the right ovarian artery.

CHOICE OF EMBOLICS

There is no consensus opinion concerning the choice of embolic agent (7,23,25,26). Small embolic particles are reported to cause more fibroid shrinkage but may also be associated with an increased risk of complications (e.g., damage to normal myometrium, cervical or ovarian ischemia) (5,11,27).

Nonspherical Polyvinyl Alcohol Particles

Nonspherical PVA particles have been widely used to perform uterine fibroid embolization (1–11). PVA has been used as an embolic agent in various vascular distributions for 20 years (28,29). The irregular shape of the material is associated with a larger granulometric range of the particles than is advertised (26,30,31). In addition, there is a risk of

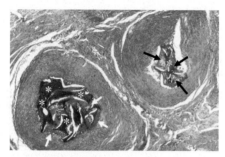

FIGURE 9-8. A 38-year-old woman with uterine fibroids treated with premyomectomy embolization of the uterine arteries using 355- to 500-μm nonspherical PVA particles. Photomicrograph of high-power section through the periphery of a resected intramural fibroid immediately after embolization. The two arteries shown contain aggregates of PVA particles *(stars)*. Thrombus is seen within the interstices *(arrows)* (hematoxylin safran and eosin, magnification ×400).

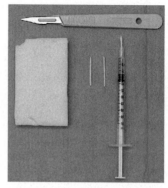

FIGURE 9-9. Gelatin sponge pledgets manually cut into strips with a scalpel, rolled, and placed into 1-mL syringes with saline and contrast are particularly suitable for pelvic embolization.

injection of particles smaller than the theoretical size in conjunction with aggregates (5,26,30–32). This potential adverse effect of PVA particles has been reported several times (5,32). In clinical practice, clumping of PVA particles can lead to obstruction of the catheter or microcatheter and potentially to an uncontrolled level of arterial occlusion (31). With nonspherical particles, clumping of the embolic material may result in a false angiographic endpoint at the conclusion of embolization. The mechanism of arterial occlusion induced by nonspherical PVA particles has been reported (26). The particles do not completely occlude the lumen of the occluded arteries (28,29). The initial incomplete lumen occlusion by the particles is associated with thrombus formation within the interstices (Fig. 9-8). Subsequent luminal recanalization may allow perfusion of normal myometrium in most patients, although uterine ischemic injury necessitating hysterectomy has been reported (3,27). Recanalization of the vessel is usually observed after several months or years (26,29). Several mechanisms may be responsible for recanalization: distal migration, fragmentation or extravascular migration of PVA particles, and resorption of thrombus (26,29,33). Calcification of PVA particles has also been reported (33,34). The histologic effects observed after fibroid embolization are interstitial edema followed by ischemic necrosis of the fibroids (26,29,33,35). In the long term, there is progressive replacement of myomatous tissue by hyalinized scar tissue (33). Small fragments of PVA particles may cause nontarget embolization of normal tissue, such as the ovaries (11).

To reduce clumping of particles, each vial of PVA foam particles is usually diluted in 20 or 30 mL of a 50% iodinated contrast medium and 50% saline solution (36). Prior to each injection, the mixture is agitated to maintain homogeneous particle suspension. Embolization to stasis is usually performed (1–5,7,11). Embolization is stopped when there is no proximal arterial flow and/or reflux of contrast material. The quantity of embolic agent used for a typical case ranges between 200 and 400 mg, corresponding to two to four vials (37).

Gelatin Sponge

Gelatin sponge has been extensively used for 30 years to perform embolization, particularly in the management of obstetric hemorrhage (26,38–40). Gelatin sponge is a foamlike material initially used to obtain hemostasis during surgery. It is a biodegradable material considered to be a resorbable agent. Three forms are available from different companies: a powder containing small fragments, a sheet from which sections of different sizes can be cut, and thicker blocks from which large pledgets can be obtained. The gelatin sponge powder is associated with a high risk of ischemia and should not reasonably be used for fibroid embolization (40). Pledgets measuring 1 × 2 to 3 × 3 mm that are manually cut into strips with scissors or scalpel and then rolled are particularly suitable for pelvic embolization (Fig. 9-9). The pledgets are placed into 1- or 2-mL syringes with saline and contrast material. A gelatin sponge slurry can also be obtained by mixing small pledgets with contrast. Mechanical arterial occlusion is obtained, followed by acute necrotizing arteritis (26,41). Thrombus formation is also associated. Arterial recanalization is observed within days to weeks after embolization, even if long-term occlusions have also been reported (26,41). Until now, only a small number of patients with fibroids have been treated with gelatin sponge (42–44). Short-term results are encouraging, but it can be hypothesized that a higher rate of clinical failures or recurrence will be observed (42).

Tris-Acryl Microspheres

Tris-acryl gelatin microspheres were developed in France and have been used in various European territories since

1994 (12,45). Microspheres are spherical, precisely calibrated, microporous, cross-linked acrylic beads embedded with gelatin (12,45,46). The tris-acryl polymer has been used for many years as a base material for chromatographic filtration and is well characterized and understood. There is a large experience with the use of tris-acryl microspheres in the neuroradiology field, where calibration of the embolization agent is crucial to prevent complications (45,47). We started using calibrated microspheres in 1998 to perform uterine artery embolization in selected cases (13,14). The spheres are compressible, which allows easy passage through a microcatheter with a luminal diameter smaller than that of the microspheres (46). A better distribution of tris-acryl microspheres than nonspherical particles has been observed after injection into the rete mirabile of pigs or into the uterine arteries of sheep (46,48). Angiographically, apparent clumping may occur with microspheres, and the embolic material may redistribute depending on the infusion rate and the concentration (23). Each vial (1 or 2 mL) of microspheres is diluted in a total of 20 mL of contrast material and saline solution (13,14). Typically, 4 to 8 mL of microspheres are used to perform bilateral uterine artery embolization (13,14,49).

Various types and sizes of embolic particles have been compared in an experimental model of embolization in sheep uterus (48). It was demonstrated that the degree of penetration of the particles into the vascular system was different for nonspherical PVA particles and tris-acryl microspheres (48). A significant correlation between the level of arterial occlusion and the diameter of the particles used was observed for all sizes of tris-acryl microspheres (48). Thus, a deeper penetration of embolic particles can be advantageous, leading to more effective tumoral devascularization of many hypervascularized lesions, including meningiomas (47). In a renal artery embolization animal model, blood flow was more quickly and reliably reduced using tris-acryl microspheres than with nonspherical PVA particles (50). Because the mechanism of occlusion is different from that of nonspherical PVA particles with a small number of microspheres occluding a vessel of the corresponding size, a more segmental arterial occlusion is obtained (Fig. 9-10) (47,48). In the long term, there is no chronic inflammatory reaction and no degradation of the polymer (51). In a series of preoperative embolizations of uterine fibroids, a correlation between the level of arterial occlusion and the diameter of the microspheres used was found (52). Choosing a size of calibrated microspheres solely on the basis of experience with nonspherical PVA particles could result in significant complications. Because the diameter of occluded arteries correlates well with microsphere size, the investigator should carefully choose the optimal size for a specific procedure. Currently, it is recommended to use tris-acryl microspheres larger than 500 μm for uterine fibroid embolization (13,14,53). Tris-acryl microspheres were recently approved by the US

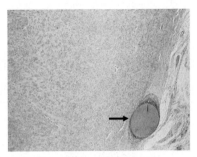

FIGURE 9-10. A 33-year-old woman with uterine fibroids treated with premyomectomy embolization of the uterine arteries using 500- to 700-μm tris-acryl microspheres. Photomicrograph of high-power section through the periphery of a resected intramural fibroid immediately after embolization. The artery shown is occluded by one microsphere of the same diameter *(arrow)* (hematoxylin safran and eosin, magnification ×200).

Food and Drug Administration for use in uterine fibroid embolization.

Polyvinyl Alcohol Microspheres

Because of the unpredictable behavior of nonspherical PVA particles during uterine fibroid embolization and in light of the theoretical and published advantages of tris-acryl microspheres for neurologic and gynecologic interventions, PVA spheres have been recently introduced (15,16). The decision to use PVA as the core constituent was based on the long track record of safety and efficacy of this material in embolization procedures. Like tris-acryl microspheres, even large PVA spheres were easy to inject through microcatheters. Initial animal studies demonstrated that PVA microspheres were effective embolization particles associated with a degree of targeted renal parenchymal infarction similar to that of tris-acryl microspheres (15). PVA spheres were associated with a mild inflammatory reaction compared to the irregular PVA particles (15). Initial experimental studies suggested that PVA spheres tended to travel more distally than the irregular PVA particles (15). In addition, it has been demonstrated that the degree of penetration of the particles into the vascular system was different for PVA spheres and tris-acryl spheres (54). PVA spheres always occluded at a more distal level than the tris-acryl spheres, probably because of different compressibility properties (54). Even if the clinical experience with PVA spheres is limited, the interventional radiologist should consider upsizing particles when PVA spheres are used instead of tris-acryl spheres.

OPTIMAL EMBOLIC SIZE FOR UTERINE FIBROID EMBOLIZATION

The perifibroid vascular plexus surrounding the fibroid (with arteries ranging from 500 to 900 μm in diameter)

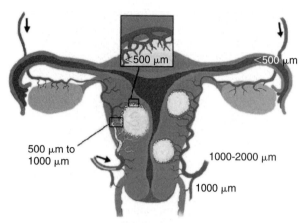

FIGURE 9-11. Anatomic drawing showing the arterial blood supply to the uterus and the fibroids. The perifibroid plexus is composed of arteries ranging from 500 to 1,000 μm in most cases. Branches supplying normal myometrium are usually smaller. The size of the uteroovarian anastomosis is usually less than 500 μm. (From Pelage JP, Le Dref O, Beregi JP, et al. Limited uterine artery embolization with tris-acryl gelatin microspheres for uterine fibroids. *J Vasc Interv Radiol* 2003;14:15–20, with permission.)

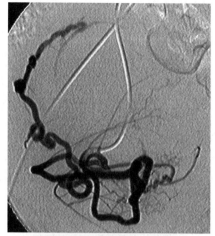

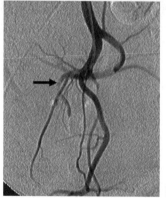

FIGURE 9-12. A 39-year-old woman with multiple uterine fibroids. **A:** Digital subtraction angiogram of selective injection into an enlarged right uterine artery. **B:** After embolization to stasis using three vials of nonspherical 300- to 600-μm PVA particles, the right uterine artery is completely occluded at its origin *(arrow)*.

seems to be a logical target for embolization (Fig. 9-11) (14,33). The center of the fibroid itself is relatively hypovascular. In addition, because of potentially dangerous pelvic anastomoses and the lack of specific tumoral feeding arteries, small particles should not be used (13,14). From experimental and clinical reports, it has been suggested that tris-acryl microspheres larger than 500 μm are the best compromise between safety and efficacy (Figs. 9-10 and 9-11) (13,14,48). Because PVA spheres are more compressible than tris-acryl spheres, the level of arterial occlusion seems to be more distal. Therefore, the use of 700- to 900-μm PVA spheres is currently recommended for fibroid embolization (54). Conversely, because of a more proximal occlusion than with microspheres, nonspherical PVA particles larger than 355 to 500 μm can be used (2–4,11,17). The use of 150- to 250-μm nonspherical PVA particles promoted in the initial studies has been abandoned because of increased complication rates (1,5,11). In addition, because of the different mechanism of occlusion of nonspherical particles, the angiographic endpoint should be different (4,5,13,14,23).

ANGIOGRAPHIC ENDPOINT FOR UTERINE FIBROID EMBOLIZATION

Complete occlusion of the uterine artery with stasis of contrast material is the usual angiographic endpoint when nonspherical PVA particles are injected (2,3,5,11). Embolization is stopped when a standing column of contrast is present in the uterine artery or when reflux of contrast toward the uterine artery origin or into the hypogastric artery is observed (Fig. 9-12).

Recently, the use of a different angiographic endpoint when microspheres are used has been investigated (13,14,53). Because the target of embolization is the perifibroid arterial plexus, the main uterine artery should be spared (13,14,27,53). Limited embolization of the uterine arteries should be performed to reduce ischemic injury to normal myometrium/endometrium due to complete occlusion of collateral flow (Fig. 9-13). Becoming comfortable with this angiographic endpoint may require the experience of several cases (57). Different reliable angiographic criteria have been developed to indicate that the embolization is sufficient (14,23). The curvilinear enlarged arteries of the perifibroid plexus should be occluded (14,23). Typically, a "pruned tree" appearance is seen on the final angiogram, with the proximal portion of the primary trunks still patent and all distal portions occluded (Fig. 9-13). This endpoint usually coincides with sluggish forward flow remaining in the main uterine artery (23). To help identify the endpoint, the rule of thumb popularized by Shlansky-Goldberg can be used. A small amount of contrast material injected in the main uterine artery should move slowly forward and remain visible for five heartbeats before disappearing into distal

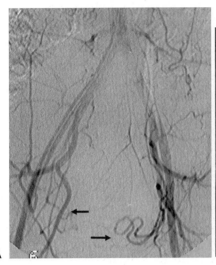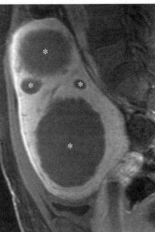

A

B

FIGURE 9-13. A 45-year-old woman with multiple intramural uterine fibroids. **A:** Flush pelvic aortogram obtained after limited embolization of both uterine arteries using a total of 8 ml of 500- to 700-µm tris-acryl microspheres (late arterial phase). No vascularization to the fibroids is visible, whereas both proximal portions of the uterine arteries are patent *(arrows)*. **B:** Dynamic T1-weighted sagittal image after gadolinium injection obtained 24 hours after embolization shows normal myometrial perfusion and complete devascularization of all the fibroids.

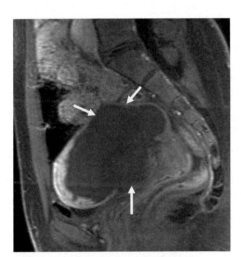

FIGURE 9-14. A 44-year-old woman with uterine fibroids. Dynamic T1-weighted sagittal image after gadolinium injection performed 24 hours after embolization because of intractable postprocedural pain. Embolization to stasis using nonspherical PVA particles was performed. Areas of myometrial devascularization are identified *(arrows)*, and only the fundal region is normally perfused.

branches. Secondary signs of embolization completion include flow redistribution with identification of normal myometrial branches, easy reflux into the ovarian artery when it had not been present earlier, and filling of cross-uterine branches.

Many of the early studies were based on the use of nonspherical PVA particles with stasis of uterine flow (2,3,5,11). Although the reported risk of uterine necrosis is far less than 1%, steps such as avoiding complete stasis during embolization may help reduce this risk even more. In addition, postprocedure pain is related not only to fibroid infarction but also to myometrial ischemia (Fig. 9-14) (14,25).

Even if clinical results with the use of calibrated microspheres are good, it is not clear how frequently the

fibroids are completely infarcted and if the risks of uterine ischemic injury are significantly reduced (14,55,56). Embolization of both uterine arteries to stasis with calibrated microspheres may result in severe myometrial injury (57). However, preliminary results using large calibrated microspheres and incomplete embolization of the uterine arteries demonstrate similar clinical success rates (13,14,49,53). Larger studies are needed to confirm the value of this alternative strategy.

OVARIAN PROTECTION DURING UTERINE ARTERY EMBOLIZATION

It appears likely that embolic particles entering the ovaries during uterine artery embolization may account for premature ovarian failure (11,48,58,59). The collateral vessel from the uterine artery to the ovary usually arises from the mid to distal portion of the ascending segment of the uterine artery (18,60,61). The diameter of the uteroovarian anastomosis is smaller than 500 µm in most cases (14). Therefore, it has been suggested that use of spherical particles larger than the anastomosis may be sufficient to protect the ovary (14). When a large uteroovarian anastomosis is identified, the particles should be upsized in order to avoid nontarget embolization. Another option to protect the ovary is to embolize with the catheter tip placed distal to the anastomosis, although this is not commonly feasible. An alternative is to perform microcoil embolization of the anastomosis, which may protect the ovary during uterine artery embolization (Fig. 9-15) (61,62). One important consideration is the direction of flow in the tuboovarian anastomosis. If it is enlarged because of ovarian inflow to supply fibroids, then it may be visualized during initial arteriography, but during careful embolization the anastomosis may not be visualized because the flow is from

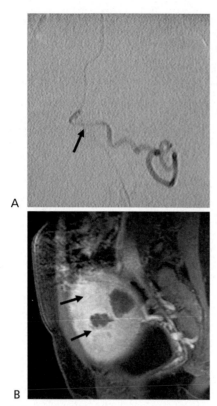

FIGURE 9-15. A 39-year-old woman with three intramural uterine fibroids who presented with menorrhagia. **A:** Digital subtraction angiogram of selective injection into the right uterine artery shows proximal spasm *(arrow)* despite the use of a microcatheter. **B:** Dynamic T1-weighted sagittal image after gadolinium injection performed 3 months after embolization shows persistent perfusion of two fibroids *(arrowheads)*. The patient reported no clinical improvement after embolization.

the ovary to the uterus rather than the opposite direction. This is discussed in greater detail in the chapter on pitfalls (Chapter 10).

SECONDARY EMBOLIZATION AGENTS

In initial reports of uterine fibroid embolization, injection of PVA particles was followed by injection of gelatin sponge pledgets to ensure durable occlusion of the uterine artery (1,5). Other interventional radiologists used supplemental metal coils to reach the angiographic endpoint (stasis or near stasis) (Fig. 9-16) (11,17). The use of secondary embolization agents is still a source of debate. Similar clinical results have been reported using PVA particles only. Most groups are not currently using any type of secondary embolization agent (4,10). Use of coils increases the cost of the procedure and may prevent reembolization at a later date (7,11).

OVARIAN ARTERY EMBOLIZATION

Uterine fibroids derive their main peripheral blood supply almost exclusively from the uterine arteries (5,7,25,63,64). However, the presence of residual fibroid blood supply from the ovarian artery has been reported as the potential cause of failure of uterine artery embolization (18,65,66). The assessment and significance of ovarian flow are covered in detail in the chapter on pitfalls during embolization. Only the technique of embolization will be discussed here.

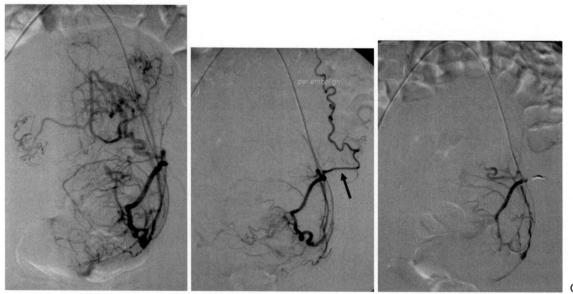

FIGURE 9-16. A 31-year-old woman with multiple uterine fibroids. **A:** Preembolization digital subtraction angiogram of selective injection into the left uterine artery shows diffuse uterine hypervascularization consistent with multiple fibroids. **B:** Preembolization digital subtraction angiogram of selective injection into the left uterine artery shows a large collateral vessel to the left ovary *(arrow)* arising from the distal ascending portion of the left uterine artery, while some fibroid branches are still patent. **C:** After coil embolization (2-mm × 3-mm coil) of the left uteroovarian anastomosis, reduced flow to the ovary is seen. With the ovary protected, uterine artery embolization was completed using 500- to 700-μm tris-acryl microspheres.

In the past decades, superselective catheterization of the ovarian arteries was used for angiographic diagnosis of malignant or benign adnexal tumors (67). Significant ovarian artery supply to the fibroids is easily identified on a preembolization or postembolization pelvic aortogram (68,69). Then, superselective catheterization of the origin of the ovarian artery can be successfully performed using a 4-French cobra-shaped catheter. A reverse curve given to the 4-French catheter after forming a Waltman loop allows easier catheterization of the ovarian artery (69). A Simmons 2 catheter or a Mickaelsson catheter is also helpful. After catheterization using the 4- or 5-French catheter, a microcatheter can be used to perform a more stable embolization (Fig. 9-17). Embolization from the origin with the 4- or 5-French catheter is ill advised because there is a significant chance of misembolization down the aorta. Because of the tortuosity of the vessel and the high incidence of vasospasm, it is usually difficult to catheterize the distal segment of the ovarian artery. If distal catheterization of the ovarian artery is achieved, injection of embolization particles downstream from the ovary can be performed (68,69). Otherwise, free-flow embolization of the fibroids can be performed successfully with the tip of the catheter positioned 3 to 4 cm from the origin of the ovarian artery.

Particulate embolization agents (nonspherical PVA particles, tris-acryl microspheres) have been used in most reported ovarian embolization cases (69,70). When high flow to the fibroids is demonstrated, the particles will be carried beyond the ovary. Nonspherical PVA particles larger than 355 μm and tris-acryl microspheres larger than 500 μm have been chosen (69,70). Others have used coils or gelatin sponge pledgets embolizing more proximally (71,72). Limited ovarian artery embolization leaving some sluggish forward flow at the end of embolization should be performed with particles (Fig. 9-18) (69,70).

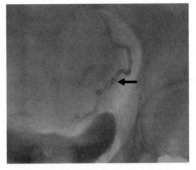

FIGURE 9-17. A 42-year-old woman with multiple uterine fibroids. Digital subtraction angiogram of selective injection into the left uterine artery performed after embolization using 355- to 500-μm nonspherical PVA particles and two 3-mm coils shows complete arterial occlusion *(arrow)*.

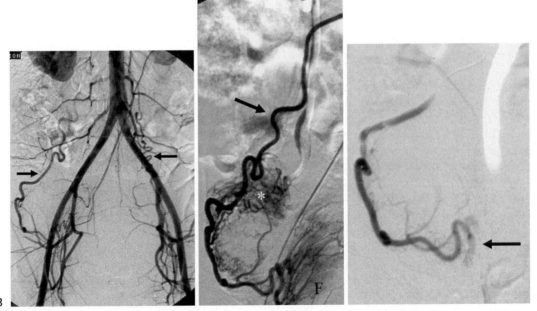

A, B   F   C

FIGURE 9-18. A 41-year-old para 2 gravida 4 woman with multiple uterine fibroids. **A:** Flush aortogram demonstrates a large right ovarian artery and a thin left ovarian artery, both originating below the renal arteries *(arrows)*. **B:** Digital subtraction angiogram of selective injection into the right ovarian artery using a 5-French Simmons 2-type catheter confirms that the fibroids *(F)* are supplied by the right ovarian artery *(arrow)*. The ovary is well identified *(star)*. **C:** Superselective embolization is performed using a small amount of 355- to 500-μm nonspherical PVA particles in order to obtain fibroid devascularization. Note that the main ovarian artery is patent after embolization *(arrow)*.

FERTILITY AND EMBOLIZATION AGENTS

Several pregnancies have been reported after uterine artery embolization with gelatin sponge in women treated for severe postpartum hemorrhage (49). Reports describing pregnancy after uterine fibroid embolization with PVA particles or calibrated microspheres have accumulated slowly, mainly because embolization was offered to women who had already accomplished their childbearing (5,11,14,73,74). Because of the complications associated with uterine fibroid embolization using nonspherical PVA particles (i.e., emergent infection leading to hysterectomy, ovarian failure, chronic vaginal discharge), it has been stated that gelatin sponge could be an alternative agent (42,43). However, there are insufficient data available to advocate the use of gelatin sponge in young patients desiring to preserve fertility options (42). In addition, long-term arterial occlusion has been reported even when embolization had been performed with gelatin sponge pledgets (26).

RADIATION EXPOSURE

Fluoroscopy time during embolization should be kept at a low level because the ovaries are in the fluoroscopic field during the procedure. The difficult procedure may rapidly increase radiation dose, and it is important to recognize those circumstances where success is unlikely. A bilateral femoral approach with simultaneous embolization of both uterine arteries may be useful in order to decrease the amount of radiation exposure (21). Catheterization from the contralateral side using a cross-over technique is usually easier, and once the two catheters are in place, simultaneous injection of both uterine arteries is performed before and after embolization. This effectively reduces the number of angiographic images by 50% (75,76). In addition, the fluoroscopy time is dramatically reduced because simultaneous embolization of both uterine arteries is performed. It is important to keep the fluoroscopy time to a minimal level because the majority of the absorbed ovarian dose during the procedure is related to fluoroscopy (75–77). The average fluoroscopy time when the unilateral approach is used ranges from 18.9 to 30.6 minutes (17,77,78). A significant decrease in fluoroscopy time is noted with increased experience (11,17,78). In our practice, we use the two-catheter technique only in young women seeking to conceive after embolization (Fig. 9-3). With the unilateral approach, coning carefully, minimizing the distance between the patient and image intensifier, embolizing in the anteroposterior projection, and using low-dose or pulsed fluoroscopy can reduce radiation exposure (75,76,78). With pulsed fluoroscopy, a rate of no more than 15 pulses per second should be used, but even rates of 7.5 pulses per second are acceptable for uterine fibroid embolization. Even

if road-mapping technique allows easier catheterization of the uterine artery, its use may convert the fluoroscopy to continuous mode with many systems (76).

It is clear that, with experience, the potential risk of radiation exposure to this patient population can be reduced to the point where it should no longer be of concern to any patient. However, patients actively seeking to become pregnant should not engage in unprotected intercourse during the menstrual cycles prior to the procedure in order to reduce the incidence of radiation-induced injury to an undetected developing embryo.

CONCLUSION

Although much has already been published on fibroid embolization, there are still many unanswered questions. There is no consensus opinion concerning the choice of embolization agent. Small embolization particles are reported to cause more fibroid shrinkage but may also be associated with an increased risk of complications (e.g., damage to normal myometrium, cervical or ovarian ischemia). Complete occlusion of both uterine arteries with stasis of contrast material may cause more myometrial and ovarian ischemia. Therefore, a more limited devascularization of the perifibroid plexus seems to become an attractive alternative option. These changes have been adopted by most radiologists. Spherical embolization agents now widely available on the market are easy to deliver through microcatheters and allow more targeted tumoral devascularization. Special attention should be paid to the choice of the diameter used for each indication. For uterine fibroid embolization, microspheres larger than 500 μm should be used. Microcatheters may lead to more effective devascularization of all uterine fibroids than large 4- or 5-French catheters because of a reduced incidence of flow-limiting arterial spasm. Radiation exposure should be a priority consideration, particularly in young patients.

REFERENCES

1. Ravina JH, Herbreteau D, Ciraru-Vigneron N, et al. Arterial embolization to treat uterine myomata. *Lancet* 1995;346: 671–672.
2. Goodwin SC, Vedantham S, McLucas B, et al. Preliminary experience with uterine artery embolization for uterine fibroids. *J Vasc Interv Radiol* 1997;8:517–526.
3. Worthington-Kirsch RL, Popky GL, Hutchins FL. Uterine arterial embolization for the management of leiomyomas: quality-of-life assessment and clinical response. *Radiology* 1998; 208:625–629.
4. Spies JB, Scialli AR, Jha RC, et al. Initial results from uterine fibroid embolization for symptomatic leiomyomata. *J Vasc Interv Radiol* 1999;10:1149–1157.

5. Pelage JP, Le Dref O, Soyer P, et al. Fibroid-related menorrhagia: treatment with superselective embolization of the uterine arteries and mid-term follow-up. *Radiology* 2000;215:428–431.

6. Worthington-Kirsch RL, Andrews RT, Siskin GP, et al. Uterine fibroid embolization: technical aspects. *Tech Vasc Interv Radiol* 2002;5:17–34.

7. Walker WJ, Sutton C, Pelage JP. Fibroid embolisation [Review]. *Clin Radiol* 2002;57:325–331.

8. Pelage JP, Soyer P, Le Dref O, et al. Uterine arteries: bilateral catheterization using a single femoral approach and a single 5-French catheter. *Radiology* 1999;210:573–575.

9. Hutchins FL, Worthington-Kirsch R, Berkowitz RP. Selective uterine artery embolization as primary treatment for symptomatic leiomyomata uteri. *J Am Assoc Gynecol Laparosc* 1999;6:279–84.

10. Goodwin SC, Mc Lucas B, Lee M, et al. Uterine artery embolization for the treatment of uterine leiomyomata: mid-term results. *J Vasc Interv Radiol* 1999;10:1159–1165.

11. Walker WJ, Pelage JP. Uterine artery embolisation for symptomatic fibroids: clinical results in 400 women with imaging follow up. *Br J Obstet Gynaecol* 2002; 109:1262–1272.

12. Laurent A, Beaujeux R, Wassef M, et al. Trisacryl gelatin microspheres for therapeutic embolization, I: development and in vitro evaluation. *Am J Neuroradiol* 1996;17:533–540.

13. Spies JB, Benenati JE, Worthington-Kirsch RL, et al. Initial experience with the use of trisacryl gelatin microspheres for uterine artery embolization for leiomyomata. *J Vasc Interv Radiol* 2001;12:1059–1063.

14. Pelage JP, Le Dref O, Beregi JP, et al. Limited uterine artery embolization with tris-acryl gelatin microspheres for uterine fibroids. *J Vasc Interv Radiol* 2003;14:15–20.

15. Siskin GP, Dowling K, Virmani R, et al. Pathologic evaluation of a spherical polyvinyl alcohol embolic agent in porcine renal model. *J Vasc Interv Radiol* 2003;14:89–98.

16. Redd D, Chaouk H, Shengelaia G, et al. Comparative study of PVA particles, Embospheres and Gelspheres in a rabbit renal artery embolization model [Abstract]. *J Vasc Interv Radiol* 2002;13:S57.

17. Pron G, Bennett J, Common A, et al. Technical results and effects of operator experience on uterine artery embolization for fibroids: the Ontario uterine fibroid embolization trial. *J Vasc Interv Radiol* 2003;14:545–554.

18. Pelage JP, Le Dref O, Soyer P, et al. Arterial anatomy of the female genital tract: variants and relevance to transcatheter embolization of the uterus. *AJR Am J Roentgenol* 1999;172: 989–994.

19. Waltman AC, Courey WR, Athanasoulis C, et al. Technique for left gastric artery catheterization. *Radiology* 1973;109:732–734.

20. Shlansky-Goldberg R, Cope C. A new twist on the Waltman loop for uterine artery for fibroids. *J Vasc Interv Radiol* 2001; 12:997–1000.

21. Levy EB, Spies JB, Wood BJ, et al. Two-catheter technique for uterine fibroid embolisation. *Min Invas Ther Allied Technol* 1999; 8:411–414.

22. Spies JB, Spector A, Roth AR, et al. Complications of uterine artery embolization for leiomyomata. *Obstet Gynecol* 2002;100: 873–880.

23. Spies JB. Uterine artery embolization for fibroids: understanding the technical causes of failure. *J Vasc Interv Radiol* 2003; 14:11–14.

24. Keyoung JA, Levy EB, Roth AR, et al. Intraarterial lidocaine for pain control after uterine artery embolization for leiomyomata. *J Vasc Interv Radiol* 2001;12:1065–1069.

25. Burbank F, Hutchins FL. Uterine artery occlusion by embolization or surgery for the treatment of fibroids: a unifying hypothesis-transient uterine ischemia. *J Am Assoc Gynecol Laparosc* 1999;7[Suppl]:S1–S49.

26. Siskin GP, Englander M, Stainken BF, et al. Embolic agent used for uterine fibroid embolization. *AJR Am J Roentgenol* 2000;175: 767–773.

27. Godfrey CD, Zbella EA. Uterine necrosis after uterine artery embolization for leiomyoma. *Obstet Gynecol* 2001;98: 950–952.

28. Kerber CW, Bank WO, Horton JA. Polyvinyl alcohol foam: prepackaged emboli for therapeutic embolization. *AJR Am J Roentgenol* 1978;130:1193–1194.

29. Castaneda-Zuniga WR, Sanchez R, Amplatz K. Experimental observations on short and long-term effects of arterial occlusion with Ivalon. *Radiology* 1978;126:783–785.

30. Derdeyn CP, Moran CJ, Cross DT AI, et al. Polyvinyl alcohol particle size and suspension characteristics. *Am J Neuroradiol* 1995;16:1031–1036.

31. Barr JD, Lemley TJ, Petrochko CN. Polyvinyl alcohol foam particle sizes and concentrations injectable through microcatheters. *J Vasc Interv Radiol* 1998;9:113–118.

32. Repa I, Moradian GP, Dehrer LP, et al. Mortalities associated with use of a commercial suspension of polyvinyl alcohol. *Radiology* 1989;170:395–399.

33. Kardache M, Soyer P, Le Dref O, et al. Uterine leiomyoma: histopathological features after superselective transcatheter embolization of the uterine arteries [Abstract]. *AJR Am J Roentgenol* 1998;170[Suppl]:40.

34. Nicholson TA, Pelage JP, Ettles DF. Fibroid calcification after uterine artery embolization: ultrasonographic appearance and pathology. *J Vasc Interv Radiol* 2001;12:443–446.

35. McCluggage WJ, Ellis PK, McClure N, et al. Pathologic features of uterine leiomyomas following uterine artery embolization. *Int J Gynecol Pathol* 2000;19:342–347.

36. Goodwin SC, Lai AC. Uterine embolization technique [Abstract]. *J Vasc Interv Radiol* 2000;11:26–32.

37. Subramanian S, Spies JB. Uterine artery embolization for leiomyomata: resource use and cost estimation. *J Vasc Interv Radiol* 2001;12:571–574.

38. Brown BJ, Heaston DK, Poulson AM, et al. Uncontrollable postpartum bleeding: a new approach to hemostasis through angiographic arterial embolization. *Obstet Gynecol* 1979;54: 361–365.

39. Stancato-Pasik A, Mitty H, Richard HM III, et al. Obstetric embolotherapy: effects on menses and pregnancy. *Radiology* 1997;204:791–793.

40. Greenwood LH, Glickman MG, Schwartz PE, et al. Obstetric and nonmalignant gynecologic bleeding: treatment with angiographic embolization. *Radiology* 1987;164:155–159.

41. Gold RE, Grace DM. Gelfoam embolization of the left gastric artery for bleeding ulcer: experimental considerations. *Radiology* 1975;116:563–567.

42. Stancato-Pasik A, Katz R, Mitty HA, et al. Uterine artery embolisation of myomas: preliminary results of gelatin sponge pledgets as the embolic agent. *Min Invas Ther Allied Technol* 1999;8:393–396.

43. Rana T. Uterine artery embolisation for symptomatic fibroids: experience of a cost effective approach in a developing country using Gelfoam only [Abstract]. *J Vasc Interv Radiol* 2001;12:S17.

44. Katsumori T, Nakajima K, Mihara T, et al. Uterine artery embolization using gelatin sponge particles alone for symptomatic uterine fibroids: midterm results. *AJR Am J Roentgenol* 2002;178:135–139.

45. Beaujeux R, Laurent A, Wassef M, et al. Trisacryl gelatin microspheres for therapeutic embolization, II: clinical evaluation in tumors and arteriovenous malformations. *Am J Neuroradiol* 1996;17:541–548.

46. Derdeyn CP, Graves VB, Salamat MS, et al. Collagen-coated acrylic microspheres for embolotherapy: in vivo and in vitro characteristics. *Am J Neuroradiol* 1997;18:647–653.

47. Bendszus M, Klein R, Burger R, et al. Efficacy of trisacryl gelatin microspheres and polyvinyl alcohol particles in the preoperative embolization of meningiomas. *Am J Neuroradiol* 2000;21:255–261.

48. Pelage JP, Laurent A, Wassef M, et al. Acute effects of uterine artery embolization in the sheep: comparison between polyvinyl alcohol particles and calibrated microspheres. *Radiology* 2002; 224:436–445.

49. Joffre F, Tubiana JM, Pelage JP, and the FEMIC group. FEMIC Fibromes Embolisés aux Microsphères calibrées. Uterine fibroid embolization using tris-acryl microspheres: a French multicentric study. *Cardiovasc Interv Radiol* 2004 *(in press)*.

50. Andrews TA, Binkert CA. Relative rates of blood flow reduction during transcatheter arterial embolization with tris-acryl gelatin microspheres or polyvinyl alcohol: quantitative comparison in a swine model. *J Vasc Interv Radiol* 2003;14:1311–1316.

51. Pelage JP, Wassef M, Namur J, et al. Uterine artery embolization in sheep using tris-acryl microspheres and non spherical PVA: comparison of pathological findings at 2 years [Abstract]. Presented at the annual meeting of the Radiological Society of North America, Chicago, Illinois, November 30–December 3, 2003.

52. Pelage JP, Ferrand J, Wassef M, et al. Combined embolization and myomectomy for symptomatic uterine fibroids: clinical and pathological aspects [Abstract]. *Radiology* 2001;221[P]:265

53. Lampmann LEH, Smeets AJ, Lohle PNM. Uterine fibroids: targeted embolization, an update on technique. *Abdom Imaging* 2004;29:128–131.

54. Saint-Maurice JP, Wassef M, Namur J, et al. Vascular distribution of two types of microspheres (Embosphere and Contour SE): a comparative study [Abstract]. Presented at the annual meeting of the Cardiovascular and Interventional Radiological Society of Europe, Antalya, Turkey, September 20–24, 2003.

55. Banovac F, Ascher S, Jones DA, et al. Magnetic resonance imaging outcome after uterine artery embolization for leiomyomata with use of tris-acryl gelatin microspheres. *J Vasc Interv Radiol* 2002;13:682–687.

56. Ryu RK, Omary RA, Sichlau MJ, et al. Comparison of pain after uterine artery embolization using tris-acryl gelatin microspheres versus polyvinyl alcohol particles. *Cardiovasc Interv Radiol* 2003;26:375–378.

57. de Blok S, de Vries C, Prinssen HM, et al. Fatal sepsis after uterine artery embolization with microspheres. *J Vasc Interv Radiol* 2003;14:779–783.

58. Payne JF, Robboy SJ, Haney AF. Embolic microspheres within ovarian arterial vasculature after uterine artery embolization. *Obstet Gynecol* 2002;100:883–886.

59. Ryu RK, Chrisman HB, Omary RA, et al. The vascular impact of uterine artery embolization: prospective sonographic assessment of ovarian arterial circulation. *J Vasc Interv Radiol* 2001;9:1071–1074.

60. Razavi MK, Wolanske KA, Hwang GL, et al. Angiographic classification of ovarian artery-to-uterine artery anastomoses: initial observations in uterine fibroid embolization. *Radiology* 2002;224:707–712.

61. Marx M, Wack JP, Baker EL, et al. Ovarian protection by occlusion of uteroovarian collateral vessels before uterine fibroid embolization. *J Vasc Interv Radiol* 2003;14:1329–1332.

62. Wolanske KA, Gordon RL, Wilson MW, et al. Coil embolization of a tuboovarian anastomosis before uterine artery embolization to prevent nontarget particle embolization of the ovary. *J Vasc Interv Radiol* 2003;14:1333–1338.

63. Sampson J. The blood supply of uterine myomata. *Surg Gynecol Obstet* 1912;14:215–234.

64. Holmgren B. Some observations on the blood vessels of the uterus under normal conditions and in myoma. *Acta Obstet Gynecol Scand* 1938;18:192–213.

65. Nikolic B, Spies JB, Abbara S, et al. Ovarian artery supply of uterine fibroids as a cause of treatment failure after uterine artery embolization. *J Vasc Interv Radiol* 1999;10:1167–1170.

66. Matson M, Nicholson A, Belli AM. Anastomoses of the ovarian and uterine arteries: a potential pitfall and cause of failure of uterine embolization. *Cardiovasc Interv Radiol* 2001;23: 393–396.

67. Frates RE. Selective angiography of the ovarian artery. *Radiology* 1969;92:1014–1019.

68. Binkert CA, Andrews RT, Kaufman JA. Utility of non selective abdominal aortography in demonstrating ovarian artery collaterals in patients undergoing uterine artery embolization for fibroids. *J Vasc Interv Radiol* 2001;12:841–845.

69. Pelage JP, Walker WJ, Le Dref O, et al. Ovarian artery: angiographic appearance, embolization and relevance to uterine fibroid embolization. *Cardiovasc Interv Radiol* 2003;26:227–233.

70. Barth MM, Spies JB. Ovarian artery embolization supplementing uterine embolization for leiomyomata. *J Vasc Interv Radiol* 2003;14:1177–1182.

71. Pelage JP, Le Dref O, Jacob D, et al. Ovarian artery supply of uterine fibroid [Letter]. *J Vasc Interv Radiol* 2000;11:535.

72. Andersen PE, Lund N, Justesen P, et al. Uterine artery embolization of symptomatic uterine fibroids. Initial success and short-term results. *Acta Radiol* 2001;42:234–238.

73. Ravina JH, Ciraru-Vigneron N, Aymard A, et al. Pregnancy after embolization of uterine myoma: report of 12 cases. *Fertil Steril* 2000;73:1241–1243.

74. McLucas B, Goodwin S, Adler L, et al. Pregnancy following uterine fibroid embolization. *Int J Gynaecol Obstet* 2001; 74:1–7.

75. Nikolic B, Abbara S, Levy E, et al. Influence of radiographic technique and equipment on absorbed ovarian dose associated with uterine artery embolization. *J Vasc Interv Radiol* 2000;11: 1173–1178.

76. Nikolic B, Spies JB, Campbell L, et al. Uterine artery embolization: reduced radiation with refined technique. *J Vasc Interv Radiol* 2001;12:39–44.

77. Nikolic B, Spies JB, Lundsten MJ, et al. Patient radiation dose associated with uterine artery embolization. *Radiology* 2000;214: 121–125.

78. Andrews RT, Brown PH. Uterine arterial embolization: factors influencing patient radiation exposure. *Radiology* 2000;217: 713–722.

10

THE PITFALLS OF UTERINE EMBOLIZATION: AVOIDING THE FAILED PROCEDURE

JAMES B. SPIES

INTRODUCTION

With several years of experience with uterine embolization, sufficient data are now available to allow some perspective on the outcome of this procedure. One thing we have learned is that not every patient improves after treatment: if 90% of patients are symptomatically improved, then 10% are not. The reasons for these failures are becoming clearer as research advances. The causes of gynecologic symptoms are myriad and may be unrelated to fibroids that may be present. As discussed in the chapter on patient selection (Chapter 7), it is important to be certain that a patient's symptoms are due to (or at least likely due to) fibroids.

Even in the presence of symptoms caused by fibroids, the procedure may fail to control them. The subject of this chapter is how to optimize the outcome from embolization. Before we can consider the potential causes of a failed procedure, we need to define failure.

DEFINING FAILURE

From a technical perspective, failure is when the fibroids do not infarct after the embolization. The goal of embolization is to cause ischemic infarction of the fibroids, which, from both a pathologic (1,2) and an imaging perspective (3,4), is what occurs after a successful embolization.

Beyond a short-term improvement in symptoms, the acceptance of this procedure depends on the durability of symptom control. This must be understood in the context of other uterine-sparing therapies, such as myomectomy.

Most uterine fibroid embolization series indicate that 80% to 95% of patients will have symptomatic improvement in the short term (5–8), but the real question is how long the symptom improvements will last. Durability depends on completely treating the fibroids that are present at the time of embolization. Even in instances when uterine volume decreases and the fibroids shrink, recurrence can be predicted when other substantial fibroids do not infarct, as the residual viable tissue is likely to regrow (Figs. 10-1 and 10-2) (9). Although it is likely that some patients will develop new fibroids over time, this is presently beyond the control of uterine embolization.

Finally, there are two uterine comorbidities that may adversely affect outcome that require specific attention. These are adenomyosis (10) and leiomyosarcoma (11) and are discussed at the end of this chapter.

UNDERSTANDING THE CAUSES OF FAILURE

There are several potential causes of failure, and we will consider each in turn. These potential causes are failure to catheterize the uterine artery, false endpoint leading to underembolization, spasm resulting in underembolization, supplemental blood supply to the fibroids from the ovarian arteries, and the uterine comorbidities adenomyosis and leiomyosarcoma.

Failed Catheterization of the Uterine Artery

For nearly all patients, bilateral embolization is necessary for the procedure to succeed. In most operators' experience, fibroids usually derive a portion of their vascular supply from both uterine arteries. If only one artery is embolized, it is likely that at least a portion of the fibroids will not infarct. Rarely, all of the apparent blood supply to the fibroids will be from one side (Fig. 10-3). In this case, a unilateral embolization is all that is necessary, but there has been no study published to corroborate this opinion.

Based on the preceding discussion, an obvious cause of a technical failure is the failure to catheterize the uterine artery, either on one or both sides. With experience, this type of catheterization failure is very unusual, occurring in about 1% of the patients (8,12,13). However, failures will occur early in the experience of most physicians. Emboliza-

FIGURE 10-1. Fibroids completely treated after uterine embolization. **A:** Sagittal contrast enhanced magnetic resonance image of a multifibroid uterus demonstrating numerous enhancing fibroids. **B:** Three months after embolization, all of the visible fibroids are infarcted and are shrinking in volume. **C:** One year after embolization, there is continued reduction in the fibroids. **D:** Three years after embolization, the fibroids continue to reduce in size, and there has been no regrowth of fibroid tissue.

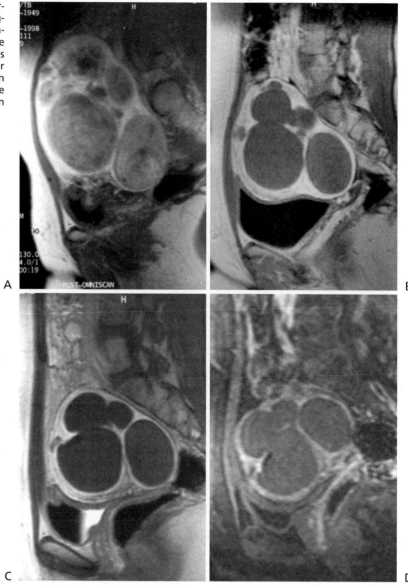

tion should not be performed unless the uterine artery has been selectively catheterized and test injections ensure that embolization can proceed without reflux into other branches. A failure is better than a complication from misembolization. Techniques to avoid a failed catheterization are provided in Chapter 9.

Beyond the technical failure to catheterize a uterine artery that is present, the artery may, in fact, be absent on one or both sides. In a patient who has undergone a previous myomectomy, this condition may be iatrogenic, the opposite uterine artery may provide all of the supply to the uterus, and unilateral embolization may be effective. However, there may also be ovarian flow, and these arteries should be surveyed routinely to detect additional collateral flow. In almost all cases, absence of the uterine artery indicates replacement of that flow by the ipsilateral ovarian

artery or the opposite uterine artery (Fig. 10-4). We have also seen one patient in whom the uterine artery was replaced by the round ligament artery, which arose from the inferior epigastric artery (Fig. 10-5) (14). There may also be rare cases of multiple uterine arteries, none of which may be large enough to cannulate and thus allow embolization. The variations in ovarian flow are discussed in detail in the following.

False Endpoint

Contrary to early thought about uterine embolization, there are nuances to the technique of embolization that have real consequences to the outcome of the procedure. Both underembolization and overembolization can occur, with the consequence of a failure of the procedure in the former

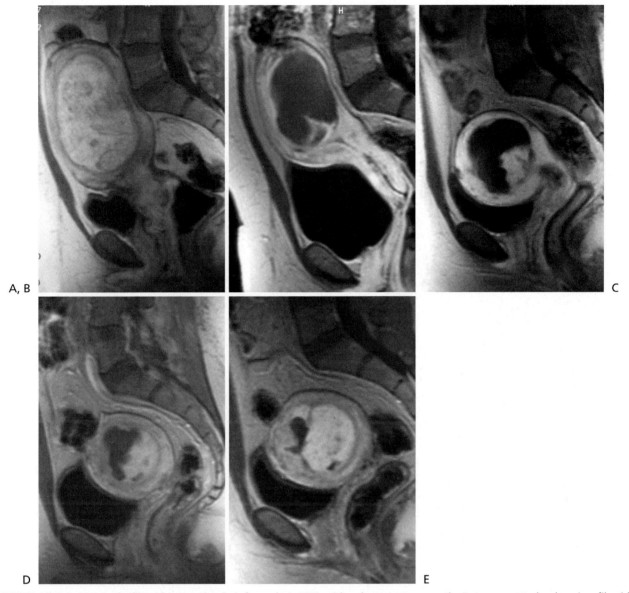

FIGURE 10-2. Large single fibroid incompletely infarcted on MRI, with subsequent regrowth. **A:** Large central enhancing fibroid on contrast-enhanced sagittal MRI. **B:** Three months after embolization, nearly 90% of the fibroid is completely avascular, with only a wedge of residual enhancement at the base of the tumor. There has been substantial reduction in fibroid volume. **C:** One year after embolization, there has been a dramatic reduction in fibroid volume, but there is some increase in the size of the enhancing portion. **D:** Two years after treatment, there is continued reduction in overall fibroid size but an increase in the degree of enhancement. **E:** Three years after embolization, there is near complete revascularization of the fibroid, and the patient has recurrent symptoms. She went on to have a hysterectomy. It is interesting to note that the size of the fibroid is smaller on each succeeding image, but symptom recurrence appears tied not to fibroid size but to the extent of viable tissue.

or a complication in the latter. For these reasons, careful attention to the details of the procedure is important for all practitioners.

Although there may be some variation in the flow dynamics of the different embolic materials currently in use, in our experience they all can clump in the uterine artery. It appears that this clumping is related to the rate at which the embolic agent is injected and is more likely to occur with rapid injection. This can be confirmed by waiting a few minutes after the apparent conclusion of embolization and retesting the endpoint with an additional injection of contrast. Commonly, we have seen reacceleration of flow in the vessel with partial restoration of flow to the fibroids. This appears to be less common with slower injection of embolic agent and with a greater dilution of the embolic. Each allows the material to flow further before lodging in an occlusive position. The theoretical goal is to have embolic particles line up singly in the fibroid arteries and occlude the branches completely. This should provide a more stable occlusion than a clump located more proximally, which

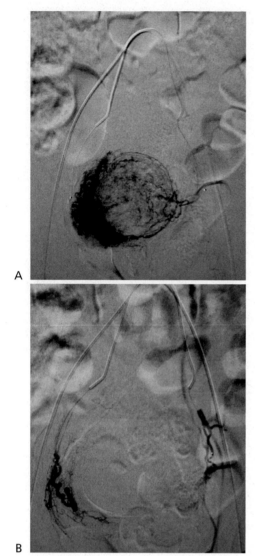

FIGURE 10-3. Unilateral uterine supply to single intramural and submucosal fibroid. **A:** Bilateral simultaneous injections of the uterine arteries reveal that all of the blood supply to the fibroid arises from left uterine branches. This is confirmed on several images from the angiographic series. **B:** Postembolization of the left side only, with no residual fibroid flow identified.

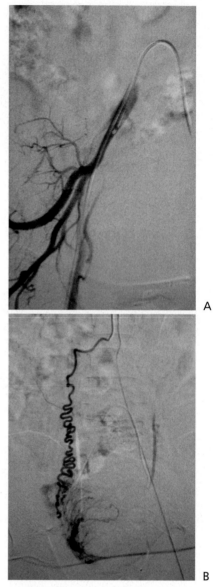

FIGURE 10-4. Uterine artery replaced by ovarian artery. **A:** Right hypogastric arteriogram fails to reveal a uterine artery. **B:** Right ovarian arteriogram in the same patient shows the entire right uterine blood supply arising from the ovarian artery.

may redistribute more distally in the first minutes to hours after the procedure is complete.

Uterine Artery Spasm

Spasm in the uterine artery may contribute to the phenomenon of a false endpoint, with apparent occlusion being relieved by resolution of spasm within minutes or hours after catheter removal. For this reason, in recent years we have become much more attentive to the presence of spasm.

Our attention was first focused on this issue because of an unexpected observation during a randomized study evaluating the use of intraarterial lidocaine as a means of reducing

the pain associated with uterine embolization (15). This was a double-blind, placebo-controlled study that involved injecting either lidocaine or saline solution. Initially planned for 50 patients, we noted that a high percentage of patients appeared to develop severe uterine arterial spasm after injection of the test material. The spasm was severe and often took 10 to 15 minutes or longer to resolve sufficiently to allow embolization. In all cases, embolization was completed in what we believed at the time to be a satisfactory manner. With such a high frequency of spasm, we stopped the study early and learned that of the nine patients treated with lidocaine, seven developed significant spasm. Among this group, at least three patients had incomplete infarction of the fibroids based on assessment of

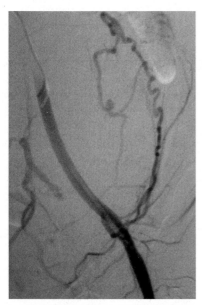

FIGURE 10-5. Absent left uterine artery replaced by round ligament artery. Injection of contrast into the left inferior epigastric artery, which supplies a markedly enlarged round ligament artery, supplying the left half of the uterus.

contrast-enhanced MRI studies 3 months later. One patient underwent attempted repeat embolization, during which both uterine arteries were found to be occluded completely. The ovarian arteries had taken over supply of the uterus and fibroids. Because of the potential risk of ovarian injury if ovary artery embolization were undertaken, the patient elected to have a simple hysterectomy. In this case, it appeared as if the only reasonable explanation for the failed procedure was spasm of the uterine arteries. The embolic material did not migrate into the fibroid branches but instead occluded the uterine arteries, apparently proximal to the ovarian anastomoses. The patient had only minimally enlarged ovarian arteries at the time of initial embolization, but at the repeat procedure, the ovarian arteries had enlarged significantly to provide the fibroid flow.

We have subsequently graded and recorded the severity of spasm in both uterine arteries in more than 300 patients and have other cases in which the presence of severe spasm corresponds with failure of some of the ipsilateral fibroids to infarct, in the absence of other apparent causes.

Although we have not completed a formal analysis of the data set, we have taken away two lessons from this experience. One, intraarterial lidocaine should not be used in uterine embolization. Second, where possible, spasm should be avoided to try to optimize the effectiveness of embolization.

Early in our experience, we routinely used a 4- or 5-French nonbraided hydrophilic catheter for nearly all embolizations. Only in those cases with severe spasm with stasis did we consider using a microcatheter (16). Other early investigators used a similar method, although they used braided standard angiographic catheters (17,18). With

growing experience with this procedure, we now routinely use a coaxial microcatheter. In the past, we placed a 5-French guiding catheter into the origin of the uterine artery and then through the catheter advanced the microcatheter farther into the vessel. Even this seemed to cause unnecessary spasm in some cases, so at this time we most commonly leave the 5-French outer catheter in the hypogastric trunk and use a microwire and microcatheter to enter the uterine artery. The uterine arteries are commonly tortuous, and the farther the microcatheter is advanced into the vessel, the more likely spasm is to occur. Therefore, we limit the distance that the catheter is advanced to the proximal portion of the uterine artery prior to any severe angles that may be present. On the other hand, it is important that the catheter be well within the vessel to prevent inadvertent reflux of embolic material back out the vessel origin. Ideally, several centimeters of vessel should be catheterized. If this results in spasm, we gently retract the microcatheter, which reduces the angular distortion of the vessel and often helps relieve the spasm. However, one of the most common causes of spasm we have encountered is a severe kink or loop in the uterine artery near its origin. This type of arterial angle can cause nearly flow-stopping spasm and can be difficult to relieve.

One issue that has been of concern to some is performing embolization with the tip of the catheter proximal to the cervicovaginal branch, because of potential concerns regarding sexual function after embolization. Such problems have been very rare, and spasm is frequently caused by the attempt to advance a catheter beyond it. Therefore, we would position the catheter beyond the cervicovaginal branch only if it can be done without significant spasm.

We have used both intraarterial nitroglycerin (in 100- to 200-μg aliquots) and, on occasion, tolazoline (Priscoline; 25 to 50 mg diluted in 10 mL of saline) delivered slowly through the catheter. We have had mixed results with both. Part of the problem may be that the spasm occurs as a result of the catheter irritating the proximal descending portion of the vessel. When intraarterial medications are given, they are delivered distal to the site of the actual spasm. In recent years, we have learned that slowly retracting the microcatheter while injecting contrast often reveals a kink in the proximal few centimeters of the vessel, and that the spasm resolves once the catheter is above that level. If the catheter is in the uterine artery a sufficient distance to prevent reflux and possible misembolization, then the procedure can proceed. Some operators have suggested that systemic vasodilators, such as nifedipine, might be useful in preventing or treating uterine artery spasm. Although it has a theoretical basis, to our knowledge its use has not been evaluated in a clinical study.

Ovarian Artery Supply to Fibroids

Even in the presence of two apparently normal uterine arteries, additional supply to the fibroids may come from

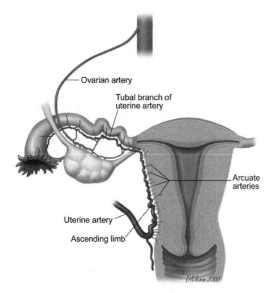

FIGURE 10-6. Normal uterine and ovarian arterial anatomy. In the normal relationship of uterine and ovarian artery flow in a patient without fibroids, the uterus derives its flow from the uterine arteries, while its terminal tubal branch anastomoses with the ovarian artery.

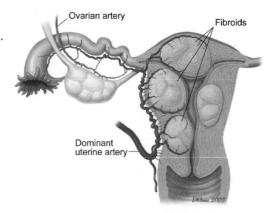

FIGURE 10-7. Uterine and ovarian flow in a patient with fibroids. In most cases, the uterine artery alone enlarges to supply the fibroids, without significant contribution from the ovarian arteries.

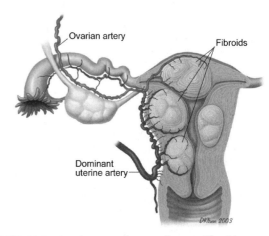

FIGURE 10-8. Ovarian contributory flow to fibroids. In a small minority of cases, likely less than 15%, uterine artery flow to fibroids is supplemented by additional recruited flow from the ovarian artery. In many cases, this type of arterial supply can be treated during the uterine embolization (see text).

the ovarian arteries, which may occur in about 5% to 10% of patients. In a recent study (19), ovarian blood supply to at least the margin of the uterus was discovered at the conclusion of embolization in 14% of patients. Perhaps only half of these had sufficient flow to potentially impact the success of the procedure. The degree of ovarian supply varies, but in our experience, a potential predictor of a failed procedure is the presence of ovarian supply not just to the uterus but also to fibroids or portions of fibroids not supplied by the uterine arteries.

The extent of ovarian artery supply to the fibroids should be assessed by aortogram. This may be done before or after the uterine embolization is completed. The injection is made at the level of the renal arteries to ensure that the ovarian vessels are opacified. They normally arise from the anterior aorta below the renal arteries, although infrequently the ovarian artery arises from an inferior polar branch of the renal artery or an accessory polar branch. Although the presence of enlarged ovarian arteries supplying the uterus may be detected both before and after the embolization, there is an advantage to performing the aortogram after embolization of the uterine arteries is completed. The reasons are as follows.

In the normal case, the ovarian artery communicates with tubal branches of the uterine artery (Fig. 10-6). When fibroids are present, in most cases they are supplied only by the uterine arteries, which enlarge to meet the increased demand for blood flow (Fig. 10-7). The uterine supply to fibroids may be supplemented by flow recruited from the ovarian arteries (contributory flow) (Fig. 10-8). When initial arteriography of the uterine arteries is performed, the presence of contributory flow can occasionally be detected

by reflux into the ovarian arteries, which may show those arteries to be enlarged. Although the contrast will initially reflux into the ovarian arteries, once the uterine injection is stopped but filming is continued, the contrast in the ovarian artery will be seen to flow progressively toward the uterus, showing a backwash of contrast from the unopacified flow from the ovarian artery. If the flow from the ovarian arteries is substantial, it is unlikely that they will be visualized during preembolization angiography. This type of flow may be detected during initial arteriography, with a dilution of the contrast within vessels distal to the ovarian inflow of unopacified blood. During embolization, ovarian inflow can be detected as a speeding and dilution of the contrast-laden embolic mix at the point where the ovarian artery joins the uterine artery. There can even be reversal of flow in the main uterine artery if the ovarian contribution is sufficiently large.

As can be seen in Figure 10-8, contributory flow mixes with uterine flow to feed the fibroids. If recognized, this fact

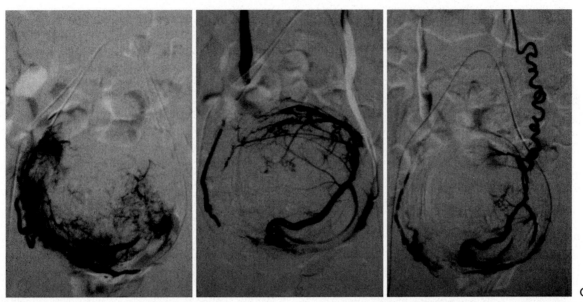

A, B

C

FIGURE 10-9. Competitive contributory ovarian supply. **A:** Initial arteriogram (bilateral injection) showing major defect in perfusion to the left upper portion of the uterus. Serial image revealed slight retrograde flow of contrast in the left ascending uterine artery from ovarian inflow. **B:** After partial embolization, forcible injection reveals branches not previously opacified. They are now visualized as the distal flow to the fibroid has decreased and along with it the inflow from the left ovarian artery. **C:** Final image with minimal filling of fibroid branches and reflux up a substantially enlarged ovarian artery. Selective ovarian arteriogram (not shown) did not show any additional flow to the fibroids and had very sluggish flow.

can be used at the time of embolization. The key is to embolize in a manner that delivers the particles to at least the level of the ovarian inflow so that flow can help carry embolics to the fibroids. What will assure a failed procedure is if the proximal transverse and ascending uterine artery is occluded by embolic material without sufficiently occluding the perifibroid vessels. If the path to those fibroids from the ovarian arteries is not occluded, those fibroids will not infarct. This concept is demonstrated in Figure 10-9.

If contributory flow is treated successfully from the uterine side, then ovarian embolization is not needed. This can be confirmed with an abdominal aortogram obtained after uterine embolization. An enlarged ovarian artery might be seen, but it would have very sluggish flow because the distal outflow to the fibroids will have been successfully occluded from the uterine side.

There are several variations of isolated (noncontributory) ovarian arterial flow to fibroids, ranging from minor flow to complete replacement of the uterine artery by the ovarian artery (Fig. 10-10A–C). As the proportion of fibroid arterial supply from the ovarian arteries increases, so does the likelihood of a failed procedure due to uninfarcted fibroids. Whether failure can be prevented with embolization of the affected ovarian artery in addition to the uterine arteries is not yet certain, although preliminary evidence suggests that ovarian embolization is effective (20). However, the impact on ovarian function of ovarian artery embolization as a supplement to uterine embolization is not known at this time; therefore, the procedure should be approached with caution. Unless the major portion of the uterine artery flow on a given side is replaced by ovarian flow, usually we do not

embolize any ovarian arteries on the day of the initial procedure. If the patient's symptoms do not improve and fibroids in the distribution of the ovarian supply do not infarct, then unilateral and, in some cases, bilateral ovarian embolization may be offered. In patients at or near the age of natural menopause, this may be an acceptable alternative to hysterectomy. In a younger woman interested in maintaining her fertility, other alternatives such as myomectomy may be preferred to the chance of ovarian injury due to embolization of these arteries.

IMPACT OF FIBROID POSITION ON OUTCOME OF EMBOLIZATION

As yet there is no clear evidence on whether fibroid position is a clear predictor of success or failure. Although the rate of fibroid shrinkage after embolization is influenced by the position of the dominant fibroids, this fact does not necessarily correspond to a difference in symptom improvement (21). What can be said is that certain subtypes of fibroids may be less likely to completely infarct after embolization. These include pedunculated serosal fibroids and cervical fibroids. Although no studies have yet documented this clinical opinion, we have observed this phenomenon on a number of occasions. Two potential causes appear to contribute to this tendency: false endpoint and/or collateral sources of blood supply. Small pedunculated serosal fibroids (Fig. 10-11) may have very small vessels supplying them that may be temporarily occluded and reperfuse subsequently. Alternatively, they may be more

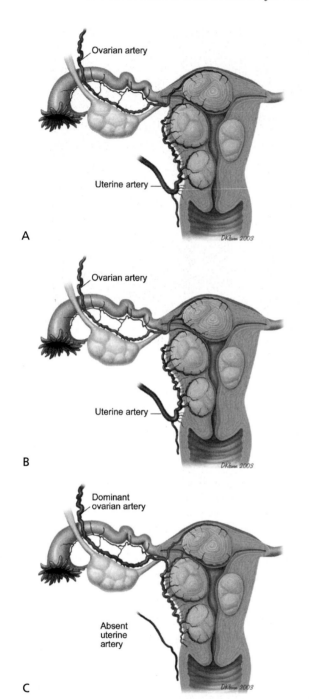

FIGURE 10-10. Variations in isolated fibroid flow from the ovarian artery. There is considerable variability in the extent of additional flow to the fibroids, from marginal **(A)** through moderate **(B)** to complete **(C)** replacement of the uterine artery by the ovarian artery. Whether embolization of the ovarian artery is necessary depends on the degree to which the fibroids depend on that flow (see text).

likely than other types to have collateral sources of blood supply parasitized from nonuterine sources. Similarly, cervical fibroids commonly do not infarct, which may be due to collateral supply. In addition, underembolization may contribute, as shown in Figure 10-12.

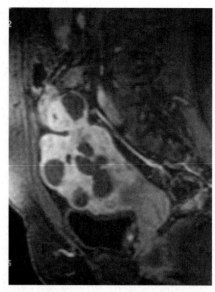

FIGURE 10-11. Incompletely infarcted pedunculated serosal fibroid. A small fibroid at the fundus of the uterus did not completely infarct after embolization, with retention of perfusion in its anterior portion.

UTERINE ARTERY EMBOLIZATION FOR ADENOMYOSIS

It is not yet clear what embolotherapy may have to offer in terms of controlling the symptoms from adenomyosis. There have been some reports of experience with embolization in patients with adenomyosis. Two small studies reported in 2000 demonstrated that in patients with fibroids and adenomyosis, embolization had similar rates of symptomatic improvement. In a small group (N = 13) at Georgetown (22), 92% had symptomatic improvement in both menorrhagia and pelvic pain and pressure at 3 months after treatment. In this series, there was a 52% reduction in fibroid volume and a 39% reduction in uterine volume. There was not a significant change in the internal appearance of the adenomyosis. At Albany Medical School, Siskin (23) treated 14 patients with focal adenomyomas or diffuse adenomyosis. There was symptom improvement in 90% of patients. Regression in uterine volume, focal adenomyoma volume, and thickness of the junctional zone was noted in all cases.

Ahn et al. (24) from Korea presented a much larger series (N = 65) at the Society of Cardiovascular and Interventional Radiology (SCVIR) annual meeting in 2000. Twenty-nine percent of the group had both myomas and adenomyomas, with the remainder having adenomyosis alone. Among all patients, 93.8% reported improvement in symptoms. The authors used varying sizes of polyvinyl alcohol particles and commented that coagulation necrosis only occurred when particles 355 to 500μm or smaller were used. They suggested that this finding is necessary to assure clinical improvement. The group at Georgetown used 500-

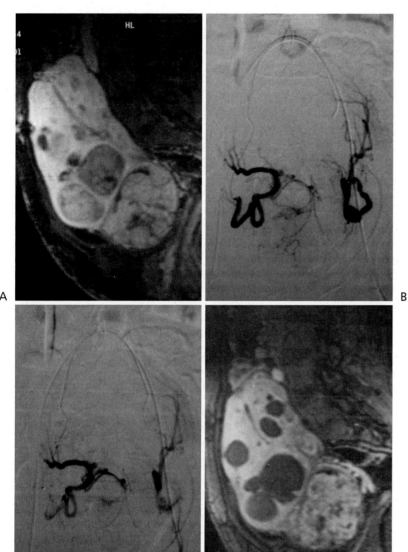

FIGURE 10-12. Cervical fibroid with failure to infarct. **A:** Multifibroid uterus with large cervical fibroids. **B:** Bilateral uterine arteriogram before embolization, with prominent cervical vaginal branch on the right. **C:** After embolization, there was stasis in the cervical vaginal branch, and the distal branches were occluded. **D:** Despite symptom relief and infarction of most of the fibroids, the cervical fibroid did not infarct as noted by magnetic resonance study 3 months later.

to 710-μm particles and did not observe infarction of the adenomyosis, but they noted similar rates of symptomatic improvement. None of the studies have yet documented the long-term outcome.

Although these limited series are encouraging, there have been cases in which the presence of adenomyosis has been implicated as the cause of failure of uterine embolization (10).

Additional study is needed to determine the role that UAE will play in the treatment of adenomyosis, but these initial reports are very encouraging. The optimal method for embolization has yet to be determined, and validated outcome measures have yet to be used in assessing embolotherapy.

LEIOMYOSARCOMA

Leiomyosarcoma deserves special consideration because it is both a cause of failure and a source of considerable morbidity and mortality in patients in whom it is undiagnosed (11). The imaging appearance is described in the imaging chapter (Chapter 5). Detecting those embolization patients in whom a leiomyosarcoma may have been treated is a challenge. Many of them will have the typical dramatic improvement in symptoms and initial shrinkage of their tumor(s). In order to be certain that this is not temporary regression of a leiomyosarcoma, our current practice (and that of others) is to perform a contrast-enhanced MRI of the pelvis 3 months after embolization. If there is a major fibroid that is incompletely infarcted, we usually recommend a follow-up MRI examination 3 to 9 months later, depending on the level of suspicion regarding the lesion. If there is a smoothly defined fibroid that has a regular minor area of incomplete infarction, then a follow-up study 12 months after the embolization is usually recommended. If the lesion is more suspicious, then a shorter-term follow-up is needed. Obviously, if there is regrowth of the fibroid with major areas of incomplete infarction, then a recommendation of immediate surgery may be the most appropriate course. Uterine artery embolization nearly always causes major or complete infarction of fibroids. Unless there is a clear technical explanation, such as untreated ovarian supply, for failure to achieve major infarction of a large fibroid, then the diagnosis of leiomyosarcoma should at least be considered. If there is to be no surgical intervention, then very close follow-up is indicated to ensure that there is a benign course and that a malignancy is not missed.

From a clinical perspective, the interventionalist must be attuned to the symptoms and signs that suggest that the fibroid that has been treated may be malignant. As suggested previously, there may be initial improvement in symptoms. Although there has been little published experience after embolization, one clinical sign might be initial shrinkage of a fibroid or uterus on physical examination but regrowth over a period of months. Early recurrence of symptoms related to regrowth is another possible clinical indicator of malignancy. Because temporary recurrence of fibroid symptoms and "regrowth" are not rare complaints, any suspected recurrence must be confirmed with an imaging study to document the rapid regrowth.

Detecting a missed malignancy or preventing embolization of a malignancy remains a difficult task, but fortunately it is a rare one. It is also a problem for many new uterine-sparing therapies, such as cryomyolysis and high-frequency ultrasound. Until an accurate noninvasive means of diagnosing leiomyosarcoma is developed, vigilance and an appropriately high index of opinion remain the primary tools for detecting these tumors.

SUMMARY

As with any new procedure, learning the basic technique is the first step. After several cases, one often has the sense that the procedure has been mastered. We once thought that ourselves. Now we are a little wiser and recognize that there are a number of potential pitfalls that can prevent a successful procedure. Anticipating them and planning for them may save the case and result in the successful outcome that all are seeking. It is hoped that this brief discussion has illuminated some of the procedure-related pitfalls so that they can be recognized and managed effectively.

REFERENCES

1. Siskin, G, Eaton L, Stainken B, et al. Pathologic findings in a uterine leiomyoma after bilateral uterine artery embolization. *J Vasc Interv Radiol* 1999;10:891–894.
2. Abbara S, Spies J, Scialli A, et al. Transcervical expulsion of a fibroid as a result of uterine artery embolization for leiomyomata. *J Vasc Interv Radiol* 1999;10:409–411.
3. Burn P, McCall JM, Chinn R, et al. Uterine fibroleiomyoma: MR imaging appearances before and after embolization of uterine arteries. *Radiology* 2000;214:729–734.
4. Jha R, Ascher S, Imaoka I, et al. Symptomatic fibroleiomyomata; MR imaging of the uterus before and after uterine arterial embolization. *Radiology* 2000;217:228–235.
5. Goodwin S, McLucas B, Lee M, et al. Uterine artery embolization for the treatment of uterine leiomyomata: midterm results. *J Vasc Interv Radiol* 1999;10:1159–1165.
6. Katsumori T, Nakajima K, Tokuhiro M. Gadolinium-enhanced MR imaging in the evaluation of uterine fibroids treated with uterine artery embolization. *AJR Am J Roentgenol* 2001;177:303–307.
7. Pelage J, LeDref O, Soyer P, et al. Fibroid-related menorrhagia: treatment with superselective embolization of the uterine arteries and midterm follow-up. *Radiology* 2000;215:428–431.
8. Spies J, Ascher SA, Roth AR, et al. Uterine artery embolization for leiomyomata. *Obstet Gynecol* 2001;98:29–34.
9. Pelage J, Guaou N, Jha R, et al. Uterine fibroid tumors: long term MR imaging outcome after embolization. *Radiology* 2004;230:803–809.
10. Smith S, Sewall L, Handelsman A. A clinical failure of uterine fibroid embolization due to adenomyosis. *J Vasc Interv Radiol* 1999;10:1171–1174.
11. Common A, Mocarski E, Kolin A, et al. Therapeutic failure of uterine fibroid embolization caused by underlying leiomyosarcoma. *J Vasc Interv Radiol* 2001;12:1449–1451.
12. Hutchins F, Worthington-Kirsch R, Berkowitz R. Selective uterine artery embolization as primary treatment for symptomatic leiomyomata uteri. *J Am Assoc Gynecol Laparosc* 1999;6:279–284.
13. Walker WJ, Pelage J. Uterine artery embolisation for symptomatic fibroids: clinical results in 400 women with imaging follow up. *Br J Obstet Gynaecol* 2002;109:1262–1272.
14. Saraiya P, Chang T, Pelage J, et al. Uterine artery replacement by the round ligament artery: an anatomic variant discovered during uterine artery embolization for leiomyomata. *J Vasc Interv Radiol* 2002; 13[9 Pt 1]:939–941.
15. Keyoung J, Levy E, Roth A, et al. Intraarterial lidocaine for pain control after uterine artery embolization for leiomyomata. *J Vasc Interv Radiol* 2002;12:1065–1069.
16. Spies J, Scialli A, Jha R, et al. Initial results from uterine fibroid embolization for symptomatic leiomyomata. *J Vasc Interv Radiol* 1999;10:1149–1157.
17. Goodwin S, Vedantham S, McLucas B, et al. Preliminary experience with uterine artery embolization for uterine fibroids. *J Vasc Interv Radiol* 1997;8:517–526.
18. Worthington-Kirsch R, Popky G, Hutchins F. Uterine arterial embolization for the management of leiomyomas: quality-of-life assessment and clinical response. *Radiology* 1998;208:625–629.
19. Bruno J, Allison S, McCullough M, et al. Recovery after uterine artery embolization for leiomyomas: a detailed analysis of its duration and severity. *J Vasc Interv Radiol* 2004 (in press).
20. Barth M, Spies JB. Ovarian embolization supplementing uterine embolization for leiomyomata. *J Vasc Interv Radiol* 2003;14:1177–1182.

21. Spies J, Roth AR, Jha R, et al. Uterine artery embolization for leiomyomata: factors associated with successful symptomatic and imaging outcome. *Radiology* 2002;222:45–52.

22. Thomas J, Gomez-Jorge J, Chang T, et al. Uterine fibroid embolization in patients with leiomyomata and concomitant adenomyosis: experience in thirteen patients. *J Vasc Interv Radiol* 2000;11:S191.

23. Siskin G. Uterine artery embolization for the treatment of adenomyosis: clinical response and evaluation with MR imaging. *AJR Am J Roentgenol* 2001;177:297–302.

24. Ahn C, Lee W, Sunwoo T, et al. Uterine arterial embolization for the treatment of symptomatic adenomyosis of the uterus. *J Vasc Interv Radiol* 2000;11:S192.

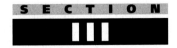

SECTION
III

OUTCOME FROM THERAPY

11

UTERINE FIBROID EMBOLIZATION: WHERE ARE WE? —AN OUTCOME ANALYSIS

MARGARET H. LEE
HSIN-YI LEE
SCOTT C. GOODWIN

Uterine fibroid embolization (UFE) has emerged as a highly effective, uterus-sparing, minimally invasive alternative to hysterectomy and is now widely accepted for the management of symptoms secondary to fibroids. The development and technical considerations of this procedure in the treatment of uterine leiomyomata have been described in earlier chapters. This chapter summarizes the reported results of UFE with respect to clinical benefits, change in health-related quality-of-life measurements, and patient satisfaction.

OVERVIEW OF UTERINE FIBROID EMBOLIZATION OUTCOME

Since the application of transcatheter UFE for the treatment of uterine leiomyomata, many case series were published between 1995 and 2003 (1–28), demonstrating the effectiveness of UFE. Table 11-1 lists case series published to date with a minimum of 50 patients (6–8,12–21,23,24). The outcomes from these studies can best be summarized by considering each outcome measure separately.

Technical Success

Technical success has generally been described as successful embolization of both uterine arteries. Although the endpoint of embolization has varied among studies, a procedure is unlikely to be successful unless both arteries are treated. In early series, complete occlusion of the uterine arteries with polyvinyl alcohol (PVA) particles, often supplemented with either a gelatin sponge plug or a coil, was the standard endpoint of embolization. With the introduction of tris-acryl gelatin microspheres (Embosphere Microspheres), the appropriate endpoint has become a subject of discussion (29–31). Regardless of the endpoint used, it appears that the effectiveness of the procedure is similar, although definitive conclusions await the results of comparative studies. The reported technical success rates range from 84% to 100% (see Table 11-1) (1–28), with most series reporting more than 95% technically successful procedures.

Increasing operator experience will likely improve the technical success and efficiency of the procedure, with concomitant reduction of procedure and fluoroscopy times, as reported from the Canadian experience (22).

Clinical Success

Clinical success has been measured by the degree of improvement or the frequency of resolution of the primary symptoms. These symptoms include bleeding, pain, and bulk-related symptoms related to the uterine leiomyomata (32). In the majority of published studies, patient outcome has been evaluated at follow-up office visits or with the use of symptom questionnaires. Studies have reported that success rates for treating menorrhagia, pelvic pain, and bulk-related symptoms ranged from 81% to 96%, 70% to 100%, and 46% to 100%, respectively (see Table 11-1) (1–28). The largest reported series to date from Ontario, Canada, consists of analysis of fibroid reduction and symptom relief in a cohort of 508 patients undergoing bilateral UFE in a multicenter (university-affiliated teaching and community hospitals), prospective, single-arm clinical treatment trial (21). Bilateral UFE was performed with PVA particles. At 3-month follow-up, significant improvements were reported for menorrhagia (83%), dysmenorrhea (77%), and urinary frequency/urgency (86%) (21). The mean menstrual duration was significantly reduced after UFE (7.6 to 5.4 days) (21). In their review of 262 patients with symptomatic fibroids, Ravina et al. (13) from France reported complete resolution of symptoms in 245 (94%) cases and disappearance of hemorrhage in 80% of cases.

TABLE 11-1. EVIDENCE OF UTERINE FIBROID EMBOLIZATION

Peer-Reviewed Published Case Series
Inclusion Criteria: Series Including a Minimum of 50 Patients

Reference	No. of Patients (Age)	Follow-up Interval (Mean)	Technical Success	Menorrhagia (Percent Improved)	Pelvic Pain/Bulk-Related Symptoms (Percent Improved)	Fibroid (Uterine) Volume Reduction	Complications/Failures/Others
Hutchins F, 1999 (6)	305 (26–52)	12 mo	96%	86% at 3 mo 85% at 6 mo 92% at 12 mo	64% at 3 mo 77% at 6 mo 92% at 12 mo	(48%)	Puncture site hematoma: 4 Readmission for pain: 2 Subsequent hysterectomy: 6; myomectomy: 5
Goodwin SC, 1999 (7)	60	16.3 mo	100%	81%	93%	48.4 at 10.2 mo	Hysterectomy (infection): 1 Fibroid expulsion: 6
Ravina JH, 1999 (8)	188	20 mo		90%		50%–100% in 87% of patients at 6 mo	Hysterectomy (uterine necrosis and bowel obstruction): 1
Pelage JP, 2000 (12)	76 (44.7)			95%		20% at 2 mo 52% at 6 mo	Hysterectomy (septic uterine necrosis): 1 Myomectomy: 5/80 (6%), including 3 unil. Amenorrhea: 4 Fibroid passage: 4 Full-term pregnancy: 3; prospective
Ravina JH, 2000 (13)	262 (21–53)	6 mo		80% immediately		60% at 6 mo	Failures: 17/262 Pregnancy: 13; 0 recurrence
Chrisman HB, 2000 (14)	66 (30–55)	21 wk	100%	91%	87%		External iliac artery dissection: 1 Hysterectomy: 0
Brunereau, 2000 (15)	58 (33–65)	12 mo	84%	90% at 3 mo 92% at 6 mo 93% at 12 mo		23% at 3 mo 43% at 6 mo 51% at 12 mo	New fibroids: 1 at 24 mo
McLucas B, 2001 (16)	167	6 mo	98%	88% at 6 mo		(49%) at 6 mo (52%) at 12 mo	Hysterectomy: 6 (3.5%), 1 infection Premature menopause: 4 Fibroid passage: 5%
Andersen PE, 2001 (17)	62	6 mo	97%	96% (29/30)	70%	68% at 6 mo	Fibroid expulsion: 2 Endometritis: 1 Hysterectomy: 1
Spies JB, 2001 (18)	200	21 mo	99%	87% at 3 mo 90% at 12 mo	93% at 3 mo 91% at 12 mo	42% at 3 mo 60% at 12 mo	Pulmonary embolus: 1 Deep vein thrombosis: 1 Endometrial infection: 2 Fibroid expulsion: 1 Hysterectomy: 0 Subsequent gynecologic interventions: 10.5%

Study	N (age)	Follow-up					Complications / Notes
Katsumori T, 2002 (19)	60 (32–52)	10.6 mo		98% at 4 mo / 100% at 12 mo	97% at 4 mo / 100% at 12 mo	55% at 4 mo / 70% at 12 mo	No major
Walker WJ, 2002 (20)	400	16.7 mo (mean)	99%	84%	79%	73% at 9.7 mo (mean)	Fibroid expulsion: 2 / Amenorrhea: 1 / Hysterectomy: 0 / Recurrence: 0 / Gelatin sponge particles alone
Pron G, 2003 (21)	508	3 mo		83%	86%	42% (35%)	Hysterectomy (infection): 3 / Amenorrhea: 26 (7%) / Chronic vaginal discharge: 13 (4%) / Clinical failure or recurrence: 23 (6%) (hysterectomy: 9 [2%]) / Pregnancy: 13 in 12 patients / 97% pleased with outcome / PVA and coils
Marret H, 2003 (23)	80 (31–65)	30 mo		83.5% clinical improvement		73% at 36 mo (61%) at 36 mo	Amenorrhea (age dependent): 3% / Median fibroid life-impact scores sig reduced (8.0 to 3.0, 10-point scale) / 91% satisfaction
Ravina JH, 2003 (24)	454 (21–68)	3, 6, 12 mo		86% symptom-free at 6 mo		55% at 6 mo / 70% at 1 yr	External iliac artery dissection: 1 / Adenomyosis: 2 / Subserosal fibroids: 2 / Endometrial carcinoma: 1 / Progression fibroid: 1 / Recurrent fibroids: 7 / Failures: 42 (9.6%) / Surgery: 3 / Amenorrhea and fibroid sloughs

Reports of mid-term efficacy after UFE is likewise favorable. Walker and Pelage (20) reported on their experience with UFE in the evaluation of 400 women with symptomatic fibroids with a mean clinical follow-up of 16.7 months. Menstrual bleeding improved in 84% of women and menstrual pain was improved in 79%. In a prospective longitudinal study of 305 patients, Hutchins et al. (10) reported successful control of menorrhagia and satisfactory control of bulk symptoms in 92% of their patients at 12 months. Spies et al. (18) reported similar results at 12-month post-UFE follow-up. Most recently, Marret et al. (23) reported 83.5% overall clinical improvement at median follow-up of 30 months in 80 treated patients.

Most of the published literature report on outcomes of patients with symptomatic fibroids who underwent uterine artery embolization that was completed using PVA particles as the embolic material. UFE using gelatin sponge particles alone shows comparable results as those obtained with PVA particles, as reported by Katz et al. (33) and Katsumori et al. (19). Katsumori et al. (19) reported markedly or moderately improved menorrhagia in 41 (98%) of 42 patients 4 months after embolization and in 20 of 20 patients 1 year after embolization. Bulk-related symptoms improved markedly or moderately in 31 (97%) of 32 patients 4 months after embolization and in 19 of 19 patients 1 year after embolization (19). Mean volume reduction of the largest tumor was 55% at 4 months and 70% at 1 year; mean uterine volume reduction was 40% at 4 months and 56% at 1 year (19).

Similarly, the outcome from the use of tris-acryl gelatin microspheres does not appear to differ from early studies using PVA particles. Banovac et al. (30) reported their experience with microspheres in a retrospective review of 23 patients with 61 leiomyomata. Median volume of all leiomyomata was decreased by 52%, whereas median uterine volume was decreased by 32% (30). Thus, early experience with the use of calibrated tris-acryl gelatin microspheres appears promising (29–31), and comparative studies are under way that should provide more definitive answers regarding the relative effectiveness of each embolic type.

Subsequent Gynecologic Intervention

Another measure of outcome is the effectiveness of UFE in avoiding other treatments for fibroids, as measured by subsequent medical therapies or surgery. For example, hysterectomy after UFE is an important measure of safety and a key outcome measure of UFE. The results in terms of safety are discussed in Chapter 12, although it appears that the need for hysterectomy because of complications within 30 days of therapy is less than 1%. The results reported to date are highly variable. In a small study, Du et al. (27) reported the highest rate of reintervention in the short term, with 5 of 38 patients requiring hysterectomy or myomectomy 1 to 3 weeks after the procedure. This is much higher

than in any other series to date. For example, at a median follow-up of 8.1 months, 8 of the 550 women who underwent UFE required complication-related hysterectomy in the Canadian multicenter clinical trial (34). Similar results were noted by Spies et al. (18), with 9 (4.5%) of 200 patients undergoing hysterectomy within 12 months of therapy. None of the hysterectomies in this series was performed because of complications of UFE. Seven of the patients underwent hysterectomy for failure to sufficiently improve their symptoms after UFE. The other two patients underwent incidental hysterectomy—one in treatment of unilateral salpingo-oophorectomy 7 months after embolization for a tuboovarian abscess and the other for resection of an adnexal mass (18). In this study, dilation and curettage (D&C) and hysteroscopic resection were the most common interventions for acute gynecologic problems related to the treated leiomyomata (18). Most gynecologic procedures in this series were performed months after the UFE (18).

The frequency of hysterectomy for a procedure that fails is likely higher, but the true rate requires longer-term follow-up. The rate of development of new fibroids is not yet known. At least one recently published study suggests that recurrence rates are low (23). In their ongoing clinical experience of 85 UFE procedures performed in 80 patients, Marret et al. (23) reported a 10% recurrence rate at a median follow-up interval of 30 months. The incidence of other conditions requiring hysterectomy following UFE is unknown.

Imaging Outcome

The dominant tumor and uterine volume reduction rates range from 43% to 73% and from 48% to 61%, respectively, for follow-up interval of 6 months or more after UFE (see Table 11-1). Pron et al. (21) from the Ontario Uterine Fibroid Embolization Trial with the largest single cohort to date of 508 patients, published median uterine and dominant fibroid volume reduction of 35% and 42%, respectively, at 3-month follow-up. In a cohort of 262 patients, Ravina et al. (13) reported a marked 60% reduction in the size of myomata at 6 months. Walker and Pelage (20) evaluated follow-up ultrasound imaging of fibroids in 400 patients who underwent UFE demonstrating 58% and 83% median reduction of uterine and dominant fibroid volumes, respectively, at a mean clinical follow-up of 16.7 months. Most recently, Marret et al. (23) reported 61% mean reduction of uterine volume and 73% mean reduction of fibroid volume at 36 months post UFE. Similar to observed symptomatic improvement using PVA particles, the degree of tumor regression does not appear to be affected by use of alternate embolic agents, as previously discussed.

Predicting Outcome

Goodwin et al. (7) statistically analyzed multiple patient characteristics as possible prognostic factors. Patient characteristics such as age, race, size, vascularity and location of the leiomyoma, pertinent history, and medical or surgical therapies were evaluated for each failure group (7). Using various statistical analyses, Goodwin et al. (7) concluded that only age and earlier myomectomy predicted outcome. Young age was a predictor of clinical failure and those patients who underwent previous myomectomy were more likely to have a successful outcome after embolization. They noted a lack of correlation of initial uterine volume, vascularity, and postprocedural pain with outcome (7). Further studies are needed to assess the validity of these prognostic factors. Comorbid diseases may also affect the outcome of the procedure. Goodwin et al. (7,32) suggested that adenomyosis may "predispose" the patient to clinical failure after the embolization procedure. Smith et al. (35) reported a clinical failure after UFE in a patient with underlying adenomyosis.

The presence of other comorbid diseases can complicate both patient selection and assessment of outcome. Many patients have fibroids, but their symptoms may be caused by ovarian cysts, tubal inflammation, endometriosis, diverticulosis, or other conditions. Those patients with underlying diseases can have persistent pain after the procedure and therefore have a poor clinical outcome.

Leiomyoma location within the uterus may correlate with outcome. Spies et al. (36) reported that smaller baseline leiomyoma size and submucosal location are more likely to result in a positive imaging outcome. Bleeding outcome correlated with submucosal leiomyoma location and smaller baseline uterine and leiomyoma volumes (36), whereas the odds of improved bulk-related symptoms were not associated with leiomyoma volume change or location. With use of regression models, Spies et al. (36) showed that there were very significant associations between bleeding and bulk-related symptom (i.e., pain) improvements and improved symptom outcome and between these symptom improvements and satisfaction outcome. There was a weak association between symptom or satisfaction outcome and either absolute uterine or dominant leiomyoma volume or percentage volume reduction at each follow-up interval. These findings suggest that improvement in one fibroid symptom is likely to be associated with improvement in others and these correlate, as might be expected, with patient satisfaction with outcome. Perhaps surprisingly, these improvements occurred in most patients, regardless of fibroid volume reduction. This may be explained by remembering that a positive outcome depends on infarction of all or most of the fibroids (as demonstrated by contrast-enhanced MRI, as discussed in the following) rather than shrinkage.

Ultrasound has been used to try to predict the outcome of uterine embolization, but with mixed results. Fleischer et al. (37), using three-dimensional color Doppler sonography, found that hypervascular fibroids tend to decrease in size after treatment more than their isovascular or hypovascular counterparts. Weintraub et al. (38), however,

found no statistical relationship between echogenicity and vascularity before the procedure and the percentage decrease in the uterine size. In their follow-up of 188 patients 6 months after UFE, McLucas et al. (16) showed that the initial peak systolic velocity was positively correlated with the size and shrinkage of myomas and uterine volume and that high peak systolic velocity (>64 cm/s) was a significant predictor of failure.

MRI is useful for quantitative assessment of signal intensity and morphologic changes before and after UFE. Burn et al. (39) studied the MRI characteristics of fibroleiomyomas or fibroids as predictors of UFE outcome. They noted that the mean reduction in fibroleiomyoma volume was 43% at 2 months and 59% at 6 months. In addition, pretreatment MRI findings may help predict the success of the procedure. They reported that before embolization, high signal intensity on T1-weighted images was predictive of a poor response ($p = 0.008$) and high signal intensity on T2-weighted images was predictive of a good response ($p = 0.007$) in terms of volume reduction. Further, the degree of gadolinium enhancement was not correlated with fibroleiomyoma volume reduction. Similar results were reported by deSouza and Williams (40), who in their evaluation of perfusion and volume changes at MRI before and after UFE noted clear differential perfusion responses between the myometrium and the leiomyoma after UFE. They also demonstrated that leiomyomas initially high on T2-weighted images showed significantly greater volume reduction than those low in signal intensity, and preembolization perfusion characteristics (i.e., enhancement pattern) of the leiomyomas did not impact on degree of volume reduction. Further, deSouza and Williams (40) concluded that immediate reduction in leiomyoma perfusion after bilateral UFE correlates with clinical response. This indicates that devascularization of the fibroid, the MRI correlate of fibroid infarction, is the necessary precursor of symptom improvement in the long term. This has been demonstrated when viewing the long-term imaging outcome of embolization, because complete fibroid infarction does result in long-term improvement of symptoms, whereas incomplete infarction may predispose to regrowth (26). Jha et al. (41) studied the MRI characteristics before and after embolization in an attempt to predict outcome (volume, location, signal intensity characteristics, and vascularity). They found that submucosal location was a strong positive predictor of fibroleiomyoma volume reduction ($p < 0.001$) and that baseline hypervascularity was a strong indicator of success ($p < 0.005$) with a reduction in vascularity as a measure of success.

Patient Satisfaction After Uterine Fibroid Embolization

Patient satisfaction with the clinical outcome of UFE has usually been measured with follow-up questionnaires and correlates well with symptomatic improvement.

Worthington-Kirsch et al. (42) surveyed their cohort of 53 patients (age range 33–58 years) for satisfaction with the UFE procedure and reported that 41 (79%) of the patients interviewed would choose the procedure again; 8 (15%) would consider choosing the procedure again; and only 3 (6%) would choose another treatment option. Overall, patient satisfaction with outcomes ranged from 84% to 95% in the literature (19). In their treatment of 200 consecutive patients, Spies et al. (18) observed that patient satisfaction paralleled the symptom results and that these results remained stable during the course of follow-up.

Impact of Uterine Fibroid Embolization on Quality of Life

A broader measure of outcome is the change in quality of life after UFE. Health-related quality of life is a broad construct, usually measuring concepts such as energy, vitality, mood, pain, physical energy, social functioning, and sexual function and is usually determined by written questionnaire. There are two basic categories of health-related quality-of-life questionnaires: generic and disease specific. A generic instrument is usually composed of questions assessing broad categories of health status and does not contain disease-specific questions. An advantage of this approach is that these generic questionnaires have been extensively validated, have age- and sex-specific norms available, and often have extensive data available for individuals with different clinical conditions. One commonly used generic quality-of-life questionnaire is the SF-36, which was derived from the scales developed in the Medical Outcomes Study (43). It has been used to assess health status in a broad range of conditions, such as cardiac disease, renal disease, epilepsy, back pain, and many others. The availability of scores from patients with a variety of medical conditions as well as the normal population provides a means of comparing health status across the population. A disadvantage of generic instruments is that they may not be sensitive enough to detect changes in patient status or to adequately distinguish among patients with a specific medical condition. This is particularly an issue with a condition such as uterine fibroids, in which otherwise normal patients have very specific menstrual-related symptoms. There has been relatively little written about the impact of UFE on quality of life, in part because until recently there have been few validated fibroid-specific quality-of-life questionnaires. Standardized quality-of-life questionnaires such as the SF-36 and the SF-12 have also been used to a limited extent in UFE (44,45).

Using a proprietary fibroid health-related quality-of-life questionnaire, Spies et al. (44) found that there were significant improvements in health-related quality of life and fibroid-specific symptoms in 50 patients undergoing UFE and suggested that the measurement of health-related quality of life may be a useful means of comparing relative outcome of UFE with other fibroid therapies. That same questionnaire was used in the ongoing phase II study comparing uterine embolization to myomectomy, which is nearing completion. The SF-12, a 12-question generic quality-of-life questionnaire based on the SF-36, has also been reported to be sensitive to change in health-related quality of life after UFE, indicating that improvements can be detected even using relatively insensitive brief generic instruments. The SF-12 was one key measure of outcome in a recent comparative study of the outcome of UFE and hysterectomy (25). That study demonstrated dramatic improvement in the quality of life for both hysterectomy and embolization patients, and there was no statistically significant difference between the two therapies during follow-up.

A disease-specific quality-of-life instrument for fibroids has been developed with the support of the Cardiovascular and Interventional Radiology Research and Education Foundation (CIRREF) (46). It is a 37-question instrument, with eight symptom questions and 29 quality-of-life questions. It yields a score for both symptoms and quality of life. It has been used as one measure of outcome in a recent study comparing the outcome of UFE using PVA particles and Embospheres (47). In that study of 100 patients, mean scores at baseline for the entire group were dramatically improved by 3 months afterwards, indicating that the questionnaire is able to detect change in symptoms and quality of life as a result of embolization. This questionnaire is one of the key outcome measures being used in the CIRREF registry.

Quality-of-life assessments have been used in studies of gynecologic conditions, providing a model for how they might be used when comparing fibroid therapies. In one study of hysterectomy in Great Britain using the Nottingham Health Profile, the health status of subjects at 6 weeks after surgery became indistinguishable from women in the general population (48).

A number of other studies of hysterectomy and other fibroid therapies have measured outcome using health-related quality-of-life questionnaires. In a prospective cohort study of 418 women undergoing hysterectomy, Carlson (49) used a variety of quality-of-life measures, including a global rating, a mental health index, a general health index, and an activity index. Significant improvements in mental health, general health, and activity indices were reported at 6 months and sustained at 1 year. In a companion study, the same researchers also evaluated the nonsurgical management of leiomyomas, abnormal bleeding, and chronic pelvic pain (50). Therapies included oral contraceptives, cyclic progestins, nonsteroidal antiinflammatory medications, iron supplements, and, in 7%, D&C. Using the same questionnaires as in the hysterectomy study, significant improvements in symptoms were detected using medical management. However, 25% of the patients eventually underwent hysterectomy. At 1 year, 25% of patients with abnormal bleeding and 50% of patients with chronic pelvic pain reported substantial levels of residual symptoms, impacting their quality-of-life scores.

Health-related quality-of-life instruments have also been used in comparative trials in gynecology. In one, endometrial resection was compared with abdominal hysterectomy for the treatment of menorrhagia (51). A number of outcome measures were used, including the General Health Questionnaire. In this study, a statistically significant difference in favor of hysterectomy was detected at 4 months after the procedure. This appeared to be a result of a high early recurrence rate in patients with endometrial resection.

These published studies confirm the usefulness of measures of quality of life in assessing outcome and have particular utility when comparing differing therapies. The measurement of quality of life is a clearly accepted adjunct to outcome assessment, which will be central in determining the effectiveness of this therapy in the future.

Comparative Evaluation with Alternative Treatment of Fibroids

Most of the current data on UFE are based on cases series without control groups, rendering it difficult to accurately determine the comparative risks and benefits of the procedure. Broder et al. (52) developed a research agenda for UFE for the treatment of symptomatic leiomyomata.

They identified outcomes as either "important to measure" or "essential to measure" (death, reoperation, operative injury, menorrhagia, premature menopause, recurrence of myomata, and satisfaction) and four areas for research: randomized trial, prospective registry, disease-specific quality-of-life instrument, and cost analysis (52). At the time of this writing, there are four published papers comparing relative efficacy of UFE compared to alternative therapies, summarized in Table 11-2 (53–56).

In their analysis of consecutive 111 patients who underwent uterus-sparing abdominal myomectomy or fibroid embolization, Razavi et al. (53) reported success rates of 64% vs. 92% for menorrhagia ($p < 0.05$), 54% vs. 74% for pain (not significant), and 91% vs. 76% for mass effect ($p < 0.05$), and complication rates of 25% and 11% ($p < 0.05$). Moreover, they found 2.9 vs. 0 days of mean hospital stay, 8.7 vs. 5.1 days of narcotic use, and 36 vs. 8 days until resumption of normal activities (all statistically significant) (53). They concluded that efficacy appears to be greater with embolization in treatment of menorrhagia, and surgery may be a better choice for symptoms related to mass effect of fibroids.

Pinto et al. (54) reported the results of a prospective clinical trial in patients assigned to two groups: those given the option of UFE or hysterectomy and those not informed of alternative treatment. The primary variables considered for evaluation were effectiveness, efficiency, safety as

TABLE 11-2. COMPARATIVE STUDIES OF UTERINE FIBROID EMBOLIZATION AND SURGICAL ALTERNATIVES

Reference	Study Design	Alternative Treatment	Comparative Results (UFE vs. Alternative Treatment)	Comments
Broder MS, 2002 (56)	Retrospective	Myomectomy	51/59 patients vs. 30/38 patients follow-up available: UFE older patients (48 yr vs. 38 yr); UFE more likely prior surgical procedures; symptoms improved 92% vs. 90%; 94% vs. 79% at least somewhat satisfied with choice of procedure	Patients with UFE more likely to need further invasive treatment 3–5 years after index procedure; those who did not, similar satisfaction and relief of symptoms
Park KH, 2003 (55)	Prospective	Laparoscopic UAL	23 vs. 17 patients: uterine volume reduction at 3 mo (UFE) vs. 3–6 mo (UAL) (58.5%)	Mechanism of volume reduction evaluated with biopsy specimen: cell necrosis vs. physiologic cell death or apoptosis
Pinto I, 2003 (54)	Prospective	Hysterectomy	UFE clinical success 86%; UFE mean hospital stay 4.14 days shorter; UFE 25% minor complications vs. 20% major complications in hysterectomy	Primary variables evaluated: bleeding cessation, length of stay, and associated complications
Razavi MK, 2003 (53)	Retrospective	Abdominal myomectomy	92% vs. 64% for menorrhagia ($p < 0.05$); 74% vs. 54% for pain (not significant); 76% vs. 91% for mass effect ($p < 0.05$); 11% vs. 25% for complication rates ($p < 0.05$); 0 vs. 2.9 days mean hospital stay; 5.1 vs. 8.7 days of narcotic use; 8 vs. 63 days until resumption of normal activities	

UAL, Uterine artery ligation; UFE, uterine fibroid embolization.

measured by bleeding control, total length of hospital stay, and complications. The overall clinical success of UFE is 86% (31/36 patients). The hospital stay for patients treated with UFE was shorter than for those who underwent hysterectomy. Of those who underwent UFE, 25% had minor complications, in contrast to 20% of those who underwent hysterectomy having major complications (54).

In their analysis of treatment outcomes of 23 patients who underwent UFE and 17 who underwent laparoscopic uterine artery ligation, Park et al. (55) concluded that both procedures are equally effective in relieving symptoms caused by uterine myoma, and that both procedures can be used in place of hysterectomy or myomectomy. However, the follow-up is limited.

In their retrospective review of subgroups of patients undergoing UFE and myomectomy, Broder et al. (56) found that overall symptoms improved in 33 (92%) of 36 UFE patients and 26 (90%) of 29 myomectomy patients, respectively, and that 34 (94%) of 36 UFE patients were at least somewhat satisfied with the choice of their procedure compared to 23 (79%) of 29 myomectomy patients. Reintervention rates among myomectomy patients were much lower than in embolization patients (3% vs. 29%, $p < 0.001$) A recent multicenter study comparing embolization to hysterectomy has been completed by Spies et al. (25). For embolization patients, there were marked reductions in blood loss scores ($p < 0.001$) and menorrhagia questionnaire scores ($p < 0.001$) compared to baseline. At 12 months, a larger proportion of hysterectomy patients had improved pelvic pain ($p = 0.021$), and there was a trend toward greater improvement of pelvic pressure among hysterectomy patients. There was no difference in the proportion of patients with improvement in urinary symptoms. Both groups had marked improvement in other symptoms and quality-of-life scores, with no difference between groups. Complications were more frequent in hysterectomy patients (50% vs. 27.5%, $p = 0.01$). Serious complications were infrequent in both groups, although complications were twice as likely with hysterectomy as with embolization, and there was a trend toward more frequent serious complications among hysterectomy patients. This study indicates that UFE is effective in most patients, and patient satisfaction and quality-of-life improvement outcomes are similar to those of hysterectomy, which is the gold standard of fibroid therapies.

Cost Analysis

Admittedly, measuring medical costs is difficult. Nevertheless, in the current health care environment, in which cost considerations are important when evaluating new treatments, careful study of the costs of UFE should be a priority. The cost information can be used to analyze the cost effectiveness of UFE compared to other therapies for fibroids. An initial analysis by Subramanian and Spies (57)

published in 2001 assessed the facility cost associated with UFE. They found that the facility cost of UFE ($3,080) compared favorably with that of hysterectomy, which ranged in cost from $3,100 to $4,900 depending on the type of procedure performed. A subsequent comparative study at the same institution reported by Baker et al. (58) concludes that procedure-related costs are lower with UFE than with abdominal myomectomy despite higher physician costs. Other cost analyses estimating and comparing UFE against surgical procedures yield similar results. Through a decision model comparing the costs and effectiveness of UFE and hysterectomy and performing the analysis from a societal perspective, Beinfeld et al. (59) deduced that UFE is more effective and less expensive than hysterectomy such that UFE is a cost-effective alternative to hysterectomy across a wide range of assumptions about the costs and effectiveness of the two procedures. Al-Fozan et al. (60) in Canada report that UFE is associated with a lower hospital cost and a shorter hospital stay compared with abdominal myomectomy, abdominal hysterectomy, and vaginal hysterectomy. These authors noted that hospitalization after UFE was mainly for postprocedural abdominal pain and suggested improved pain control methodology as a strategy to reduce the rate of hospitalization and its associated cost (60).

CONCLUSION

Symptomatic uterine leiomyomata are a significant source of distress to many women and place a substantial burden on the health care system (52). Novel techniques such as UFE warrant further consideration as it is a minimally invasive procedure for the treatment of uterine leiomyomas. The short-term and mid-term outcomes for UFE have been excellent. Future studies should clearly define patient selection with use of predetermined inclusion and exclusion criteria. Further prospective randomized controlled trials are necessary to further validate the efficacy of UFE compared to the traditional surgical technique of hysterectomy or myomectomy.

REFERENCES

1. Ravina JH, Herbreteau D, Ciraru-Vigneron N, et al. Arterial embolisation to treat uterine myomata. *Lancet* 1995;346: 671–672.
2. Ravina JH, Bouret JH, Ciraru-Vigneron N, et al. Recourse to particular arterial embolization in the treatment of some uterine leiomyoma. *Bull Fr Natl Acad Med* 1997;181:233–243.
3. McLucas B, Goodwin SC, Vedantham S. Embolic therapy for myomata. *Min Invas Ther Allied Technol* 1996;5:336–338.
4. Goodwin SC, Vedantham S, McLucas B, et al. Preliminary experience with uterine artery embolization for uterine fibroids. *J Vasc Interv Radiol* 1997;8:517–526.

5. Bradley EA, Reidy JF, Forman RG, et al. Transcatheter uterine artery embolisation to treat large uterine fibroids. *Br J Obstet Gynaecol* 1998;105:235–240.

6. Hutchins FL, Worthington-Kirsch R, Berkowitz RP. Selective uterine artery embolization as primary treatment for symptomatic leiomyomata uteri. *J Am Assoc Gynecol Laparosc* 1999;6: 279–284.

7. Goodwin SC, McLucas B, Lee M, et al. Uterine artery embolization for the treatment of uterine leiomyomata: midterm results. *J Vasc Interv Radiol* 1999;19:1159–1165.

8. Ravina J, Ciraru-Vigneron N, Aymard A, et al. Uterine artery embolisation for fibroid disease: results of a 6 year study. *Min Invas Ther Allied Technol* 1999;8:441–447.

9. Spies JB, Scialli AR, Jha RC, et al. Initial results from uterine fibroid embolization for symptomatic leiomyomata. *J Vasc Interv Radiol* 1999;10:1149–1157.

10. Hutchins F, Worthington-Kirsch R, Berkowitz R. Selective uterine artery embolization as primary treatment for symptomatic leiomyomata uteri. *J Am Assoc Gynecol Laparosc* 1999;6: 279–284.

11. Siskin GP, Stainken BF, Dowing K, et al. Outpatient uterine artery embolization for symptomatic uterine fibroids: experience in 49 patients. *J Vasc Interv Radiol* 2000;11:305–311.

12. Pelage J, LeDref O, Soyer P, et al. Fibroid-related menorrhagia: treatment with superselective embolization of the uterine arteries and midterm follow-up. *Radiology* 2000;215:428–431.

13. Ravina JH, Aymard A, Ciraru-Vigneron N, et al. [Arterial embolization of uterine myoma: results apropos of 286 cases]. *J Gynecol Obstet Biol Reprod* 2000;29:272–275.

14. Chrisman HB, Saker MB, Ryu RK, et al. The impact of uterine fibroid embolization on resumption of menses and ovarian function. *J Vasc Interv Radiol* 2000;11:699–703.

15. Brunereau L, Herbreteau D, Gallas S, et al. Uterine artery embolization in the primary treatment of uterine leiomyomas: technical features and prospective follow-up with clinical and sonographic examinations in 58 patients. *AJR Am J Roentgenol* 2000;175:1267–1272.

16. McLucas B, Adler L, Perrella R. Uterine fibroid embolization: nonsurgical treatment for symptomatic fibroids. *J Am Coll Surg* 2001;192:95–105.

17. Andersen PE, Lund N, Justesen P, et al. Uterine artery embolization of symptomatic uterine fibroids. Initial success and short-term results. *Acta Radiol* 2001;42:234–238.

18. Spies JB, Ascher SA, Roth AR, et al. Uterine artery embolization for leiomyomata. *Obstet Gynecol* 2001;98:29–34.

19. Katsumori T, Nakajima K, Mihara T, et al. Uterine artery embolization using gelatin sponge particles alone for symptomatic fibroids: midterm results. *AJR Am J Roentgenol* 2002;178:135–139.

20. Walker WJ, Pelage JP. Uterine artery embolisation for symptomatic fibroids: clinical results in 400 women with imaging follow up. *BJOG* 2002;109:1262–1272.

21. Pron G, Cohen M, Soucie J, et al., Ontario Uterine Fibroid Embolization Collaboration Group. The Ontario Uterine Fibroid Embolization Trial. Part 2. Uterine fibroid reduction and symptom relief after uterine artery embolization for fibroids. *Fertil Steril* 2003;79:120–127.

22. Pron G, Bennett J, Common A, et al. Technical results and effects of operator experience on uterine artery embolization for fibroids: the Ontario uterine fibroid embolization trial. *J Vasc Interv Radiol* 2003;14:545–554.

23. Marret H, Alonso AM, Cottier JP, et al. Leiomyoma recurrence after uterine artery embolization. *J Vasc Interv Radiol* 2003;14: 1395–1399.

24. Ravina JH, Aymard A, Ciraru-Vigneron N, et al. [Uterine fibroids embolization: results about 454 cases]. *Gynecol Obstet Fertil* 2003;31:597–605.

25. Spies JB, Cooper JM, Worthington-Kirsch R, et al. Outcome from uterine embolization and hysterectomy for leiomyomas: results of a multi-center study. *Am J Obstet Gynecol* 2004 *(in press)*.

26. Pelage JP, Guaou NG, Jha RC, et al. Long-term imaging outcome after embolization for uterine fibroid tumors. *Radiology* 2004;230:803–809.

27. Du J, Zuo Y, Chen X, et al. [Clinical observation of transcatheter uterine artery embolization for uterine myoma]. *Zhonghua Fu Chan Ke Za Zhi* 2002;37:12–15.

28. Golfieri R, Muzzi C, De Laco P, et al. [The percutaneous treatment of uterine fibromas by means of transcatheter arterial embolization]. *Radiol Med (Torino)* 2000;100:48–55.

29. Spies JB, Benenati JF, Worthington-Kirsch RL, et al. Initial experience with use of tris-acryl gelatin microspheres for uterine artery embolization for leiomyomata. *J Vasc Interv Radiol* 2001;12:1059–1063.

30. Banovac F, Ascher SM, Jones DA, et al. Magnetic resonance imaging outcome after uterine artery embolization for leiomyomata with use of tris-acryl gelatin microspheres. *J Vasc Interv Radiol* 2002;13:681–688.

31. Pelage JP, Le Dref O, Beregi JP, et al. Limited uterine artery embolization with tris-acryl gelatin microspheres for uterine fibroids. *J Vasc Interv Radiol* 2003:14:11–14.

32. Goodwin SC, Bonilla SM, Sacks D, et al. Reporting standards for uterine artery embolization for the treatment of uterine leiomyomata. *J Vasc Interv Radiol* 2001;12:1011–1020.

33. Katz RN, Mitty HA, Stancata-Pasik A, et al. Comparison of uterine artery embolization for fibroids using gelatin sponge pledgets and polyvinyl alcohol [Abstract]. *J Vasc Interv Radiol* 1998;9[Suppl]:184.

34. Pron G, Mocarski E, Cohen M, et al. Hysterectomy for complications after uterine artery embolization for leiomyoma: results of a Canadian multicenter clinical trial. *J Am Assoc Gynecol Laparosc* 2003;10:99–106.

35. Smith SJ, Sewall LE, Handelsman A. A clinical failure of uterine fibroid embolization due to adenomyosis. *J Vasc Interv Radiol* 1999;10:1171–1174.

36. Spies JB, Roth AR, Jha RC, et al. Leiomyomata treated with uterine artery embolization: factors associated with successful symptom and imaging outcome. *Radiology* 2002;222:45–52.

37. Fleischer AC, Donnelly EF, Campbell MG, et al. Three-dimensional color Doppler sonography before and after fibroid embolization. *J Ultrasound Med* 2000;19:701–705.

38. Weintraub JL, Romano WJ, Kirsch MJ, et al. Uterine artery embolization: sonographic imaging findings. *J Ultrasound Med* 2002;21:633–637.

39. Burn PR, McCall JM, Chinn RJ, et al. Uterine fibroleiomyoma: MR imaging appearances before and after embolization of uterine arteries. *Radiology* 2000;214:729–734.

40. deSouza NM, Williams AD: Uterine arterial embolization for leiomyomas: perfusion and volume changes at MR imaging and relation to clinical outcome. *Radiology* 2002;222:367–374.

41. Jha RC, Ascher SM, Imaoka I, et al. Symptomatic fibroleiomyomata: MR imaging of the uterus before and after uterine arterial embolization. *Radiology* 2000;217:228–235.

42. Worthington-Kirsch RL, Popky GL, Hutchins FL. Uterine arterial embolization for the management of leiomyomas: quality-of-life assessment and clinical response. *Radiology* 1998; 208:625–629.

43. Ware JE Jr, Sherbourne CD. The MOS 36-item short-form health survey (SF-36), 1. Conceptual framework and item selection. *Med Care* 1992;30:473–483.

44. Spies JB, Warren EH, Mathias SD, et al. Uterine fibroid embolization: measurement of health-related quality of life before and after therapy. *J Vasc Interv Radiol* 1999;10:1293–1303.

45. Kim J, Spies JB, Zorn JG, et al. Use of the SF-12 health survey for general health status assessment after uterine fibroid embolization: preliminary findings [Abstract]. *J Vasc Interv Radiol* 2000;11[Suppl]:309.

46. Coyne K, Sasane M, Walsh SM, et al. Developing a symptom and health-related quality of life questionnaire for uterine fibroids. Presented at the 7th annual Conference of the International Society for Quality of Life Research, October 29–31, 2000, Vancouver, BC, Canada.

47. Spies JB, Allison S, Flick PA, et al. Polyvinyl alcohol particles and tris acryl gelatin microspheres for uterine artery embolization for leiomyomas: results of a randomized comparative study *(in press)*.

48. Clarke A, Black N, Rowe P, et al. Indications for and outcome of total abdominal hysterectomy for benign disease: a prospective cohort study. *Br J Obstet Gynaecol* 1995;102:611–620.

49. Carlson K, Miller B, Fowler F. The Maine Women's Health Study: I. outcomes of hysterectomy. *Obstet Gynecol* 1994;83:556–565.

50. Carlson K, Miller B, Fowler F. The Main Women's Health Study: II. Outcomes of nonsurgical management of leiomyomas, abnormal bleeding, and chronic pelvic pain. *Obstet Gynecol* 1994;83:566–572.

51. Dwyer N. Hutton J, Stirrat G. Randomised controlled trial comparing endometrial resection with abdominal hysterectomy for the surgical treatment of menorrhagia. *Br J Obstet Gynaecol* 1993;100:237–243.

52. Broder MS, Landow WJ, Goodwin SC, et al. An agenda for research into uterine artery embolization: results of an expert panel conference. *J Vasc Interv Radiol* 2000;11:509–515.

53. Razavi MK, Hwang G, Jahed A, et al. Abdominal myomectomy versus uterine fibroid embolization in the treatment of symptomatic uterine leiomyomas. *AJR Am J Roentgenol* 2003;180:1571–1575.

54. Pinto I, Chimeno P, Romo A, et al. Uterine fibroids: uterine artery embolization versus abdominal hysterectomy for treatment—a prospective, randomized, and controlled clinical trial. *Radiology* 2003;226:425–431.

55. Park KH, Kim JY, Shin JS, et al. Treatment outcomes of uterine artery embolization and laparoscopic uterine artery ligation for uterine myoma. *Yonsei Med J* 2003;44:694–702.

56. Broder MS, Goodwin S, Chen G, et al. Comparison of long-term outcomes of myomectomy and uterine artery embolization. *Obstet Gynecol* 2002;100:864–868.

57. Subramanian S, Spies JB. Uterine artery embolization for leiomyomata: resource use and cost estimation. *J Vasc Interv Radiol* 2001;12:571–574.

58. Baker CM, Winkel CA, Subramanian S, et al. Estimated costs for uterine artery embolization and abdominal myomectomy for uterine leiomyomata: a comparative study at a single institution. *J Vasc Interv Radiol* 2002;13:1207–1210.

59. Beinfeld MT, Bosch JL, Isaacson KB, et al. Cost-effectiveness of uterine artery embolization and hysterectomy for uterine fibroids. *Radiology* 2004;230:207–213.

60. Al-Fozan H, Dufort J, Kaplow M, et al. Cost analysis of myomectomy, hysterectomy, and uterine artery embolization. *Am J Obstet Gynecol* 2002;187:1401–1404.

12

MANAGEMENT OF COMPLICATIONS

GARY SISKIN

INTRODUCTION

Since the first reports of its use as a therapeutic option for women with symptomatic uterine fibroids, uterine artery embolization has become increasingly accepted as therapy for this patient population. With the increasing frequency of its use in this setting, a greater understanding of both the potential risks and the potential benefits of this procedure has developed. This has provided interventionalists with the knowledge to convey information to both patients and gynecologists concerning the complications that can occur as a result of the UAE procedure and strategies to manage these complications.

Frequency of Complications

In trying to determine the frequency of complications that occur during and after UAE, it quickly becomes apparent how difficult it is to obtain these data because of inconsistent reporting of complications and inherent differences in how physicians define complications or, more specifically, the significance of complications. This difficulty can be addressed by considering the classification systems established by the Society of Cardiovascular and Interventional Radiology (SCVIR) (Table 12-1), as well as a modified system established by the American College of Obstetrics and Gynecology (ACOG) for perioperative complications (Table 12-2). Using the SCVIR system, one can distinguish between minor (classes A–C) and major (classes D–F) complications. In a review of outcomes after UAE in 400 patients, Spies et al. (1) reported a minor complication rate of 10% and a major complication rate of 1.25%, with no complications resulting in either permanent adverse sequelae or death. A majority of the complications reported in this series required either no or nominal therapy without consequences using the SCVIR classification system. When the modified ACOG system was used, Spies et al. (1) reported that the overall morbidity after UAE was 5%. This highlights the low short-term complication rate seen in association with UAE.

TABLE 12-1. SOCIETY OF CARDIOVASCULAR AND INTERVENTIONAL RADIOLOGY CLASSIFICATION SYSTEM DEFINITIONS OF POSTPROCEDURAL COMPLICATIONS

Class	Description
A	No therapy, no consequences
B	Nominal therapy, observation, no consequences
C	Required therapy, minor hospitalization (<48 hr)
D	Major therapy, unplanned increase in level of care, prolonged hospitalization (>48 hr)
E	Permanent adverse sequelae
F	Death

In trying to determine the actual complication rate during and after UAE, it is just as important to understand how these rates compare with accepted surgical therapy for uterine fibroids, including hysterectomy and myomectomy. With techniques for both hysterectomy and myomectomy continuously evolving, it seems that the reported complication rates are evolving as well; therefore, it may not be appropriate to dwell on complication rates associated with open surgery when so many of the procedures performed today are utilizing vaginal, hysteroscopic, and laparoscopic approaches. In 2000, Sawin et al. (2) reported on the complications of abdominal hysterectomy and myomectomy for the treatment of uterine fibroids. Using the modified ACOG criteria, the overall morbidity rate for myomectomy was 38.6%, and the overall morbidity rate for hysterectomy was 40.1%. Fever was the most commonly reported complication in association with these procedures, accounting for 85% of myomectomy complications and 60% of hysterectomy complications. Sawin et al. (2) reported a 1.5% incidence of life-threatening events associated with myomectomy and a 1.0% incidence associated with hysterectomy. This is similar to the 0.5% incidence of life-threatening events reported by Spies et al. (1). In similar studies, Shen et al. (3) reviewed their experience with laparoscopically assisted vaginal hysterectomy and reported a major complication rate of 1.3%, and Takamizawa et al. (4) reported a major complication rate of

TABLE 12-2. MODIFIED AMERICAN COLLEGE OF OBSTETRICS AND GYNECOLOGY CLASSIFICATION SYSTEM FOR POSTPROCEDURAL COMPLICATIONS

Morbidity Indicator	Definition
Febrile morbidity	Occurrence of infection not present on admission or initiation of antibiotics >24 hr after surgery
Hemorrhage	Gynecologic surgery with >2 units of blood, postoperative hematocrit <24% of postoperative hemoglobin concentration <8 g/dL
Unintended procedure	Unplanned removal, injury, or repair of organ during operative procedure or unplanned return to operating room for surgery during the same admission
Life-threatening events	Cardiopulmonary arrest, resuscitation, unplanned admission to special (intensive) care unit, or death
Readmission	Unplanned readmission within 14 days or admission after return visit to the emergency department for the same problem

1.4% in association with hysterectomy. These results demonstrate that the risk of major complications is similar for these procedures.

Few studies have directly compared the risks associated with hysterectomy and/or myomectomy with UAE. McLucas and Adler (5) compared patients undergoing myomectomy and embolization and found a higher rate of blood transfusions and longer length of hospital stay for patients undergoing myomectomy. The requirement for blood transfusions is a well-established risk of myomectomy that remains with the use of laparoscopic techniques (6,7). Razavi et al. (8) presented similar findings, concluding that myomectomy required a longer length of stay and had a higher complication rate (25% vs. 11%) compared with myomectomy. Pinto et al. (9) reported the results of a prospective, randomized study comparing hysterectomy with UAE and found that hysterectomy was associated with both a longer hospital stay and a higher rate of major complications. The specific major complications reported in association with hysterectomy included deep venous thrombosis (DVT), abscess, and bleeding requiring transfusion, whereas DVT was the only major complication associated with UAE. All of these studies consisted of small patient populations, thereby limiting the power of their conclusions, but they are consistent in reporting fewer major complications in association with UAE than with abdominal hysterectomy and myomectomy. Comparisons between embolization and less invasive surgical techniques including hysteroscopic myomectomy and laparoscopically assisted vaginal hysterectomy are not yet available.

INTRAPROCEDURAL COMPLICATIONS
Angiographic Complications

The intraprocedural complications associated with the UAE procedure are in large part related to the fact that this is an angiographic procedure. As such, patients are at risk for the complications typically associated with arterial catheterization procedures. Complications that can occur at the common femoral artery puncture site include formation of a hematoma, pseudoaneurysm, or arteriovenous fistula, dissection or thrombosis of the common femoral artery, and infection. In patient populations more likely to undergo femoral catheterization procedures, such as patients with coronary or peripheral arterial disease, the most commonly encountered puncture site complication is formation of a hematoma. Although hematomas large enough to require operative repair are rare after angiography, occurring in 0.5% of patients, the incidence of minor hematomas has been reported to be as high as 11% for diagnostic angiographic studies and as high as 18% for arterial interventional procedures (10–12). The other puncture site complications are also rare, with a less than 1% incidence similar to that of major hematomas (10). Fortunately, the population of patients undergoing the uterine fibroid embolization procedure tends to be a healthier group of patients than those studied to determine these complication rates. Kruse and Cragg (13) demonstrated that the complication rate during outpatient angiographic (both diagnostic and interventional) procedures increases in patients with poorly controlled diabetes mellitus, uncontrolled hypertension, significant renal insufficiency, cardiopulmonary failure, and coagulopathy. Although the incidence of angiographic complications in patients undergoing uterine fibroid embolization has not been specifically studied, it is likely that the absence of significant systemic arterial disease and the previously mentioned risk factors in these patients will lead to an even lower incidence of these complications.

Infection at the femoral puncture is a similarly rare occurrence that has been demonstrated to be more common in patients undergoing repeat femoral artery punctures over a short period or in patients with femoral sheaths in place for an extended period (10). Although use of prophylactic antibiotics has not been recommended for routine diagnostic angiography (14), their common use prior to uterine fibroid embolization, in addition to the universal use of aseptic technique, helps to minimize the incidence of puncture site infection (15).

Manipulation of a catheter and guidewire as they pass through the arterial system on the way to selectively catheterizing the uterine arteries can potentially lead to arterial dissection, arterial perforation, and vasospasm. Subintimal passage of the guidewire or catheter results in arterial dissection, which can ultimately lead to vessel occlusion. This can potentially prohibit both selective catheterization and effective embolization of the target vessel. This is a rare complication, but it can occur given the tortuous nature of the uterine arteries. If this occurs, options include proceeding with embolization if the catheter has been positioned in the uterine artery and antegrade flow is present or returning to the vessel at a later time (either after contralateral UAE or on a different day) for selective catheterization and embolization (15). Vessel perforation is even more unusual than arterial dissection but may be problematic because it can cause either occlusion of the uterine artery prior to embolization or bleeding from the perforated vessel, which may itself require embolization as treatment.

Nontarget Embolization

Nontarget embolization can occur if embolic material enters a vessel other than the uterine artery. This can occur due to either catheterization of a vessel other than the uterine artery or reflux of embolic material in a retrograde fashion out of the uterine artery and subsequently into a vessel originating more distal than the uterine artery from the anterior division of the internal iliac artery. Appropriate knowledge of pelvic arterial anatomy should help eliminate the first potential cause of nontarget embolization. Careful fluoroscopic monitoring during the administration of embolic material into the uterine artery should eliminate the second.

The potential effects of nontarget embolization warrant this type of monitoring and concern during UAE procedures. An awareness of nontarget embolization was established more than two decades ago in association with pelvic arterial embolization procedures performed for a variety of different indications. Early reports demonstrated the potential risks of paresis as well as bladder and muscle necrosis during pelvic embolization procedures (16,17), risks that still exist in association with UAE because all vessels arising from the internal iliac artery are potentially at risk for nontarget embolization. This risk was highlighted by Yeagley et al. (18) in their report of a patient who developed labial necrosis after UAE. The patient in their report presented 5 days after embolization with vulvar pain and a tender, hypopigmented, necrotic-appearing area on the labium. Ultimately, this patient's pain was successfully managed with medication, and the labial lesion was self-limited, resolving completely within 4 weeks. This finding was attributed to nontarget embolization into the internal pudendal artery, possibly due to retrograde reflux of embolic particles. Although reports of misembolization to date have been limited to pelvic structures, it is possible that the arterial circulation to the lower extremity is also at risk in extreme cases of nontarget embolization, potentially resulting in dysesthesias and digital ischemia (15).

In 2000, Lai et al. (19) reported on a patient who experienced sexual dysfunction, that is, a loss of orgasm response to sexual stimulation, after UAE. The finding was potentially attributed to embolization of the cervicovaginal branch of the uterine artery, again highlighting the potential risk of nontarget embolization during this procedure. The cervicovaginal branch can often be visualized angiographically arising from the distal descending segment or proximal transverse segment of the uterine artery. It is believed that this vessel is responsible for supplying the uterovaginal plexus, which consists of the nerves surrounding and innervating the cervix and upper vagina (15). Thakar et al. (20) reported sexual dysfunction after hysterectomy due to nerve injury, so it is certainly possible that ischemia induced by angiographic occlusion of this vessel can lead to reductions in sexual arousal and orgasm. Although the patient presented by Lai et al. ultimately recovered her clitoral orgasm, this case has led many practicing interventionalists to adopt the practice of positioning the angiographic catheter beyond the origin of the cervicovaginal branch during UAE procedures. By doing this, the embolic material administered through this catheter will be delivered to tissue beyond this branch, potentially sparing the uterovaginal nerve plexus from the ischemic effects of the embolization procedure.

It is important to remember that although Lai et al. theorized about this potential risk associated with UAE in their single case, there is no proof of this supposition. In addition, this case occurred early in the UCLA experience, at a time when complete occlusion of the uterine artery by polyvinyl alcohol, with a supplemental Gelfoam pledget, was the standard. It must also be stated that several published abstracts have demonstrated the potential beneficial effect that UAE may have on female sexuality. In 2001, Ammann et al. (21) and Wysoki et al. (22) reported that UAE had no adverse effects on sexual function, and some patients reported improvement after embolization. Similar findings were reported by Lvoff et al. (23) and Watkinson et al. (24) in 2002. These preliminary reports speak well for UAE with regard to preservation of female sexual function, but it is important to recognize the potential harm of embolization in terms of sexual function. Additional research is needed in this area.

A final area of concern is in other branches of the uterine artery to the bladder and the distal ureter. There are no published reports, but there are anecdotal rare reports of injuries to these structures, so care is needed to prevent misembolization into these structures.

Radiation Injury

Because UAE requires the use of fluoroscopic guidance, the potential effects of radiation exposure to the uterus and ovaries must be taken into account when determining the risks of this procedure. To date, there have been no published reports of radiation-induced injury in association with UAE. However, given that a significant percentage of patients undergoing UAE have a desire to preserve their fertility in hopes of having children, the true effects of radiation exposure in this population may not be known for several years.

As yet there is no consensus as to the true radiation dose experienced by patients during the UAE procedure. Although the techniques used by Nikolic et al. (25) and Andrews et al. (26,27) differed in the methodology used to measure radiation exposure during UAE, both agree that this exposure is far below the thresholds required to cause either clinically detectable skin injury or ovarian failure. Skin injury and ovarian failure have been reported at thresholds of 200 and 400 cGy, respectively (28). Even with the knowledge that typical fluoroscopy times are not associated with radiation-induced injury, it remains the responsibility of the interventionalist performing the procedure to limit radiation exposure to the patient whenever possible. Techniques such as utilizing low-dose or pulsed fluoroscopy, raising the patient away from the beam source, minimizing the distance between the patient and image intensifier, minimizing the use of oblique projections, magnification, and road mapping, and limiting the number of images acquired can all be helpful in reducing radiation exposure to the patient during embolization or any angiographic procedure (27,29). Techniques specific to UAE, such as bilateral common femoral artery access and elimination of an initial flush aortogram to search for collateral supply to the uterus, can be utilized as well (29).

Another method to consider as a way to reduce radiation exposure during embolization is to gain experience with the UAE procedure. It is well established that increasing one's experience with this procedure can and does lead to significant reductions in overall procedure time (27% reduction in procedure time with experience) and fluoroscopy time (24% reduction in fluoroscopy time with experience) (25,26,30). It is clear that, with experience, the potential risk of radiation exposure to this patient population can be reduced to the point where it should no longer be of concern to any patient. However, patients actively seeking to become pregnant should be counseled not to engage in unprotected intercourse during the menstrual cycle prior to the procedure in order to reduce the incidence of radiation-induced injury to a developing embryo.

POSTPROCEDURAL COMPLICATIONS

Ovarian Failure

Onset of amenorrhea and other symptoms of menopause are well-documented complications following UAE, occurring in fewer than 5% of patients but reported to be as high as 14% in at least one report (31–34). Symptoms commonly associated with the onset of menopause, including vaginal dryness, hot flashes, mood swings, and night sweats, have been reported after UAE. Often, these symptoms are temporary and resolve spontaneously in a few weeks.

However, both temporary and permanent amenorrhea, although rare, can occur after this procedure. Although the incidence of this complication can be considered low based on these data, the impact of this complication can be quite significant, especially in patients wishing to preserve fertility options after embolization.

Temporary amenorrhea has been attributed to endometrial ischemia induced by the UAE procedure, most commonly in patients near the age of menopause. At the present time, the mechanism for permanent ovarian failure after embolization has not been definitively demonstrated. However, several theories have been proposed as explanations for this complication. Current theory begins with the known occurrence of anastomoses between the arterial blood supply of the uterine and the ovaries (35). As a result of these anastomoses, embolic material administered within the uterine arteries can potentially make their way into the ovarian arterial circulation, increasing the risk of reduced ovarian perfusion and subsequent ischemia. This theory is supported by the demonstration of angiographically visible anastomoses between these two arterial beds by Razavi et al. (36). In addition, Payne et al. (37) described the presence of ovarian ischemia and tris-acryl gelatin microspheres in the ovarian arterial vasculature, within an oophorectomy specimen obtained after UAE. Adjusting the size of the embolic agent so that it will not traverse the ovarian arcades is one approach to preventing ovarian injury. Pelage et al. (38) observed microspheres smaller than 500 μm in diameter within the ovarian arterial circulation after UAE performed in sheep, which may offer some guidance as to particle size selection for this procedure.

Data from a small study reported by Ryu et al. (39) may shed some light on the impact of UAE on ovarian arterial flow. Using ovarian Doppler flow measurements, Ryu et al. demonstrated that 50% of patients have decreased ovarian arterial flow after UAE. Given the high incidence of diminished ovarian perfusion after UAE, one might expect an equally high incidence of ovarian failure in this patient population. However, this is not the case based on the reported incidence of this complication as described previously. Certainly, the degree to which the ovaries rely on the uterine arteries as a source of arterial blood flow is variable and likely represents a contributing factor (albeit a difficult one to measure) to the occurrence of ovarian failure after UAE.

It is more likely that the answer to this question lies with the observation that this complication is age related. Chrisman et al. (31) reported results from 66 patients undergoing UAE and reported a 14% incidence of ovarian failure in this population. When stratified by age, Chrisman et al. found that all of the patients who experienced ovarian failure after embolization were older than 45 years, leading to an ovarian failure rate of 43% after UAE in this patient population. Spies et al. (32) reported that patients older than 45 years are at higher risk for experiencing significant increases in follicle-stimulating hormone (FSH) levels compared to baseline. Based on this study, Spies et al. concluded that there is an approximately 15% chance of a significant change in FSH levels after UAE in patients older than 45 years. FSH levels are commonly used to measure ovarian function, with higher serum levels corresponding to reduced ovarian function. Ahmad et al. (40) observed no significant changes in menstruation or FSH levels in 30 patients younger than 45 years. However, these investigators also observed that two patients with higher FSH levels and irregular menses prior to the procedure experienced transient amenorrhea after the procedure, highlighting the increased risk in older patients. All of these studies suggest a direct relationship between increasing age and an increased risk for developing permanent ovarian failure after UAE.

Thirty-five years ago, Beavis et al. (41) theorized that functional ovarian reserve decreases with age, specifically with regard to the function of residual ovarian tissue after oophorectomy. The ovaries of younger patients have a greater degree of functional reserve than the ovaries of older patients and may recover without significant functional impairment after embolization. Payne et al. (37) theorized that the sequelae of UAE may depend on the number of oocytes lost as a result of the procedure. Amenorrhea results from a complete loss of oocytes, transient or long-term oligomenorrhea results from a significant depletion of oocytes, and early menopause results when the number of oocytes is reduced below a critical threshold (37). Similarly, Chrisman and Sterling (15) theorized that vascular flow in older ovaries may differ from that in younger ovaries, making them potentially more susceptible to the effects of the embolic material used during UAE.

Regardless of the mechanism, the risk of menopausal changes after embolization appears to be negligible in patients younger than 45 years at the time of the embolization procedure. Despite this, younger patients, especially those interested in preserving fertility, must be made aware of this risk and be encouraged to seek information regarding the risks and benefits of other treatment options before considering UAE.

Uterine Infection

One of the potentially more serious complications of UAE is infection after embolization. This was one of the first complications of embolization reported by Goodwin et al. (42) in 1997. In this initial case series, Goodwin et al. described a patient who experienced increasing pelvic pain, fever to 40°C (104°F), and leukocytosis of 22,000/mm³ 3 weeks after UAE. Despite the use of intravenous antibiotics, the fever persisted, and a hysterectomy was performed, revealing endometritis with endometrial necrosis, pyometra, and chronic salpingitis. Additional reports by Robson et al. (43) and Payne and Haney (44) described cases of pelvic sepsis after UAE. However, when several of the largest

published series are considered in aggregate, the overall rate of significant infection after embolization remains low and can be estimated at <1% (33,34,45–47). It has been suggested that submucosal fibroids or intramural fibroids with a significant submucosal component may be at increased risk for infection after embolization due to the potential for bacteria from the endometrial cavity to seed ischemic tissue (47).

The severity of this particular complication was made clear by Vashisht et al. (48) in 1999 when a postembolization infection resulted in the death of a 51-year-old patient. During the embolization procedure, 355- to 500-µm polyvinyl alcohol particles were used to embolize both uterine arteries. After an immediate postprocedural period highlighted by a urinary tract infection 3 days after the procedure, the patient returned to the hospital on day 7 with abdominal pain, diarrhea, vomiting, and fever (38.5°C). Evaluation revealed pelvic tenderness, an elevated white blood cell count, and evidence of disseminated intravascular coagulation. Intravenous antibiotics were administered, but the patient ultimately became hypotensive and oliguric, prompting laparotomy, total abdominal hysterectomy, and bilateral salpingo-oophorectomy. Blood cultures ultimately were positive for *Escherichia coli*. Two weeks later, the patient died of a massive hemothorax and multiorgan failure.

It is often difficult to know exactly how to manage patients who present with signs that might indicate the presence of a uterine infection after embolization. The diagnosis is made even more difficult by the fact that fever is often seen during the normal postprocedural recovery period (49,50). When patients present with these symptoms after embolization, interventionalists must differentiate between the onset of a uterine infection and either a prolonged or delayed postembolization syndrome. The case reported by Vashisht et al. (48), however, indicates the potential severity of this complication and the need to be proactive in addressing any symptoms potentially indicative of infection. Even the initial report of Goodwin et al. (42) in 1997 recommended that any patient presenting with delayed fever or pelvic pain should be carefully evaluated and that both cross-sectional pelvic imaging and initiation of antibiotic therapy should be considered. Therefore, patients with a fever, purulent discharge, or other symptoms suggestive of a uterine infection should be evaluated with a pelvic examination, laboratory tests including a complete blood count and blood and urine cultures, and imaging. In the presence of significant uterine infection, cervical motion tenderness is often present on pelvic examination. Caution is advised when using pelvic computed tomography in this scenario because gas bubbles are often seen within the embolized fibroid, even in patients without signs and symptoms suggestive of infection (15,45).

When a patient presents with potential infection, the initial selection of intravenous antibiotics should be broad spectrum in coverage until culture results indicate more directed therapy. These infections may be mixed flora, although Gram-negative aerobes and anaerobes should be considered likely pathogens.

With the risk of infection always present in these patients, one should consider the use of prophylactic antibiotics prior to embolization; however, a consensus has not yet been reached regarding prophylactic antibiotics (15). Whereas some centers do not use antibiotics because of the rarity of infectious complications, those centers that do use antibiotics administer either cefazolin for cutaneous prophylaxis or a regimen of gentamicin and clindamycin to address the organisms most likely to cause this type of infection (50,51). In patients who receive antibiotics, there is a small but real risk of *Clostridium difficile* infection, as previously reported (1).

Uterine Infarction

Transcatheter occlusion of the uterine arteries during UAE clearly increases the risk of global uterine ischemia and subsequent infarction in patients undergoing the procedure. In fact, it is fair to assume that transient uterine ischemia occurs in most patients undergoing this procedure and that this ischemia likely contributes to the postprocedural pain commonly experienced by most patients after embolization. However, in rare cases, this transient ischemia worsens to the point where the uterus becomes globally infarcted, most likely because an extensive collateral network exists within the pelvis in general and within the uterus more specifically. It has been well established that the uterus is able to draw arterial supply from a variety of vessels, including the ovarian arteries, vaginal arteries, and round ligament arteries (36,52,53). Imaging studies have been helpful in confirming myometrial perfusion and the absence of myometrial ischemia in patients after UAE (1,54,55). In addition, the gradual shift in embolization endpoint from complete stasis of uterine arterial flow to slow but persistent flow in the main uterine artery may be responsible for leaving sufficient arterial flow to support the normal portions of the myometrium (56).

Despite all of the factors limiting the risk of ischemia in the normal myometrium, there have still been rare reports of diffuse uterine ischemia and necrosis after UAE. The typical, benign presentation of uterine ischemia consists of long-standing pelvic pain that persists for several weeks beyond the expected postembolization syndrome, fever, and an elevated white blood cell count (15). Contrast-enhanced pelvic MRI may be useful in this setting to confirm the presence of uterine perfusion after embolization (15,57). Ultimately, these patients may require a hysterectomy for pain relief. This has been the clinical scenario reported in association with this complication (50,58,59). One possible sequela of uterine ischemia and necrosis is uterine rupture, which was reported by Shashoua et al. (60). Although the reported risk of uterine necrosis and subsequent rupture is

far less than 1%, steps such as preventing complete stasis during embolization may help reduce this risk even more.

Vaginal Discharge and Transcervical Fibroid Expulsion

A commonly reported complication after UAE is persistent vaginal discharge (1,34). This discharge, which is often brown or red-brown, can begin within days of the embolization procedure and can last for several months. Khilnani et al. (61) reported a mean discharge duration of 7 months (range 0.8–25 months) in patients having submucosal fibroids or intramural fibroids with a significant submucosal component. Patients should be advised that a purulent-appearing discharge associated with pelvic pain and fever can be suggestive of a uterine infection, and these patients should be evaluated appropriately.

The more commonly occurring brown or red-brown discharge, however, is a potential sign of impending transcervical passage of an embolized fibroid. This event has been well described and frequently reported both in case reports and larger case series studying UAE (33,34,47,62–65). This has been reported to occur both immediately after the embolization procedure and after a period as long as 1 year or more (1). Typically, patients experiencing passage of a fibroid report symptoms including discharge (with or without bleeding), crampy pelvic pain, and possibly urinary retention (45); these symptoms are often severe enough to require hospitalization (1). Patients with an increased risk for expulsion include those with submucosal fibroids and those with intramural fibroids that have significant contact with the endometrial cavity (1).

Transcervical fibroid passage often occurs without incident, but it may become complicated. Arrested passage of the fibroid with retention of fibroid fragments within the endometrial cavity or cervical canal can increase the risk of infection after embolization. It is often possible to identify arrested passage with the use of magnetic resonance imaging, which is often performed in this scenario given that the symptoms presented by patients in this setting are similar to those of patients experiencing a uterine infection after embolization (Fig. 12-1). With the assistance of imaging, it may be possible to identify an unattached fibroid fragment or even pyometra due to uterine obstruction (15). If retention of a fibroid fragment is suspected, a prompt gynecologic referral is indicated so that the fibroid can be resected hysteroscopically or by cervical dilation and evacuation of the uterine cavity before the fragment is seeded and an infection develops.

OTHER COMPLICATIONS
Allergic Reactions

The most common complication reported by Spies et al. (1) was rashes and allergic reactions after embolization, which

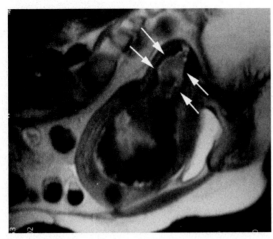

FIGURE 12-1. Sagittal nonenhanced T2-weighted magnetic resonance image of the pelvis reveals a large submucosal fibroid. The patient had undergone uterine embolization several weeks earlier when she presented with sudden onset of significant uterine cramping. The image shows the fibroid is being expelled into the cervical canal, which has started to dilate *(arrows).*

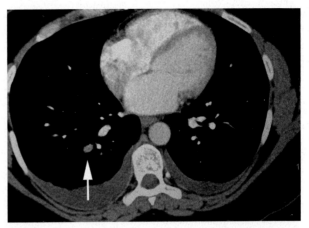

FIGURE 12-2. Axial contrast computed tomographic image of the thorax demonstrates a small pulmonary embolus *(arrow)* in a patient 3 days after uterine embolization.

occurred in 2.5% of their study population. In most cases, these reactions could be explained by allergies to medications given before, during, or after the procedure for pain control or antibiotic prophylaxis. These reactions were easily treatable with medications such as diphenhydramine or corticosteroids. In other cases, the cause of the reaction remained unexplained. Potential causes include latex allergies, unrecognized medication allergies, or reactions to the embolic material used during the embolization procedure. Late rashes have been reported, and, in particular, an allergic-type, noninfective endometritis linked to gold-colored tris-acryl gelatin microspheres (Embogold) (66). For this reason, this product is no longer recommended for use in uterine fibroid embolization. Standard tris-acryl gelatin microspheres (Embosphere) have not been associated with this complication and remain one of the primary embolics used for this procedure.

Pulmonary Embolus

As is the case with most invasive procedures, DVT and pulmonary embolus are rare but potential complications of the UAE procedure (1,67). This may be especially true in this patient population in which oral contraception, which is known to be associated with an increased risk for venous thromboembolic disease (68), is commonly used. This fact, combined with the prevalence of smoking in the general population and the fact that these patients are undergoing an invasive procedure, increases the risk of thromboembolic disease in this population (69). It has been suggested that diminished flow in pelvic veins may lead to stasis (70), prompting thrombus formation, but there is no documen-

tation that this occurs. It is known that operative procedures in which tissue injury occurs can trigger a transient hypercoagulable state, and this has been demonstrated with UAE (71). Although the hypercoagulability associated with UAE is not as severe as that seen with surgery and the duration of immobility after UAE is brief, these patients are temporarily at increased risk for thromboembolic events (Fig. 12-2).

At least two deaths have been reported in association with pulmonary embolic disease after UAE. One of these cases was presented at the Society for Minimally Invasive Therapy meeting in 1999 (67). It is not clear if prophylactic measures will reduce the risk, given that the apparent incidence of pulmonary embolus is less than 1 in 250 (1). Simple automated venous compression devices are used by some, although the efficacy is unclear. The risk of routine prophylactic antithrombotics may outweigh the risk of thrombotic complications. Thus, no clear recommendation can be made without further study.

It is important to obtain a medical history prior to embolization in order to uncover risk factors for venous thromboembolic disease. Once these risk factors are revealed, consideration can be given to initiate prophylactic measures, such as administration of heparin or use of lower extremity compression stockings, to reduce the risk of venous thromboembolic disease. If a patient has a personal or family history of hypercoagulability, then consultation with a hematologist or internist regarding the best means of prophylaxis in the periprocedural period should be considered.

Embolization of Leiomyosarcoma

It is inevitable that interventionalists will perform the UAE procedure on a patient with a leiomyosarcoma instead of the more common benign leiomyomata. Leiomyosarcoma of the uterus is a very uncommon tumor, with an incidence of less than 0.5% (72,73). This type of uterine cancer is extremely aggressive, with spread outside of the uterus commonly seen in the liver, lungs, and bone. Once extrauterine disease is present, the 5-year survival rates decrease from 50% to 20% (74).

Given the aggressive nature of leiomyosarcoma, interventionalists should always consider this diagnosis in every patient being evaluated for the UAE procedure. The difficulty in distinguishing between a leiomyoma and leiomyosarcoma is that there are no clinical or imaging features that clearly allow differentiation between these two entities. It is tempting to say that rapid fibroid growth may be indicative of sarcomatous transformation, but this is not necessarily the case. In fact, Parker et al. (73) reviewed patients known to have uterine sarcomas and found that only 2.6% of these patients experienced rapid growth of their tumors prior to diagnosis, making this a poor method to distinguish between benign fibroids and malignant leiomyosarcomas. Because most patients undergo either pelvic MRI or ultrasound prior to embolization, one can hope that imaging findings may distinguish between these entities, but this is not the case. Early ultrasound data revealed that hypoechoic changes within a uterine mass, indicating degeneration, is present in more than 70% of uterine leiomyosarcomas, but these changes are commonly seen within benign fibroids as well (75). Hata et al. (76) have reported that peak systolic velocities within leiomyosarcomas are significantly higher than those detected within benign fibroids but that there is no significant difference in the resistive indices obtained from within these two tumors. Although most agree that needle biopsy is not a useful technique to differentiate these two tumors, there are studies that support the use of a biopsy in this setting. Barbazza et al. (77) and Shibata et al. (78) reported sensitivity rates of 92.5% and specificity rates of 100% for needle biopsy as a test to diagnose uterine leiomyosarcoma. McLucas et al. (79) have been consistent advocates of laparoscopy and biopsy prior to UAE, but it is not yet clear whether this approach can be justified because of its inconsistent ability to diagnose leiomyosarcoma (15).

Cases of UAE performed in patients who were suspected of having benign fibroids but actually had a leiomyosarcoma have been reported (74,80). Al-Badr and Faught (80) reported a case in which UAE resulted in a fibroid fragment being passed out of the vagina. Biopsy of this fragment revealed a poorly differentiated, high-grade leiomyosarcoma. The timely diagnosis in this case allowed for a prompt hysterectomy to be performed in this patient. The situation was different in the case reported by Common et al. (74). In their case, UAE was successfully performed, but continued growth of the fibroid prompted hysterectomy 6 months after embolization. During surgery, adhesions between the mass and mesentery and extensive parasitization of blood from the adjacent ligaments and mesentery were noted.

Eventually, this patient required radiation therapy as treatment for leiomyosarcoma, which was diagnosed from the hysterectomy specimen.

In light of the difficulty in diagnosing leiomyosarcoma prior to embolization, one must take the lesson learned from Common et al. and apply it to the routine follow-up of patients after embolization. This case alone supports the use of follow-up imaging after embolization because failure to respond to embolization warrants consideration of a malignant diagnosis and a subsequent recommendation for surgical exploration (15).

CONCLUSION

UAE is a safe and effective procedure to offer to patients with symptomatic uterine fibroids. The risk of major complications, including pulmonary embolus, uterine infection, uterine infarction, and arterial injury associated with femoral catheterization, is low, and many of these complications are potentially treatable without surgery. By gaining an understanding of these complications and the other minor complications described in this chapter, practicing interventionalists can properly counsel patients regarding the risks associated with the procedure. In addition, this understanding enables interventionalists to effectively manage patients after embolization and to direct the additional care required in a small number of patients.

REFERENCES

1. Spies JB, Spector A, Roth AR, et al. Complications of uterine artery embolization for leiomyomata. *Obstet Gynecol* 2002;100: 873–880.
2. Sawin SW, Pilevsky ND, Berlin JA, et al. Comparability of perioperative morbidity between abdominal myomectomy and hysterectomy for women with uterine leiomyomas. *Am J Obstet Gynecol* 2000;183:1448–1455.
3. Shen CC, Wu MP, Kung FT, et al. Major complications associated with laparoscopic-assisted vaginal hysterectomy: ten-year experience. *J Am Assoc Gynecol Laparosc* 2003;10:147–153.
4. Takamizawa S, Minakami H, Usui R, et al. Risk of complications and uterine malignancies in women undergoing hysterectomy for presumed benign leiomyomas. *Gynecol Obstet Invest* 1999;48: 193–196.
5. McLucas B, Adler L. Uterine fibroid embolization compared with myomectomy. *Int J Gynaecol Obstet* 2001;74:297–299.
6. Boyd ME. Myomectomy. *Can J Surg* 1986;29:161–163.
7. Landi S, Zaccoletti R, Ferrari L, et al. Laparoscopic myomectomy: technique, complications, and ultrasound scan evaluations. *J Am Assoc Gynecol Laparosc* 2001;8:231–240.
8. Razavi MK, Hwang G, Jahed A, et al. Abdominal myomectomy versus uterine fibroid embolization in the treatment of symptomatic uterine leiomyomas. *AJR Am J Roentgenol* 2003;180: 1571–1575.
9. Pinto I, Chimeno P, Romo A, et al. Uterine fibroids: uterine artery embolization versus abdominal hysterectomy for treatment: a prospective, randomized, and controlled clinical trial. *Radiology* 2003;226:425–531.

10. Singh H, Cardella JF, Cole PE, et al. Quality improvement guidelines for diagnostic angiography. *J Vasc Interv Radiol* 2002;13:1–6.

11. Cragg AH, Nakagawa N, Smith TP, et al. Hematoma formation after diagnostic arteriography: effect of catheter size. *J Vasc Interv Radiol* 1991;2:231–233.

12. Young N, Chi KK, Asaka J, et al. Complications with outpatient angiography and interventional procedures. *Cardiovasc Interv Radiol* 2002;25:123–126.

13. Kruse JR, Cragg AH. Safety of short stay observation after peripheral vascular intervention. *J Vasc Interv Radiol* 2000;11:45–49.

14. McDermitt VG, Schuster MG, Smith TP. Antibiotic prophylaxis in vascular and interventional radiology. *AJR Am J Roentgenol* 1997;169:31–38.

15. Sterling KM, Vogelzang RL, Chrisman HB, et al. Uterine fibroid embolization: management of complications. *Tech Vasc Interv Radiol* 2002;5:56–66.

16. Hare WSC, Holland CJ. Paresis following internal iliac artery embolization. *Radiology* 1983;146:47–51.

17. Lang EK. Transcatheter embolization of pelvic vessels for control of intractable hemorrhage. *Radiology* 1981;140:331–339.

18. Yeagley TJ, Goldberg J, Klein TA, et al. Labial necrosis after uterine artery embolization for leiomyomata. *Obstet Gynecol* 2002;100:881–882.

19. Lai AC, Goodwin SC, Bonilla SM, et al. Sexual dysfunction after uterine artery embolization. *J Vasc Interv Radiol* 2000;11:755–758.

20. Thakar R, Manyonda I, Stanton SL, et al. Bladder, bowel, and sexual function after hysterectomy for benign conditions. *Br J Obstet Gynaecol* 1997;104:983–987.

21. Ammann AM, Gomez-Jorge JT, Spies JB. Sexual function after uterine embolization. *J Vasc Interv Radiol* 2001;12[Pt 2]:S76.

22. Wysoki M, Byrd BP, Onze K, et al. Sexual function after uterine fibroid embolization. *J Vasc Interv Radiol* 2001;12[Pt 2]:S77.

23. Lvoff NM, Omary RA, Chrisman HB, et al. Uterine artery embolization and female sexual function. *J Vasc Interv Radiol* 2002;13[Pt 2]:S65–S66.

24. Watkinson A, Robertson FJ, Babar S, et al. Impact of uterine artery embolization on sexual function. *J Vasc Interv Radiol* 2002;13[Pt 2]:S66.

25. Nikolic B, Spies JB, Lundsten MJ, et al. Patient radiation dose associated with uterine artery embolization. *Radiology* 2000;214:121–125.

26. Andrews RT, Brown PH. Uterine arterial embolization: factors influencing patient radiation exposure. *Radiology* 2000;217:713–722.

27. Worthington-Kirsch RL, Andrews RT, Siskin GP, et al. Uterine fibroid embolization: technical aspects. *Tech Vasc Interv Radiol* 2002;5:17–34.

28. Nikolic B, Spies JB, Campbell L, et al. Uterine artery embolization: reduced radiation with refined technique. *J Vasc Interv Radiol* 2001;12:39–44.

29. Wagner LK, Eifel PJ, Geise RA. Potential biological effects following high X-ray dose interventional procedures. *J Vasc Interv Radiol* 2000;11:25–33.

30. Pron G, Bennett J, Common A, et al. Technical results and effects of operator experience on uterine artery embolization for fibroids: the Ontario Uterine Fibroid Embolization Trial. *J Vasc Interv Radiol* 2003;14:545–554.

31. Chrisman HB, Saker MB, Ryu RK, et al. The impact of uterine fibroid embolization on resumption of menses and ovarian function. *J Vasc Interv Radiol* 2000;11:699–703.

32. Spies JB, Roth AR, Gonsalves SM, et al. Ovarian function after uterine artery embolization for leiomyomata: assessment with use of serum follicle stimulating hormone assay. *J Vasc Interv Radiol* 2001;12:437–442.

33. Spies JB, Ascher SA, Roth AR, et al. Uterine artery embolization for leiomyomata. *Obstet Gynecol* 2001;98:29–34.

34. Walker WJ, Pelage JP. Uterine artery embolization for symptomatic fibroids: clinical results in 400 women with imaging follow-up. *BJOG* 2002;109:1262–1272.

35. Sampson J. The blood supply of uterine myomata. *Surg Gynecol Obstet* 1912;14:215–234.

36. Razavi MK, Wolanske KA, Hwang GL, et al. Angiographic classification of ovarian artery-to-uterine artery anastomoses: initial observations in uterine fibroid embolization. *Radiology* 2002;224:707–712.

37. Payne JF, Robboy SJ, Haney AF. Embolic microspheres within ovarian arterial vasculature after uterine artery embolization. *Obstet Gynecol* 2002;100:883–886.

38. Pelage JJ, Laurent A, Wasset M, et al. Uterine fibroid embolization: choice of an embolic particle. *J Vasc Interv Radiol* 2000;11[Pt 2]:S189.

39. Ryu RK, Chrisman HB, Omary RA, et al. The vascular impact of uterine artery embolization: prospective sonographic assessment of ovarian arterial circulation. *J Vasc Interv Radiol* 2001;12:1071–1074.

40. Ahmad A, Qadan L, Hassan N, et al. Uterine artery embolization treatment of uterine fibroids: effect on ovarian function in younger women. *J Vasc Interv Radiol* 2002;13:1017–1020.

41. Beavis EL, Brown JB, Smith MA. Ovarian function after hysterectomy with conservation of the ovaries in pre-menopausal women. *J Obstet Gynaecol Br Commonw* 1969;76:969–978.

42. Goodwin SC, Vedantham S, McLucas B, et al. Preliminary experience with uterine artery embolization for uterine fibroids. *J Vasc Interv Radiol* 1997;8:517–526.

43. Robson S, Wilson K, Munday D, et al. Pelvic sepsis complicating embolization of a uterine fibroid. *Aust N Z J Obstet Gynaecol* 1999;39:516–517.

44. Payne JF, Haney AF. Serious complications of uterine artery embolization for conservative treatment of fibroids. *Fertil Steril* 2003;79:128–130.

45. McLucas B, Adler L, Perrella R. Uterine fibroid embolization: nonsurgical treatment for symptomatic fibroids. *J Am Coll Surg* 2001;192:95–105.

46. Hutchins FL, Worthington-Kirsch R, Berkowitz RP. Selective uterine artery embolization as primary treatment for symptomatic leiomyomata uteri. *J Am Assoc Gynecol Laparosc* 1999;6:279–284.

47. Pelage JP, Le Dref O, Soyer P, et al. Fibroid-related menorrhagia: treatment with superselective embolization of the uterine arteries and midterm follow-up. *Radiology* 2000;215:428–431.

48. Vashisht A, Stuff J, Carey A, et al. Fatal septicaemia after fibroid embolization. *Lancet* 1999;354:307–308.

49. Bradley EA, Reidy JF, Forman RG, et al. Transcatheter uterine artery embolization to treat large uterine fibroids. *Br J Obstet Gynaecol* 1998;105:235–240.

50. Siskin GP, Stainken BF, Dowling K, et al. Outpatient uterine artery embolization for symptomatic uterine fibroids: experience in 49 patients. *J Vasc Interv Radiol* 2000;11:305–311.

51. Spies JB, Scialli AR, Jha RC, et al. Initial results from uterine fibroid embolization for symptomatic leiomyomata. *J Vasc Interv Radiol* 1999;10:1149–1157.

52. Pelage JP, Le Dref O, Soyer P, et al. Arterial anatomy of the female genital tract: variations and relevance to transcatheter embolization of the uterus. *AJR Am J Roentgenol* 1999;172:989–994.

53. Saraiya PV, Chang TC, Pelage JP, et al. Uterine artery replacement by the round ligament artery: an anatomic variant

discovered during uterine artery embolization for leiomyomata. *J Vasc Interv Radiol* 2002;13:939–941.

54. Banovac F, Ascher SM, Jones DA, et al. Magnetic resonance imaging outcome after uterine artery embolization for leiomyomata with use of tris-acryl gelatin microspheres. *J Vasc Interv Radiol* 2002;13:681–688.

55. deSouza NM, Williams AD. Uterine arterial embolization for leiomyomas: perfusion and volume changes at MR imaging and relation to clinical outcome. *Radiology* 2002;222:367–374.

56. Pelage JP, Le Dref OP, Beregi JP, et al. Limited uterine artery embolization with tris-acryl gelatin microspheres for uterine fibroids. *J Vasc Interv Radiol* 2003;14:11–14.

57. Katsumori T, Nakajima K, Tokuhiro M. Gadolinium enhanced MR imaging in the evaluation of uterine fibroids treated with uterine artery embolization. *AJR Am J Roentgenol* 2001;177:303–307.

58. Worthington-Kirsch RL, Popky GL, Hutchins FL. Uterine arterial embolization for the management of leiomyomas: quality of life assessment and clinical response. *Radiology* 1998;208:625–629.

59. Godfrey CD, Zbella EA. Uterine necrosis after uterine artery embolization for leiomyoma. *Obstet Gynecol* 2001;98:950–952.

60. Shashoua AR, Stringer NH, Pearlman JB, et al. Ischemic uterine rupture and hysterectomy 3 months after uterine artery embolization. *J Am Assoc Gynecol Laparosc* 2002;9:217–220.

61. Khilnani NM, Min RJ, Golia P. The incidence and characteristics of vaginal discharge following UFE. *J Vasc Interv Radiol* 2003;14[Pt 2]:S83.

62. Kroencke TJ, Gauruder-Burmester A, Enzweiler CN, et al. Disintegration and stepwise expulsion of a large uterine leiomyoma with restoration of the uterine architecture after successful uterine fibroid embolization: case report. *Hum Reprod* 2003;18:863–865.

63. Felemban A, Stein L, Tulandi T. Uterine restoration after repeated expulsion of myomas after uterine artery embolization. *J Am Assoc Gynecol Laparosc* 2001;8:442–444.

64. Berkowitz RP, Hutchins FL, Worthington-Kirsch RL. Vaginal expulsion of submucosal fibroids after uterine artery embolization. A report of three cases. *J Reprod Med* 1999;44:373–376.

65. Abbara S, Spies JB, Scialli AR, et al. Transcervical expulsion of a fibroid as a result of uterine artery embolization for leiomyomata. *J Vasc Interv Radiol* 1999;10:409–411.

66. Richard H. Late breaking abstract. Presented at the 2003 SIR Meeting, Salt Lake City, Utah.

67. Lanocita R, Frigerio LF, Patelli G, et al. A fatal complication of percutaneous transcatheter embolization for treatment of uterine fibroids. Presented at SMIT 1999, Boston, Massachusetts.

68. Vandenbroucke JP, Rosing J, Bloemenkamp KW, et al. Oral contraceptives and the risk of venous thrombosis. *N Engl J Med* 2001;344:1527–1535.

69. Kim V, Spandorfer J. Epidemiology of venous thromboembolic disease. *Emerg Med Clin North Am* 2001;19:839–859.

70. Tanaka H, Umekawa T, Kikukawa T, et al. Venous thromboembolic diseases associated with uterine myomas diagnosed before hysterectomy: a report of two cases. *J Obstet Gynaecol Res* 2002;28:300–303.

71. Nikolic B, Kessler C, Jacobs H, et al. Changes in blood coagulation markers associated with uterine artery embolization for leiomyomata. *J Vasc Interv Radiol* 2003;14:1147–1153.

72. Leibsohn S, d'Ablaing G, Mishell DR, et al. Leiomyosarcoma in a series of hysterectomies performed for presumed uterine leiomyomas. *Am J Obstet Gynecol* 1990;162:968–976.

73. Parker WH, Fu YS, Berek JS. Uterine sarcoma in patients operated on for presumed leiomyoma and rapidly growing leiomyoma. *Obstet Gynecol* 1994;83:414–418.

74. Common AA, Mocarski EJM, Kolin A, et al. Therapeutic failure of uterine fibroid embolization caused by underlying leiomyosarcoma. *J Vasc Interv Radiol* 2001;12:1449–1452.

75. Seki K, Hoshihara T, Nagata I. Leiomyosarcoma of the uterus: ultrasonography and serum lactate dehydrogenase level. *Gynecol Obstet Invest* 1992;33:114–118.

76. Hata K, Hata A, Maruyama R, et al. Uterine sarcoma: can it be differentiated from uterine leiomyomas with Doppler ultrasonography? A preliminary report. *Ultrasound Obstet Gynecol* 1997;9:101–104.

77. Barbazza R, Chiarelli S, Quintarelli GF, et al. Role of fine needle aspiration cytology in the preoperative evaluation of smooth muscle tumors. *Diagn Cytopathol* 1997;16:326–330.

78. Shibata S, Kawamura N, Ito F, et al. Diagnostic accuracy of needle biopsy of the uterine leiomyosarcoma. *Oncol Rep* 2000;7:595–597.

79. McLucas B, Goodwin S, Vedantham S. Embolic therapy for myomata. *Min Invas Ther Allied Technol* 1996;5:336–338.

80. Al-Badr A, Faught W. Uterine artery embolization in an undiagnosed uterine sarcoma. *Obstet Gynecol* 2001;97:836–837.

13

PREGNANCY AND UTERINE ARTERY EMBOLIZATION

JEAN-PIERRE PELAGE
WOODRUFF WALKER
DENIS JACOB
OLIVIER LE DREF

INTRODUCTION

Arterial embolization is a long-established technique for the treatment of abdominal and pelvic hemorrhage but has only recently been used to treat symptomatic uterine fibroids (1–5). Since the first report of uterine artery embolization for fibroids was published, it has been estimated that approximately 50,000 women have been treated worldwide. The results of three large prospective studies have been recently published in the gynecologic literature (6–8). These reports indicate that uterine fibroid embolization appears to be effective in controlling the symptoms in 80% to 94% of women, with a rate of complications lower than that of surgery with few complications (6–9). Two studies comparing the outcomes after embolization and surgery have also demonstrated that embolization is a valuable alternative to multiple myomectomies (10,11). Whether uterine artery embolization is a safe procedure for women desiring future fertility is still controversial (12,13). Outcome data regarding fertility after uterine artery embolization to treat symptoms other than infertility are still limited. Until recently, the majority of treated women were older than 40 and not interested in future pregnancy (6–9). However, some women who have undergone fibroid embolization have become pregnant and had successful deliveries (2,4,7,14–18).

UTERINE FIBROIDS AND INFERTILITY

The decision as to when it is appropriate to treat uterine fibroids for fertility enhancement remains a subject of debate (13,19–25). In all cases, couples should complete a full infertility assessment before the role of uterine fibroids is addressed. Reproductive dysfunction is not inevitable with the myomatous uterus, but the risk of placental abruption is substantially increased if a fibroid is under the placental site

(13,23–25). In addition, if the endometrial cavity is distorted by submucous fibroids, the risk of infertility is increased (15,20,23–25). Intramural fibroids may occlude the ostia of the intramural portion of the fallopian tube, interfere with myometrial contractility, or create abnormal vascularization (13,20). Other pregnancy complications, including premature delivery, increased risk for cesarean delivery, and postpartum hemorrhage, seem to be directly related to the size of the fibroids (13,19,20,23–25).

COMPLICATIONS ASSOCIATED WITH UTERINE ARTERY EMBOLIZATION

Several potential impediments to fertility following uterine artery embolization have been identified. Transient or permanent amenorrhea associated with other symptoms of menopause is a well-documented complication following uterine artery embolization, with a reported incidence as high as 14% (26–31). Three different mechanisms have been identified as potential causes of postembolization amenorrhea: nontarget ovarian embolization through large uteroovarian anastomoses, postembolization ischemia observed when the ovaries are mainly supplied by the uterine arteries, and endometrial atrophy in case of overembolization (4,7,9,26–31). The age of the patient at the time of treatment has a direct effect on the occurrence of ovarian failure mainly reported in women older than 45 (7,30). The technique used by the interventional radiologist might also play a role in the incidence of premature menopause. Aggressive embolization, as opposed to limited arterial embolization, as well as the use of small embolic particles, may cause ovarian or endometrial ischemia or predispose to reflux of particles to the ovarian arteries (4,7,9,32–35). In some patients, transient loss of ovarian function, as evidenced by amenorrhea, menopausal symptoms, and elevated follicle-stimulating hormone levels, was followed by recurrence of cyclic menstrual bleeding and disappearance of menopausal symptoms (2,7,26,27,29).

Chronic vaginal discharge and transcervical expulsion of uterine fibroids may interfere with future fertility (7,36,37). Submucosal fibroids and intramural fibroids that have significant contact with the endometrial cavity are associated with increased risk for expulsion or chronic discharge (7,36,37).

The potential effects of radiation exposure to the uterus and ovaries must be taken into account when determining the risks of this procedure, particularly in young women seeking future pregnancy. Fluoroscopy time and subsequent radiation exposure to women vary with the technique, experience, and skill level of the interventional radiologist (7,38–40). However, the average reported radiation dose using different catheterization and embolization techniques does not indicate a significant dose of radiation (38–40).

The reported incidence of hysterectomy as a complication of uterine artery embolization is low (1%–2%) and probably even lower in a population of properly screened patients with appropriate postembolization follow-up (4–9,41). Indications for hysterectomy are pelvic infections caused by large submucosal or pedunculated subserosal uterine fibroids, misdiagnosed urinary tract infection or previous pelvic inflammatory disease, uterine necrosis, chronic postembolization pain, and intractable vaginal hemorrhage (4,7,9,41,42). Even in case of infection, early diagnosis and management using hysteroscopic resection or abdominal myomectomy may preserve future fertility (7,43).

THEORETICAL CONSIDERATIONS

In women desiring future fertility, it is important to be aware of the possible relationship between complications associated with uterine artery embolization and pregnancy. Theoretically, uterine artery embolization may cause devascularization of the endometrium and myometrium and affect its ability to successfully contract following delivery (18). Several case reports clearly show the possibility of nontarget embolization with negative impact on future fertility (31,35,42,43). However, case reports demonstrate only the possibility of events, not their probability. Encouragingly, magnetic resonance imaging examinations following embolization demonstrate rapid revascularization of the normal myometrium and an essentially normal appearance of the myometrium and endometrium after 6 months (44–46). Recanalization of the embolized uterine arteries has also been demonstrated (47). In a recent editorial, Myers (12) stated that "animal studies might provide insights into the effects of uterine artery embolization on fecundity and pregnancy." Ligation or embolization of the uterine arteries during gestation is

associated with ischemic placental damage and intrauterine growth retardation in sheep, pigs, and rats (48–50). In experimental and clinical studies, it has been demonstrated that the use of calibrated microspheres was associated with controlled myometrial devascularization (32,51). Large microspheres are associated with minimal endometrial and myometrial necrosis after embolization of the sheep uterus (51). In the same animal model, a statistically significant difference was detected between nonspherical polyvinyl alcohol (PVA) particles and microspheres of similar size with regard to the degree of uterine injury, with greater ischemic injury in PVA-treated uteri (51). In the long term, fertility rates after embolization using nonspherical PVA particles were lower than with calibrated microspheres, and the birth weight of the newborns was also significantly lower (52). Of interest, no difference was found between the control group (without embolization) and the group of animals embolized using microspheres (52).

Therefore, it can be hypothesized that pregnancy rates following uterine artery embolization may be higher in future studies than in the initial experience. Technical improvements (i.e., use of calibrated microspheres, targeted fibroid embolization sparing normal myometrium, use of large particles to reduce the risks of nontarget ovarian embolization) may play a significant role in sparing normal myometrium, endometrium, and ovaries during embolization.

PREGNANCY FOLLOWING UTERINE ARTERY EMBOLIZATION FOR OBSTETRIC AND GYNECOLOGIC CONDITIONS

Uterine fibroid embolization was developed as an extension of uterine artery embolization in other obstetric and gynecologic conditions, notably severe postpartum hemorrhage and hemorrhage from gestational trophoblastic tumors (1,53). Several publications have described pregnancies following embolization of the uterine or hypogastric arteries in this setting (53–58). To date, there is no evidence that previously fertile patients have become infertile following pelvic embolization for causes other than fibroids (53–58). However, in these cases, the embolization agent has usually been resorbable gelatin sponge, which does not produce as distal a block as nonresorbable particles and therefore may affect the uterus differently (47,53,58). With an average follow-up of 12 years in 28 women undergoing embolization of the hypogastric arteries for postpartum hemorrhage, all women who desired to become pregnant were able to do so (59). Six women reported a total of six uncomplicated pregnancies and deliveries in the years following embolization (59). However, in the majority of cases, women who suffered life-threatening postpartum hemorrhage are not seeking future pregnancy (58,59).

Stancato-Pasik et al. (58) also reported that all three patients who were trying to conceive following embolization for postpartum hemorrhage succeeded. From the literature, embolization appears to offer patients a fertility-preserving alternative to hysterectomy.

PREGNANCY FOLLOWING UTERINE ARTERY EMBOLIZATION FOR UTERINE FIBROIDS

Reports describing pregnancy after uterine fibroid embolization with gelatin sponge, PVA particles, or calibrated microspheres have accumulated slowly mainly because embolization was offered to women who had already accomplished their childbearing (2,4,5,7,14–18,20,27,32). Because of the complications associated with uterine fibroid embolization using nonspherical PVA particles (i.e., emergent infection leading to hysterectomy, ovarian failure, chronic vaginal discharge), it has been stated that gelatin sponge could be an alternative agent (47,60,61). However, there are insufficient data available to advocate the use of gelatin sponge in young patients desiring to preserve fertility options (60). In addition, long-term arterial occlusion has been reported even when embolization was performed with gelatin sponge pledgets (47). Recently, a group from Japan raised the issue of endometrial damage following embolization using gelatin sponge pledgets (62). In a group of 12 women with infertility, six developed Asherman syndrome, and four eventually required hysteroscopic resection for adhesions (62). However, despite impairment of the endometrium, the pregnancy rate in this group was 50% (5/10 women) (62). Based on the few available data, it is not yet clear whether there is any significant advantage of calibrated microspheres over nonspherical PVA particles in women of reproductive age (7,32,47). In a retrospective study reported by Ravina et al. (14), a total of 12 pregnancies were observed in women 22 to 41 years old, at an average of 13 months after embolization. However, without knowing the total number of treated women and the number of those trying to conceive after treatment (the denominator), we are unable to estimate the true pregnancy rate after embolization. In this group, seven women delivered successfully (including three premature delivery), and five had an early miscarriage (14). McLucas et al. (15) reported 17 pregnancies in 52 women, with ten successful deliveries and five miscarriages. Two additional pregnancies were ongoing at the time of publication. In the Toronto experience, a total of 17 pregnancies were reported in 15 women out of a group of 164 interested in future pregnancy after embolization (63). Most of these women (14/15) were under the age of 40 (63). A recently completed prospective study also confirmed that no woman over the age of 40 conceived successfully after embolization (16). In the group of 122 women interested in maintaining future fertility, a total of 14 pregnancies were reported in ten women. In this series, only 24 of 122 women were actively trying to conceive after embolization [pregnancy rate 58% (14/24)] (16). Most of these women were offered embolization as an alternative to hysterectomy or multiple myomectomy and presented with large-volume uteri pretreatment (mean and median volumes 1,080 and 873 cc, respectively) (Fig. 13-1) (16). Of interest, the cesarean delivery and premature delivery rates in these studies were higher than in the general population (14–16). Goldberg et al. (18) also stated that other pregnancy complications rates (low birth weight and postpartum hemorrhage) after uterine artery embolization were higher than in the general population. However, in interpreting these rates, it should be taken into consideration that it is unlikely that women undergoing uterine fibroid embolization are similar to the general obstetric population. Women undergoing embolization are generally older and have more and larger fibroids than those treated with myomectomy, which results in higher rates of spontaneous abortion, cesarean delivery, and other complications (7,12,13,16). Women treated with uterine artery embolization are older than 40 at the time of treatment in most studies, and it is well demonstrated that fertility is significantly reduced in patients of this age, irrespective of any potential adverse factors (20). Black women who have higher risks for premature or small-for-gestational age infants are also more likely to have uterine fibroids than white women (12). Black women represented more than 50% of treated patients in most studies (5,6,9,20). Without controlling for these confounding factors, one cannot draw definitive conclusions on the impact of uterine fibroid embolization on fertility (12). Table 13-1 summarizes published series of pregnancies after uterine fibroid embolization. Table 13-2 summarizes pregnancy outcomes and complications after uterine fibroid embolization.

PREGNANCY FOLLOWING MYOMECTOMY

After abdominal myomectomy, the term-pregnancy rate ranged from 10% to 46% (64,65). After laparoscopic myomectomy, the term pregnancy rate ranged between 16% and 57% (66–68). After hysteroscopic myomectomy, the term-pregnancy rate has been reported to be 10% to 35% (69–71). In comparing uterine fibroid embolization to myomectomy as a fertility-sparing procedure, we must include the known complications of surgery, such as adhesion formation, regrowth of new or treated fibroids, and conversion to hysterectomy (21,67). Spontaneous uterine rupture during pregnancy or labor has been reported several times in women who conceived after laparoscopic myomectomy (67). Overall, the uterine rupture rate during pregnancy is around 2%, raising questions regarding the safety of laparoscopic myomec-

FIGURE 13-1. A 33-year-old woman (para 0, gravida 0) with multiple uterine fibroids. Embolization was performed as an alternative to hysterectomy. **A:** Preembolization sagittal T2-weighted image demonstrates an enlarged uterus (volume 815 cc) with multiple fibroids. **B:** Preembolization axial T2-weighted image demonstrates obvious distortion of the endometrial cavity *(arrow)* due to the fibroids *(stars)*. Postembolization sagittal **(C)** and axial **(D)** T2-weighted images show significant uterine shrinkage (volume 421 cc, -48%) with reduced distortion of the endometrial cavity *(arrow)*. The woman became pregnant 22 months after embolization and delivered successfully by elective cesarean section at 39 weeks. A 4,270-g male fetus was delivered, with Apgar scores of 10 and 10 at 1 and 5 minutes, respectively. The patient had an uncomplicated recovery.

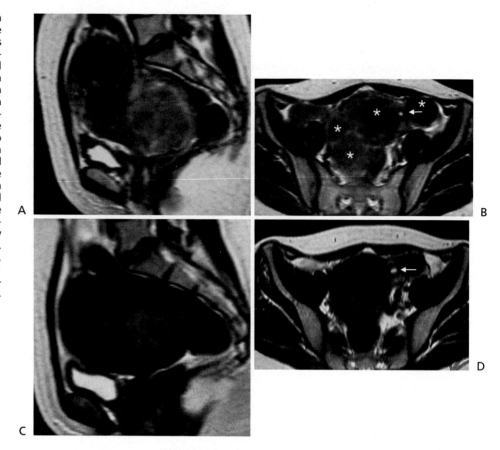

tomy, specifically, the adequacy of laparoscopic suturing of myometrium in women who desire future pregnancy (66–68). The quality of the uterine scar produced after uterine fibroid embolization is also a matter of debate, with two case reports of uterine wall defect or rupture after treatment (72,73).

SEXUALITY FOLLOWING UTERINE ARTERY EMBOLIZATION AND SURGERY

Masters and Johnson's (74) pioneering studies of the female sexual response suggested that, at least in some women, the uterus plays a role in the physiology of the vaginal orgasm. By extension, it has been suggested that hysterectomy could have a detrimental effect on orgasm by eliminating the uterine contribution. Impaired sexual function after hysterectomy has been well documented in the literature (75,76). It has been hypothesized that disturbance of the uterovaginal plexus located near the junction of the cervix and upper vagina may impair sensory and autonomic innervations to pelvic organs, including the uterus, thereby altering perceptions from these organs (75–77). Conversely, in a recent review of the literature, Farrell and Kieser (77) stated that hysterectomy did not adversely affect sexuality.

However, most of the studies utilized simplified measurement tools. Most studies only used libido and orgasm to evaluate sexuality (77). In these studies, the type of surgery performed (i.e., supracervical hysterectomy, oophorectomy) was not always discussed. Decreased libido and orgasm are not uncommon in women older than 45 regardless of their surgery (77). Reduced hormonal levels (estrogen and androgen) after oophorectomy can also account for altered sexual life (77). Therefore, the respective roles of the uterus and the ovaries, as well as overall sociopsychological well-being, should be considered together when sexual function is evaluated. Less invasive procedures, such as uterine fibroid embolization, may help preserve normal postprocedural sexual function. The impact of uterine fibroid embolization on sexual function has been evaluated in four different series and the results presented at scientific meetings (78–81). These studies showed that uterine fibroid embolization had either a neutral or enhancing effect on sexuality (78–81). Following uterine fibroid embolization, 17% to 43% of women reported increased frequency of desire or orgasm (79,80). This may be due to clinical improvement after treatment, particularly in women with bulk-related symptoms who also reported decreased pain during intercourse (79,80). However, one study reported that approximately 10% of women complained of decreased

TABLE 13-1. PUBLISHED SERIES OF PREGNANCY AFTER UTERINE FIBROID EMBOLIZATION

Study (Reference No.)	No. of Women Treated with Embolization	Mean Age of Women (Years)	No. of Women Trying to Conceive	Mean Time from Embolization to Pregnancy (Months)	No. of Pregnant Women	Total No. of Pregnancies	No. of Deliveries	No. of Term Deliveries[a]	No. of Induced Abortions	No. of Miscarriages	No. of Ectopic Pregnancies	No. of Ongoing Pregnancies
14	184	40	NA	13	9	12	7	5	0	5	0	0
15	400	41	57	NA	14	17	10	9	0	5	0	2
16	122	36	24	28	12	17	10	8	0	6	1	0
63	555	43	164	NA	15	17	11	8	1	3	0	2

[a]Premature delivery excluded.
NA, not available.

TABLE 13-2. PREGNANCY OUTCOMES AND COMPLICATIONS AFTER UTERINE FIBROID EMBOLIZATION

Study (Reference No.)	No. of Pregnant Women	Total No. of Pregnancies	No. of Deliveries	Spontaneous Abortion Rate	Premature Delivery Rate	Cesarean Delivery Rate	Smallness for Gestational Age	Postpartum Hemorrhage Rate
14	9	12	7	42% (5/12)	29% (2/7)	57% (4/7)	25% (2/8)[a]	0% (0/7)
15	14	17	10	29% (5/17)	10% (1/10)	70% (7/10)	0% (0/10)	0% (0/10)
16	12	17	10	35% (6/17)	20% (2/10)	90% (9/10)	0% (0/10)	0% (0/10)
63	15	17	11	18% (3/17)	27% (3/11)	NA	NA	NA
All	50	63	38	30% (19/63)	21% (8/38)	74% (20/27)	7% (2/28)	0% (0/27)

[a]One twin pregnancy.
NA, not available.

levels of sexual interest, sexual arousal, and sexual satisfaction (81). However, the assessment of any aspect of quality of life was not made with validated and reproducible measurement instruments. Using specific quality-of-life questionnaires before and after embolization, it has been demonstrated that energy, vitality, mental health, self-image, and sexual functioning were significantly improved after treatment (82). Significant complications interfering with sexual life, such as vaginal dryness, loss of internal orgasm, and labial necrosis, have been reported following embolization and probably are related to nontarget embolization (83,84). Lai et al. (83) reported on a patient who experienced a loss of orgasm response to sexual stimulation after uterine artery embolization. In addition, a small number of women may experience chronic vaginal discharge that interferes with their sexual life after uterine fibroid embolization (7). Finally, amenorrhea associated with symptoms of menopause, such as mood swings and vaginal dryness, may interfere with sexual life (7,30).

CONCLUSION AND PERSPECTIVES

Until recently, most authors reserved uterine fibroid embolization for women who no longer desire fertility. Other groups, such as ours, have taken a more open approach and now offer embolization to patients who desire future fertility, particularly if hysterectomy or repeat or multiple myomectomy is the only surgical alternative (2,4,7,14,16). The ability of women treated with uterine artery embolization for different types of obstetric or gynecologic hemorrhage to conceive and deliver successfully is well known, and long-term follow-up is already available (59). Even if reports of pregnancy following uterine artery embolization remain anecdotal at this time, questions of numerator (number of live births) and denominator (number of women attempting to conceive after embolization) will be determined soon by the results of large prospective registries and studies about to be published. From available prospective studies, fecundity and delivery rates are encouraging and similar to those reported after

myomectomy (16). When pregnancy occurs, the rate of intrauterine growth retardation does not seem to be increased by potential alterations in uterine blood flow after embolization. Nevertheless, in interpreting fertility rates and pregnancy outcome following uterine fibroid embolization, it should be taken into consideration that women undergoing uterine fibroid embolization are not similar to the general obstetric population. Large prospective studies, including randomized trials comparing embolization and myomectomy in women interested in future pregnancy, may answer the remaining questions.

It appears that, in the hands of experienced interventional radiologists, short- and mid-term outcomes of embolization in terms of symptom relief and complications are quite good. Before uterine fibroid embolization is performed, a pluridisciplinary evaluation with the gynecologists and interventional radiologists involved is required, particularly for women who plan future pregnancy.

REFERENCES

1. Brown BJ, Heaston DK, Poulson AM, et al. Uncontrollable postpartum bleeding: a new approach to hemostasis through angiographic arterial embolization. *Obstet Gynecol* 1979;54:361–365.
2. Ravina JH, Herbreteau D, Ciraru-Vigneron N, et al. Arterial embolization to treat uterine myomata. *Lancet* 1995;346:671–672.
3. Spies JB, Scialli AR, Jha RC, et al. Initial results from uterine fibroid embolization for symptomatic leiomyomata. *J Vasc Interv Radiol* 1999;10:1149–1157.
4. Pelage JP, Le Dref O, Soyer P, et al. Fibroid-related menorrhagia: treatment with superselective embolization of the uterine arteries and mid-term follow-up. *Radiology* 2000;215:428–431.
5. Hutchins FL, Worthington-Kirsch R, Berkowitz RP. Selective uterine artery embolization as primary treatment for symptomatic leiomyomata uteri. *J Am Assoc Gynecol Laparosc* 1999;6:279–284.
6. Spies JB, Ascher SA, Roth AR, et al. Uterine artery embolization for leiomyomata. *Obstet Gynecol* 2001;98:29–34.
7. Walker WJ, Pelage JP. Uterine artery embolisation for symptomatic fibroids: clinical results in 400 women with imaging follow up. *Br J Obstet Gynaecol* 2002;109:1262–1272.

8. Pron G, Bennett J, Common A, et al. The Ontario uterine fibroid embolization trial: uterine fibroid reduction and symptom relief after uterine artery embolization for fibroids. *Fertil Steril* 2003;79:120–127.

9. Spies JB, Spector A, Roth AR, et al. Complications of uterine artery embolization for leiomyomata. *Obstet Gynecol* 2002;100:873–880.

10. McLucas B, Adler L. Uterine artery embolization compared with myomectomy. *Int J Obstet Gynecol* 2001;74:297–299.

11. Razavi MK, Hwang G, Jahed A, et al. Abdominal myomectomy versus uterine fibroid embolization in the treatment of symptomatic uterine leiomyomas. *AJR Am J Roentgenol* 2003;180:1571–1575.

12. Myers ER. Uterine artery embolization: what more do we need to know? [Editorial] *Obstet Gynecol* 2002;100:847–848.

13. Stewart EA. Uterine fibroids. *Lancet* 2001;357:293–298.

14. Ravina JH, Ciraru-Vigneron N, Aymard A, et al. Pregnancy after embolization of uterine myoma: report of 12 cases. *Fertil Steril* 2000;73:1241–1243.

15. McLucas B, Goodwin S, Adler L, et al. Pregnancy following uterine fibroid embolization. *Int J Gynaecol Obstet* 2001;74:1–7.

16. Pelage JP, Walker WJ. Uterine artery embolisation for symptomatic fibroids and pregnancy. *J Vasc Interv Radiol* 2002;13:S65(abst).

17. D'Angelo A, Amso NN, Wood A. Spontaneous multiple pregnancy after uterine artery embolization for uterine fibroids. *Eur J Obstet Gynecol Reprod Biol* 2003;110:245–246.

18. Goldberg J, Pereira L, Berghella V. Pregnancy after uterine artery embolization. *Obstet Gynecol* 2002;100:869–872.

19. Hart R. ABC of subfertility: unexplained infertility, endometriosis, and fibroids. *Br Med J* 2003;327:721–724.

20. Forman RG, Reidy J, Nott V, et al. Fibroids and fertility. *Min Invas Ther Allied Technol* 1999;8:415–419.

21. Vollenhoven BJ, Lawrence AS, Healy DL. Uterine fibroids: a clinical review. *Br J Obstet Gynecol* 1990;97:285–298.

22. Wallach EE, Vu KK. Myomata uteri and infertility. *Obstet Gynecol Clin North Am* 1995;22:791–799.

23. Garcia CR, Tureck RW. Submucous leiomyomas and infertility. *Fertil Steril* 1984;42:16–19.

24. Donnez J, Jadoul P. What are the implications of myomas on fertility? A need for a debate? *Hum Reprod* 2002;17:1424–1430.

25. Exacoustos C, Rosati P. Ultrasound diagnosis of uterine myomas and complications in pregnancy. *Obstet Gynecol* 1993;82:97–101.

26. Amato P, Roberts AC. Transient ovarian failure: a complication of uterine artery embolization. *Fertil Steril* 2001;75:438–439.

27. Kovacs P, Stangel JJ, Santoro NF, et al. Successful pregnancy after transient ovarian failure following treatment of symptomatic leiomyomata. *Fertil Steril* 2002;77:1292–1297.

28. Tulandi T, Sammour A, Valenti D, et al. Ovarian reserve after uterine artery embolization for leiomyomata. [Letter] *Fertil Steril* 2002;78:197–198.

29. Spies JB, Roth AR, Gonsalves SM, et al. Ovarian function after uterine artery embolization for leiomyomata: assessment with use of serum follicle stimulating hormone assay. *J Vasc Interv Radiol* 2001;12:437–442.

30. Chrisman HB, Saker MB, Ryu RK, et al. The impact of uterine fibroid embolization on resumption of menses and ovarian function. *J Vasc Interv Radiol* 2000;11:699–703.

31. Tropeano G, Litwicka K, Di Stasi C, et al. Permanent amenorrhea associated with endometrial atrophy after uterine artery embolization for symptomatic uterine fibroids. *Fertil Steril* 2003;79:132–135.

32. Pelage JP, Le Dref O, Beregi JP, et al. Limited uterine artery embolization with tris-acryl gelatin microspheres for uterine fibroids. *J Vasc Interv Radiol* 2003;14:15–20.

33. Ryu RK, Chrisman HB, Omary RA, et al. The vascular impact of uterine artery embolization: prospective sonographic assessment of ovarian arterial circulation. *J Vasc Interv Radiol* 2001;9:1071–1074.

34. Ryu RK, Siddiqi A, Omary RA, et al. Sonography of delayed effects of uterine artery embolization on ovarian arterial perfusion and function. *AJR Am J Roentgenol* 2003;181:89–92.

35. Payne JF, Robboy SJ, Haney AF. Embolic microspheres within ovarian arterial vasculature after uterine artery embolization. *Obstet Gynecol* 2002;100:883–886.

36. Kroencke TJ, Gauruder-Burmester A, Enzweiler CN, et al. Disintegration and stepwise expulsion of a large uterine leiomyoma with restoration of the uterine architecture after successful uterine fibroid embolization: case report. *Hum Reprod* 2003;18:863–865.

37. Berkowitz RP, Hutchins FL, Worthington-Kirsch RL. Vaginal expulsion of submucosal fibroids after uterine artery embolization. A report of three cases. *J Reprod Med* 1999;44:373–376.

38. Nikolic B, Spies JB, Campbell L, et al. Uterine artery embolization: reduced radiation with refined technique. *J Vasc Interv Radiol* 2001;12:39–44.

39. Andrews RT, Brown PH. Uterine arterial embolization: factors influencing patient radiation exposure. *Radiology* 2000;217:713–722.

40. Nikolic B, Abbara S, Levy E, et al. Influence of radiographic technique and equipment on absorbed ovarian dose associated with uterine artery embolization. *J Vasc Interv Radiol* 2000;11:1173–1178.

41. Pron G, Mocarski E, Cohen M, et al. Hysterectomy for complications after uterine artery embolization for leiomyomata. Results of a Canadian multicenter clinical trial. *J Am Assoc Gynecol Laparosc* 2003;10:99–106.

42. Godfrey CD, Zbella EA. Uterine necrosis after uterine artery embolization for leiomyoma. *Obstet Gynecol* 2001;98:950–952.

43. Sabatini L, Atiomo W, Magos A. Successful myomectomy following infected ischaemic necrosis of uterine fibroids after uterine artery embolisation. *Br J Obstet Gynaecol* 2003;110:704–710.

44. Jha RC, Ascher SM, Imaoka I, et al. Symptomatic fibroleiomyomata: MR imaging of the uterus before and after uterine arterial embolization. *Radiology* 2000;217:228–235.

45. Banovac F, Ascher S, Jones DA, et al. Magnetic resonance imaging outcome after uterine artery embolization for leiomyomata with use of tris-acryl gelatin microspheres. *J Vasc Interv Radiol* 2002;13:682–687.

46. Burbank F, Hutchins FL Jr. Uterine artery occlusion by embolization or surgery for the treatment of fibroids: a unifying hypothesis-transient uterine ischemia. *J Am Assoc Gynecol Laparosc* 2000;7:S1–S49.

47. Siskin GP, Englander M, Stainken BF, et al. Embolic agent used for uterine fibroid embolization. *AJR Am J Roentgenol* 2000;175:767–773.

48. Gilbert M, Leturque A. fetal weight and its relationship to placental blood flow and placental weight in experimental intrauterine growth retardation in the rat. *J Dev Physiol* 1982;4:237–246.

49. Wigglesworth J. Fetal growth retardation. Animal model: uterine vessel ligation in the pregnant rat. *Am J Pathol* 1974;72:347–350.

50. Alexander G. Studies on the placenta of the sheep: effect of surgical reduction of the number of caruncles. *J Reprod Fertil* 1964;7:307–322.

51. Pelage JP, Laurent A, Wassef M, et al. Acute effects of uterine artery embolization in the sheep: comparison between polyvinyl alcohol particles and calibrated microspheres. *Radiology* 2002;224:436–445.

52. Pelage JP, Martal J, Huynh L, et al. Bilateral uterine artery embolization in the sheep: impact on fertility. *Radiology* 2002; 225[P]:306(abst).

53. Pelage JP, Le Dref O, Mateo J, et al. Life-threatening primary postpartum hemorrhage. Treatment with emergency selective arterial embolization. *Radiology* 1998;208:359–362.

54. Chapman DR, Lutz MH. Report of a successful delivery after nonsurgical management of a choriocarcinoma-related pelvic arteriovenous fistula. *Am J Obstet Gynecol* 1985;153:155–157.

55. Poppe W, VanAssche FA, Wilms G, et al. Pregnancy after transcatheter embolization of a uterine arteriovenous malformation. *Am J Obstet Gynecol* 1987;156:1179–1180.

56. Salamon LJ, de Tayrac R, Castaigne-Meary V, et al. Fertility and pregnancy outcome following pelvic arterial embolization for severe post-partum hemorrhage. A cohort study. *Hum Reprod* 2003;18:849–852.

57. Wang H, Garmel S. Successful term pregnancy after bilateral uterine artery embolization for postpartum hemorrhage. *Obstet Gynecol* 2003;102:603–604.

58. Stancato-Pasik A, Mitty H, Richard HM III, et al. Obstetric embolotherapy: effects on menses and pregnancy. *Radiology* 1997;204:791–793.

59. Ornan D, White R, Pollak J, et al. Pelvic embolization for intractable postpartum hemorrhage: long-term follow-up and implications for fertility. *Obstet Gynecol* 2003;102:904–910.

60. Stancato-Pasik A, Katz R, Mitty HA, et al. Uterine artery embolisation of myomas: preliminary results of gelatin sponge pledgets as the embolic agent. *Min Invas Ther Allied Technol* 1999;8:393–396.

61. Katsumori T, Nakajima K, Mihara T, et al. Uterine artery embolization using gelatin sponge particles alone for symptomatic uterine fibroids: midterm results. *AJR Am J Roentgenol* 2002;178:135–139.

62. Honda I, Sato T, Adachi H, et al. Uterine artery embolization for leiomyoma: complications and effects on fertility [in Japanese]. *Nippon Igaku Hoshasen Gakkai Zasshi* 2003;63:294–302.

63. Pron G, Mocarski E, Vilos G, et al. Pregnancy after fibroid uterine artery embolization: the Ontario fibroid embolization trial. *J Vasc Interv Radiol* 2003;14:S5(abst).

64. Sudik R, Hüsch K, Steller J, et al. Fertility and pregnancy outcome after myomectomy in sterility patients. *Eur J Obstet Gynecol* 1996;65:209–214.

65. Acien P, Querada F. Abdominal myomectomy: results of a simple operative technique. *Fertil Steril* 1996;65:41–51.

66. Darai E, Dechaud H, Benifla JL, et al. Fertility after laparoscopic myomectomy: preliminary results. *Hum Reprod* 1997;12:1931–1934.

67. Dubuisson JB, Fauconnier A, Deffarges JV, et al. Pregnancy outcome and deliveries following laparoscopic myomectomy. *Hum Reprod* 2000;15:869–873.

68. Landi S, Fiaccavento A, Zaccoletti R, et al. Pregnancy outcome and deliveries after laparoscopic myomectomy. *J Am Assoc Gynecol Laparosc* 2003;10:59–63.

69. Bernard G, Darai E, Poncelet C, et al. Fertility after hysteroscopic myomectomy: effect of intramural fibroids associated. *Eur J Obstet Gynecol* 2000;88:85–90.

70. Fernandez H, Sefrioui O, Virelizier C, et al. Hysteroscopic resection of submucosal myomas in patients with infertility. *Hum Reprod* 2001;16:1489–1492.

71. Varasteh NN, Neuwirth RS, Levin B, et al. Pregnancy rates after hysteroscopic polypectomy and myomectomy in infertile women. *Obstet Gynecol* 1999;94:168–171.

72. De Iaco PA, Muzzupapa G, Golfieri R, et al. A uterine wall defect after uterine artery embolization for symptomatic myomas. *Fertil Steril* 2002;77:176–178.

73. Shashoua AR, Stringer NH, Pearlman JB, et al. Ischemic uterine rupture and hysterectomy 3 months after uterine artery embolization. *J Am Assoc Gynecol Laparosc* 2002;9:217–220.

74. Masters W, Johnson V. The uterus. In: Masters W, Johnson V, eds. *Human sexual response*. Boston: Little, Brown and Company, 1966:111–126.

75. Kikku P, Gronroos M, Hirvonen T, et al. Supravaginal uterine amputation vs hysterectomy: effects on libido and orgasm. *Acta Obstet Gynecol Scand* 1983;62:147–152.

76. Thakar R, Manyonda I, Stanton SL, et al. Bladder, bowel and sexual function after hysterectomy for benign conditions. *Br J Obstet Gynaecol* 1997;104:983–987.

77. Farrell SA, Kieser K. Sexuality after hysterectomy. *Obstet Gynecol* 2000;95:1045–1051.

78. Amman AM, Gomez-Jorge JT, Spies JB. Sexual function after uterine artery embolization. *J Vasc Interv Radiol* 2001;12: S76(abst).

79. Wysoki M, Byrd BP, Onze K, et al. Sexual function after uterine fibroid embolization. *J Vasc Interv Radiol* 2001;12:S77(abst).

80. Lvoff NM, Omary RA, Chrisman HB, et al. Uterine artery embolization and female sexual function. *J Vasc Interv Radiol* 2002;13:S65(abst).

81. Watkinson A, Robertson FJ, Babar S, et al. Impact of uterine artery embolization on sexual function. *J Vasc Interv Radiol* 2002;13:S66(abst).

82. Spies JB, Warren EH, Mathias SD, et al. Uterine fibroid embolization: measurement of health-related quality of life before and after therapy. *J Vasc Interv Radiol* 1999;10:1293–1303.

83. Lai AC, Goodwin SC, Bonilla SM, et al. Sexual dysfunction after uterine artery embolization. *J Vasc Interv Radiol* 1999;11: 755–758.

84. Yeagley TJ, Goldberg J, Klein TA, et al. Labial necrosis after uterine artery embolization for leiomyomata. *Obstet Gynecol* 2002;100:881–882.

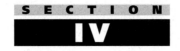

SECTION

IV

UTERINE EMBOLIZATION IN OTHER CLINICAL SETTINGS

14

EMBOLIZATION FOR THE MANAGEMENT OF OBSTETRICAL HEMORRHAGE

ANTOINETTE ROTH
SCOTT C. GOODWIN
SURESH VEDANTHAM
MICHAEL L. DOUEK
JAMES B. SPIES

Hemorrhage is a major cause of postpartum morbidity and mortality and results from a wide range of obstetric disorders. Conservative measures have been and continue to be the first line of defense, but once these measures fail, the options in the past have been few. Many patients routinely underwent bilateral hypogastric and/or uterine artery ligation. If refractory bleeding continued, a hysterectomy was needed, with subsequent loss of fertility.

The treatment algorithm has changed over the years with the emergence of transcatheter arterial embolization, which is quickly becoming the modality of choice to control and prevent pelvic hemorrhage. This chapter highlights specific causes of postpartum hemorrhage (PPH), various historic and current treatment modalities, and evolution of transcatheter embolization in the prevention and treatment of this condition.

BACKGROUND

Worldwide, PPH is one of the leading causes of maternal mortality. In the United States, PPH usually ranks among the top three causes of maternal death, along with pulmonary embolization and hypertension (1).

The traditional definition of PPH is the loss of 500 mL of blood within the first 24 hours after a vaginal delivery (2). Subsequently, more clinically relevant definitions have been proposed, including that given by the American College of Obstetrics and Gynecology, which defines PPH as a 10% drop in hematocrit between predelivery and postdelivery or the need for an erythrocyte blood transfusion (3). Using this definition, PPH occurs with a frequency of 3.9% in vaginal deliveries and 6.4% in cesarean deliveries (3,4).

One method of categorizing PPH is by its temporal relationship to delivery. Early PPH occurs in the first 24 hours postdelivery, whereas late PPH occurs more than 24 hours, but less than 6 weeks, postdelivery.

ETIOLOGY OF POSTPARTUM HEMORRHAGE

Early PPH is more common than late PPH and is associated with greater blood loss and morbidity (5). The most common cause is uterine atony. Less common causes include genital tract lacerations, retained placental fragments, uterine rupture, placenta accreta/percreta, and coagulopathies. A complete list of causes of early PPH is given in Table 14-1.

Uterine Atony

Uterine atony complicates approximately 1 in 20 deliveries and occurs when myometrial contractions fail to control blood loss after expulsion of the placenta. Risk factors include conditions that cause the uterus to be overdistended (multiple gestations and polyhydramnios), uterine fatigue (prolonged labor or chorioamnionitis), and an inhibited ability of the uterus to contract secondary to exogenous agents (use of uterine relaxing agents or general anesthesia) (5). Uterine atony is usually diagnosed by abdominal palpation, which reveals a boggy uterus.

Lacerations

Lacerations of the lower genital tract are another common cause of PPH. The cervix is lacerated in approximately 50%

TABLE 14-1. CAUSES OF EARLY POSTPARTUM HEMORRHAGE

Uterine atony
Retained placental fragments
Lower genital tract lacerations
Uterine rupture
Uterine inversion
Placenta accreta/percreta
Coagulopathy

of vaginal deliveries (6). Most of these lacerations are smaller than 5 mm and therefore do not cause significant bleeding. Occasionally, however, they can extend into the upper third of the vagina, the lower uterine segment, and/or the uterine artery. In the presence of good uterine tone, postpartum bleeding is most likely due to a lower genital tract laceration, and careful inspection of the vulva, vagina, and cervix is important. Even when uterine atony is present and steps are taken to increase myometrial contractions, the lower genital tract should be inspected in order to rule out lacerations as a concomitant source of bleeding. This is most important when specific circumstances such as instrumentation or fetal macrosomia are present, which make such trauma more likely.

Retained Placental Fragments

Retained placental fragments seldom cause immediate PPH, but a remaining piece of placenta is a common cause of bleeding late in the puerperium. Inspection of the placenta after delivery is imperative. If a portion of the placenta is missing, the uterus should be explored and the fragment removed.

Coagulopathies

Coagulopathies are rare causes of PPH. Although inherited conditions may first present as PPH, most women with these disorders have a history of abnormal bleeding. However, there are also conditions unique to pregnancy that predispose to coagulopathy. Abruption of the placenta, sepsis, massive blood transfusion, severe preeclampsia, HELLP (hemolysis, elevated liver enzymes, low platelets) syndrome, AFLP (acute fatty liver of pregnancy) syndrome, and amniotic fluid embolism can all cause disseminated intravascular coagulation (DIC).

DIC is a consumptive coagulopathy in which there is abnormal activation of platelets, clotting, and fibrinolytic mechanisms *in vivo*. In this pathologic state, coagulation may be activated by thromboplastin from tissue destruction via the extrinsic pathway and perhaps via the intrinsic pathway by collagen and other tissue components when there is loss of endothelial integrity. A common inciting

factor in obstetrics is thromboplastin from placental abruption. It is also thought that consumptive coagulopathy is associated with microangiopathic hemolysis caused by mechanical disruption of the erythrocyte membrane within small vessels in which fibrin has been deposited. This process also likely contributes to the hemolysis encountered with the HELLP syndrome (7).

As mentioned previously, the HELLP and AFLP syndromes are causes of pregnancy-induced coagulopathy and are commonly associated with DIC. The exact pathogenesis of these two syndromes has yet to be definitely established. Nevertheless, they may cause life-threatening liver dysfunction and require prompt recognition and referral/intervention in order to prevent fatal consequences.

The HELLP syndrome affects 0.1% to 0.6% of all pregnancies and 4% to 12% of pregnancies complicated by severe preeclampsia (8). This syndrome is characterized by microangiopathic hemolytic anemia and multiorgan endothelial and microvascular injury. It typically presents in the third trimester between weeks 27 and 36, although up to one third of cases may arise postpartum. Presenting signs can be mild to severe, with the most frequent signs being malaise (90%), right upper quadrant/epigastric pain (65%–90%), and nausea or vomiting (36%–50%) (8,9). The most common complication is DIC, which occurs in 20% to 40% of patients (8,10–12). Less common complications include abruptio placenta (16%), acute renal failure (7%), and pulmonary edema (6%) (8). The perinatal mortality of infants born to mothers with HELLP syndrome averages 35%, depending on the gestational age and the severity of the syndrome at the time of delivery (13). The mortality rate of the mothers is 1% to 3%, although rates as high as 25% have been reported (8). In most cases, delivery of the fetus is effective treatment.

AFLP syndrome is a rare condition estimated to occur in 1 in 13,000 deliveries (14). Again, the pathogenesis is poorly understood, but it is characterized by the accumulation of microvesicular fat within hepatocytes. Similar to HELLP syndrome, patients classically present in the third trimester with nonspecific symptoms including abdominal pain (50%–80%) and nausea and vomiting (70%) (15–17). If untreated, AFLP syndrome typically progresses to fulminant hepatic failure with encephalopathy, renal failure, uncontrollable gastrointestinal or uterine bleeding, DIC, seizures, coma, and death (17,18). DIC is a prominent feature of AFLP syndrome, occurring in more than 75% of cases (16). The mortality rate was close to 80% before 1980 (18), but current mortality rates average around 20% (16,18,19). Although some authors contend that expectant management is acceptable for mild cases (15), most believe the condition warrants prompt delivery.

Fetal death and delayed delivery are additional causes of coagulation changes. Pritchard (20,21) discovered that gross disruption of the maternal coagulation mechanism rarely develops before one month after fetal death. However, if the fetus was retained longer, approximately 25% of women developed coagulopathy.

DIC can compound all causes of hemorrhage, and in order to stop the progression, the underlying pathology must be corrected. For example, emptying the uterus in cases of sepsis or abruption or prompt delivery in cases of HELLP or AFLP syndrome is imperative to slowing or stopping the progression of DIC. In situations of massive obstetric hemorrhage, it is important to consider the involvement of a hematologist who can help guide in the appropriate investigations, resuscitation, and administration of blood products.

Placenta Accreta/Percreta

Placenta accreta/percreta will be discussed separately because the treatment algorithm differs from the etiologies mentioned previously. Specifically, in atony, lacerations, and coagulopathies, management begins after hemorrhage has started. However, with placenta accreta/percreta, PPH is very likely. Therefore, prophylactic measures are taken prior to delivery. Placenta accreta/percreta is defined and discussed in detail in a later section.

MANAGEMENT OF POSTPARTUM HEMORRHAGE

Initial therapy for PPH is fluid resuscitation with volume replacement and simultaneous search for an etiology. In order to identify the cause of hemorrhage, a bimanual examination should be performed, as well as close inspection for lacerations. Subsequently, uterine massage, suturing of lacerations, local drainage of hematomas, curettage for retained products, vaginal packing, and administration of drugs [oxytocin, methylergonovine maleate (Methergine), and prostaglandins] can be performed based on the specific etiology of bleeding. The majority of PPH cases are controlled by these conservative measures. However, if conservative management fails, the next step in the algorithm is occlusion therapy, either surgically or now transluminally. In the past, surgical ligation of the hypogastric arteries was used but, as discussed in the following section, this approach was of limited effectiveness. More recently, ligation of the uterine arteries or the corresponding angiographic embolization procedures has been the standard. A proposed treatment algorithm for PPH is shown in Figure 14-1 (22).

Hypogastric Artery Ligation

Hypogastric artery ligation was once advocated as a means to control pelvic hemorrhage. This treatment option

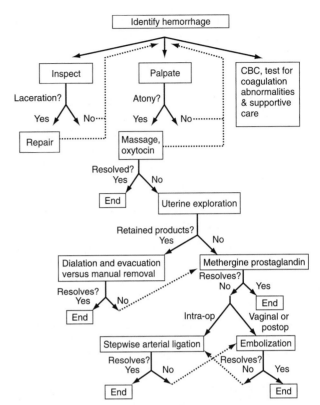

FIGURE 14-1. Algorithm for management of postpartum hemorrhage (22).

originated in 1964 when Burchell (23) proposed that ligation reduces arterial pressures, converting the pelvic arterial circulation into a venous system and creating an environment more amenable to hemostasis via clot formation. Burchell reported that bilateral hypogastric artery ligation in 13 women reduced pelvic blood flow by 49% but reduced pulse pressure by 85% distal to the ligation. The success of this technique has varied widely, ranging from 40% to 100% (24–28). One of the hypothesized explanations for the lower success rates is the rapid reconstitution of the distal hypogastric artery after ligation, which has been documented angiographically (29).

Additionally, hypogastric artery ligation has shown to be particularly poor in controlling hemorrhage due to uterine atony (25,27). A study in 1985 by Clark et al. (25) examined 19 patients with obstetric hemorrhage from uterine atony, placenta accreta, and lacerations. The success rates for hypogastric artery ligation was 40% for uterine atony compared to 50% for all other causes of PPH (25). Similarly, in 1990, Chattopadhyay et al. (27) showed that hypogastric artery ligation was successful in 50% of patients with uterine atony and 73% of patients with hemorrhage from other causes. No hypothesis explaining these findings was provided by either group of authors.

Current studies evaluating blood loss, operating time, and perioperative morbidity paint a confusing picture.

Clark et al. (25) and Chattopadhyay et al. (27) demonstrated that hypogastric artery ligation is associated with less blood loss, operating time, and morbidity compared to emergent hysterectomy when it is successful. However, Clark et al. also demonstrated that hypogastric artery ligation was successful in only 42% of cases; with the remaining 58% requiring hysterectomy. In those patients requiring hysterectomy after artery ligation, blood loss, operating time, and intraoperative morbidity were increased compared to patients undergoing emergency hysterectomy for obstetric hemorrhage without prior ligation. The authors noted that the increased blood loss and operating time associated with hypogastric artery ligation was not entirely a reflection of the time spent on arterial ligation. This was the first pregnancy for many of the women in whom hypogastric arterial ligation was attempted before hysterectomy. Thus, the increase in blood loss and operative time may reflect prolonged attempts at conservative management that included, but were not limited to, hypogastric artery ligation. Nevertheless, the decision to attempt hypogastric artery ligation rather than proceed directly to hysterectomy in the emergency setting is controversial.

There are several clear disadvantages to hypogastric artery ligation. Specifically, the procedure is technically challenging because it involves accessing the retroperitoneal space. An accurate knowledge of the iliac vessels in relation to the ureters is essential. This complex relationship may be further complicated by tissue edema and hematoma in the face of PPH. Additionally, hypogastric artery ligation precludes other hemorrhage control measures such as uterine artery embolization. In other words, when hypogastric artery ligation fails, the patient is consigned to hysterectomy, thus eliminating future fertility. Finally, as noted previously, hypogastric artery ligation has been found to be of limited success in treating uterine atony (25,27), which is one of the leading causes of PPH. In addition, the complication rate of approximately 13% remains high compared to other hemorrhage control measures (30). Complications have included wound infection (26,27), ureteral injury (25), lower extremity paresis (24), and death (26). For these reasons, hypogastric artery ligation has fallen out of favor.

Uterine Artery Ligation

Bilateral uterine artery ligation has been investigated as a fertility-preserving technique to control hemorrhage. This was a logical next step to hypogastric artery ligation, given that the uterus receives approximately 90% of its blood supply from the uterine arteries. In this procedure, the ascending branch of the uterine arteries is ligated via laparotomy. This procedure was first reported in the literature in 1952 (31), and documented success rates range from 80% to 90%, with relatively few complications (32).

In 1995, O'Leary (33) reported on 265 patients with postcesarean hemorrhage who underwent ligation of the ascending uterine artery and vein. The data were collected from 1962 to 1992. Success rates of 95% were reported, with only two minor complications. Direct comparison of this study with more modern series is somewhat limited because the conditions under which the two surgical studies were conducted have changed over time. Specifically, under the O'Leary study, 24 of the 124 procedures performed prior to 1972 were elective procedures done to educate residents and to provide additional experience with performing the procedure to staff. In addition, many of the modern pharmacologic methods of controlling hemorrhage were not available during the 1960s and 1970s. Thus, many of the patients deemed operable in the 1960s may not have had bleeding severe enough to warrant operation by today's standards.

Despite these differences, the results of the O'Leary study were substantiated in a more recent study performed by AbdRabbo (32). He described a stepwise approach to uterine artery ligation in 103 patients. The protocol called for sequential ligation of a single uterine artery, followed by the contralateral uterine artery. Subsequently, the low uterine arteries and low ovarian arteries can be ligated if the patient is not stabilized. Although only 83% successful with unilateral or bilateral uterine artery ligation alone, the entire protocol was 100% successful in controlling hemorrhage. In addition, no major complications occurred.

This technique has several advantages over hypogastric artery ligation: (i) it is a technically easier procedure because it does not involve retroperitoneal dissection; (ii) uterine artery ligation provides a more distal occlusion, thus decreasing the impact of collaterals and the likelihood of rebleeding; and (iii) injuries to other pelvic structures may be reduced.

Embolization

Selective arterial embolization has emerged as an alternative to surgical intervention in the treatment of PPH. Its origin began as a diagnostic tool in the 1960s when angiography demonstrated sites of arterial hemorrhage after surgical exploration failed (34). Its acceptance increased as percutaneous methods moved from diagnostic to therapeutic modalities in the early 1970s when embolization was first used to control gastrointestinal bleeding (35). These techniques were soon expanded to include control of hemorrhage secondary to pelvic trauma (36).

In 1979, Brown et al. (37) performed the first case of pelvic embolization as treatment for PPH. They described a case in which all local and surgical methods had failed, including transabdominal hysterectomy. Subsequently, embolization of the left internal pudendal artery with gelatin sponge (Gelfoam) powder and pledgets resulted in cessation of bleeding and stabilization of the patient.

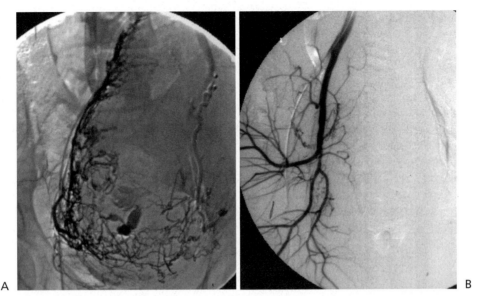

FIGURE 14-2. Focal bleeding associated with placenta accreta. **A:** Postpartum hemorrhage in a patient with placenta accreta, with a focal site of bleeding identified as being supplied by the right uterine artery. **B:** Embolization completed with Gelfoam, resulting in occlusion of the uterine artery on the right and control of the bleeding. (Images courtesy of Steven Lipman, M.D.)

Embolization Technique in the Postpartum Patient

The technique begins with a femoral artery puncture and subsequent selective catheterization of the uterine arteries. An angiogram of the uterus should be performed to identify any focal sources of bleeding (Fig. 14-2). Currently, Gelfoam pledgets or slurry are the embolic materials of choice. This material is effective for 2 to 4 weeks, which is sufficient to prevent further hemorrhage while allowing for slow development of collaterals (38,39). Even when both uterine arteries are occluded, the collateral network from other branches reconstitutes the intrauterine branches. Specifically, the ovarian arteries that arise from the anterolateral abdominal aorta may divert blood to maintain the viability of the uterus in sudden bilateral uterine artery occlusion. The round ligament artery, which arises either from the inferior epigastric artery or from the external iliac artery, can also provide blood supply to the embolized uterine artery (40).

Particulate embolics, such as Gelfoam powder, polyvinyl alcohol particles (41), and aqueous substances, are not recommended for PPH because of the likelihood of ischemic complications. These embolics may result in a more distal occlusion, making it less likely that a collateral network will form to prevent myometrial ischemia.

Although angiography is sensitive in identifying arterial bleeding, percutaneous embolization can also be effective when the specific site of bleeding is not identified. Paris et al. (29) were the first to report control of PPH despite nonvisualization of the bleeding vessel. This claim was substantiated in subsequent studies, giving angiography and

percutaneous methods an advantage over surgical treatment (42,43).

Outcome of Embolotherapy for Postpartum Hemorrhage

The success rates for percutaneous embolization are excellent, reported to be approximately 97% (30,44–47). As mentioned, there are several potential advantages of embolization over surgery. First, the exact bleeding site can often be identified, allowing more targeted therapy. For cases in which the specific bleeding site is not identified, embolization can still be effective. Second, if repeat embolization is later required to the same or different vessels, it is easier to undertake than repeat surgery. Third, the more distal occlusion that occurs with embolization minimizes the effects of collateral circulation and the likelihood of rebleeding. Fourth, the decision to proceed with arterial embolization does not preclude any other hemorrhage control measures. If necessary, arterial ligation can be performed after embolization is attempted. Finally, embolization avoids the risks of general anesthesia.

Complications after Embolization for Postpartum Hemorrhage

The complication rate for transcatheter embolization is low, reported to be 6% to 7% (30). Complications can largely be split into three categories: complications of angiography, infection, and ischemic phenomenon. Most complications are minor and include hematoma at the catheter insertion site (48) and self-limiting low-grade fever (49).

More serious complications in the postpartum setting are exceedingly rare because of the extensive collateral network in the gravid pelvis. One such complication is a single technical error in which the external iliac artery was punctured (50). Three postembolization abscesses have been reported, two in the immediate postprocedural time frame (49,51) and a third approximately 20 days later in the anterior abdominal wall, in which the patient underwent both uterine and hypogastric embolization (43).

To date, four ischemic complications have been documented. Two occurred in women with postpartum bleeding who had arterial embolization after unsuccessful internal iliac ligation (50). Subsequently, the authors speculated that hypogastric artery ligation preceding embolization may increase the likelihood of ischemic complications, but insufficient evidence exists to corroborate this conclusion. A third case occurred in a postpartum woman who underwent bilateral embolization with gelatin sponge pledgets and polyvinyl alcohol particles of 200 to 500 μm (52). The patient subsequently underwent bilateral ligation of the uterine and uteroovarian arteries because of continued bleeding. She was admitted eight weeks after surgery with sepsis and pain. Hysterectomy demonstrated uterine necrosis with polyvinyl alcohol particles in the small vessels. The only case of uterine necrosis treated with embolization alone occurred in a woman with PPH secondary to uterine atony (41). Embolization was performed with polyvinyl alcohol particles (diameter 150–250 and 300–600 μm) and gelatin sponge pledgets. Six months after embolization, she was readmitted to the hospital with bleeding and pain and subsequently had a hysterectomy that demonstrated uterine necrosis. At the junctions between the viable and nonviable tissues, vessels contained embolized foreign particles with surrounding granulomatous giant cell reaction. The authors concluded that uterine necrosis was related to the size of the polyvinyl alcohol particles; specifically, the small size of the polyvinyl alcohol particles (150–250 μm) caused the ischemia. For this reason, Gelfoam pledgets or slurry are the embolic materials of choice.

PREGNANCY AFTER POSTPARTUM HEMORRHAGE THERAPY

Hypogastric artery ligation, uterine artery ligation, and uterine artery embolization are all considered fertility-sparing procedures. Numerous successful pregnancies have been reported in women who had previously undergone bilateral hypogastric artery ligation (53). AbdRabbo (32) described ten pregnancies in patients who had undergone bilateral uterine artery ligation with or without ovarian ligation.

Pregnancies have also been reported after pelvic embolization for postpartum bleeding (50,54). Poppe et al. (55)

documented normal placental blood flow by ultrasonography in a gravid patient who previously underwent pelvic embolization. In a recent study by Ornan et al. (56), 28 patients undergoing pelvic embolization for intractable PPH between 1977 and 2002 were followed for an average of 11.7 years (±6.9 years) in order to assess subsequent fertility. This is the longest mean follow-up to date. In the six cases in which patients desired to become pregnant, all were able to do so. Of the remaining patients, none made subsequent attempts to become pregnant. Nevertheless, two patients reported unintentional pregnancies and subsequently opted for elective termination.

In conclusion, both surgical ligation and transcatheter arterial embolization spare the uterus and thus provide fertility-preserving alternatives to hysterectomy for treatment of intractable PPH.

PROPHYLACTIC USES OF OBSTETRIC EMBOLOTHERAPY

Embolization has also been used prophylactically to prevent hemorrhage in patients at high risk for severe bleeding. The original reports of embolization in this setting were in patients with ectopic pregnancy and placenta accreta/percreta.

Ectopic Pregnancy

Ectopic pregnancy has been reported to occur in the fallopian tubes, ovaries, abdominal cavity, and cervix. Surgery is considered the best treatment for tubal and ovarian pregnancies. However, surgical management of abdominal and cervical pregnancies is often associated with severe hemorrhage.

Abdominal Ectopic Pregnancy

Abdominal ectopic pregnancy is a rare condition occurring in 1 in 1,136 to 1 in 24,800 deliveries (57). The ectopic pregnancy can occur anywhere in the pelvis and is composed of richly vascular tissue. Upon removal of the gestational sac and placental tissue, there is often severe bleeding from the vessels supplying the placenta. Maternal mortality ranges from 0% to 30%, with the primary cause of morbidity and mortality being hemorrhage secondary to separation of the extrauterine placenta (58). This separation may occur before, during, or after laparotomy to remove the fetus (59). A central issue in the operative management is whether to remove the placenta with the fetus or to leave it *in situ*. When the placenta is left in the peritoneal cavity, it can cause complications. Unfortunately, removal of the placenta is associated with a large volume of blood loss. In 1993, Kerr et al. (58) reported on preoperative embolization of the placenta with Gelfoam pledgets in the management of three abdominal ectopic pregnancies. In each case, the patient underwent successful surgical removal of the nonviable pregnancy and placenta with only minor blood loss. The authors stressed the importance of evaluating the visceral blood supply to the abdominal pregnancy at angiography and of performing surgery as soon as possible after transcatheter arterial embolization to prevent the formation of collateral vessels (which can occur within hours).

Cervical Ectopic Pregnancy

Cervical ectopic pregnancy is defined as implantation of fetal tissues into the cervical canal. This rare condition has a reported incidence of 1 in 1,000 to 1 in 18,000 pregnancies (60). Prior to the widespread use of ultrasound as a means of evaluating early pregnancy, this condition typically presented with massive hemorrhage from eroded blood vessels and necessitated an emergency hysterectomy. However, with the advent of transvaginal ultrasound and quantitative serum β-human chorionic gonadotropin assays, cervical ectopic pregnancy is now often diagnosed well before the onset of bleeding. This allows for conservative management with various chemotherapeutic agents such as methotrexate or potassium chloride. Although this treatment alone can be successful, transcatheter arterial embolization is used prior to dilation and curettage in order to minimize bleeding and to treat secondary hemorrhage.

Preoperative uterine artery embolization in the management of cervical pregnancy was initially reported by Lobel et al. (61) in 1990, soon followed by Frates et al. (62) in 1994. In the two studies, a total of six patients with cervical pregnancy underwent preoperative embolization with subsequent curettage. Frates et al. did not specify the embolic material used, but Lobel et al. used Gelfoam pledgets followed by coils. In all cases, there was successful removal of the products of conception without serious bleeding. A single patient had minor vaginal bleeding treated successfully with endovaginal balloon tamponade (61). As was the case for preoperative embolization in the management of abdominal ectopic pregnancy, the need to perform curettage immediately after arterial embolization for cervical ectopic pregnancy was similarly emphasized. The obvious advantage of embolization in these patients was the avoidance of a hysterectomy and thus the subsequent preservation of fertility. Of the patients described, three later became pregnant (Figs. 14-3 and 14-4) (62).

PLACENTAL ABNORMALITIES AS A CAUSE OF POSTPARTUM HEMORRHAGE

Abnormalities of placental position and attachment predispose to abnormal bleeding at the time of delivery. In placenta previa, which is the most common abnormality of placental position, the placenta covers the internal cervical os (Fig. 14-5). Placenta accreta, placenta increta, and placenta percreta are terms used to describe a spectrum of abnormalities involving aberrant attachment of the placenta to the uterine wall, such that the chorionic villi invades into the myometrium. Three grades are described based on the pathologic assessment of myometrial invasion by the chorionic villi. Placenta accreta occurs when the chorionic villi are in contact with the myometrium, placenta increta when the villi invade into the myometrium, and placenta percreta when the villi invade into or beyond the serosa. Distinguishing among placenta accreta, placenta increta, and placenta percreta can be difficult before delivery. Their clinical behavior and radiologic appearance are similar, unless bladder involvement is present.

The optimal management strategy for these life-threatening conditions has yet to be defined. The most difficult management situation occurs with placenta percreta because the ingrowth of the placenta extends into or beyond the uterine serosa and may invade the adjacent bladder or bowel. Uterine rupture and massive hemorrhage have been associated with this type of implantation (63,64). Bleeding may occur intraabdominally, resulting in delay of diagnosis and hemodynamic instability.

It is now understood that the number of cases of placenta previa is linked to the number of previous cesarean deliveries. Specifically, there is a 0.65% risk after one prior cesarean delivery, 1.8% after two, 3% after three, and 10% after four (65). In addition, there is a strong association of placenta accreta/percreta with placenta previa. Approximately 75% of placenta percreta cases are associated with placenta previa. Approximately 25% of women with placenta previa and a single previous cesarean section have placenta accreta/percreta, and almost 50 percent of patients with placenta previa and two prior cesarean deliveries have placenta accreta/percreta (66).

Maternal morbidity and mortality are significantly increased by the presence of placenta percreta. The mortality rate secondary to hemorrhage and its complications can be as high as 10% (67,68). The average intraoperative blood loss during surgery in the face of placenta percreta is 3 to 5 L, and more than 90% of patients undergoing cesarean section with subsequent hysterectomy will require transfusion (32,65,66). Intraoperative blood loss may necessitate massive erythrocyte transfusion with subsequent complications, including disseminated intravascular coagulation, transfusion reactions, alloimmunization, and fluid overload. Potential surgical morbidity includes hysterectomy, bowel injury, ureteral injury, and bladder laceration. In addition, postoperative bleeding necessitates reexploration in up to 7% of patients with placenta accreta/percreta (69,70).

The increasing importance of placental abnormalities as a cause of PPH can be reflected in recent changes in the reported etiologies of emergency hysterectomies. Histori-

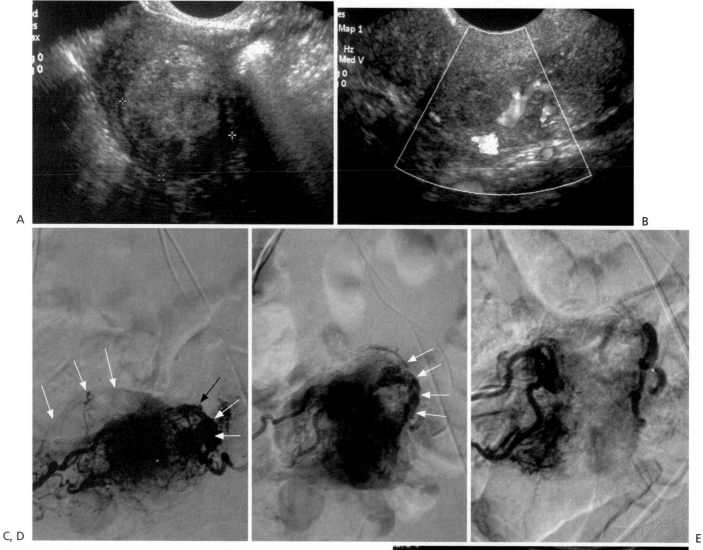

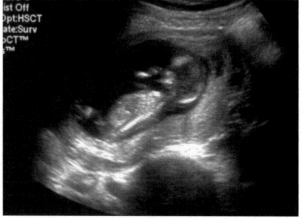

FIGURE 14-3. Cervical pregnancy. **A:** Patient with a miscarriage treated with dilation and curettage resulting in massive hemorrhage. Ultrasound reveals a mass in upper cervix. **B:** Color flow Doppler image confirms prominent venous structures associated with the lesion. **C:** Anteroposterior bilateral uterine arteriogram reveals some increase in vascularity *(white arrows)* but considerable superimposition of vessels. There is an incidental uterine fibroid *(black arrow)*. **D:** Using craniocaudal angulation of the c-arm, a hypovascular focus with surrounding vascularity is seen on the patient's left uterine artery *(arrows)*. **E:** After embolization with tris-acryl gelatin microspheres on the **left,** there is a significant reduction in vascularity. **F:** Fourteen months later, the patient had no intervening abnormal bleeding and was carrying an uncomplicated pregnancy, as demonstrated in the obstetric ultrasound study.

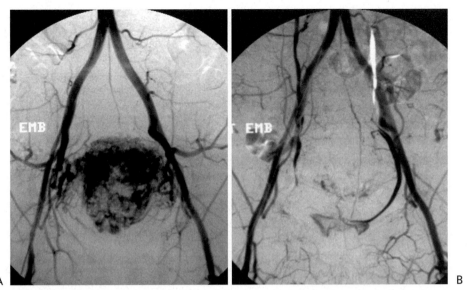

FIGURE 14-4. Cervical pregnancy treated with prophylactic embolization. **A:** Pregnant patient presented with vaginal spotting. Ultrasound revealed an 11.3-week cervical pregnancy with cardiac activity. After initial treatment with methotrexate, embolization was undertaken. The initial arteriogram demonstrated a hypervascular mass. **B:** After bilateral embolization with Gelfoam, the mass is devascularized. Dilation and curettage was subsequently performed and resulted in moderate bleeding. This required hysteroscopic endometrial ablation, which controlled the bleeding. Hysterectomy was not required. (Images courtesy of Clifton Tatum, M.D.)

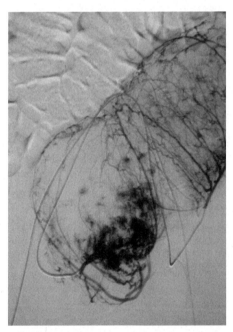

FIGURE 14-5. Fetal demise and hemorrhage from placenta previa. Sudden heavy bleeding occurred in a woman who was 18 weeks pregnant. Ultrasound revealed fetal demise and placenta previa. Bilateral catheterization of uterine arteries was performed prior to embolization.

cally, uterine atony has been the leading cause of emergent hysterectomy after delivery. More recently, however, placenta accreta/percreta has emerged as the leading indication (71–73). This change may be largely due to the introduction of noninvasive measures for treatment of uterine atony in conjunction with higher caesarean rates.

The details of diagnosing these entities are beyond the scope of this text. However, the goal is to diagnose placental implantation abnormalities early so that appropriate preoperative management can occur. More than 80% of patients with ultrasonographic diagnosis of placenta percreta will need a cesarean hysterectomy (66,67). Ideally, elective delivery is undertaken prior to spontaneous labor and severe vaginal bleeding. The optimal management of placenta percreta is complex and involves a multidisciplinary team approach involving such specialties as urology, anesthesia, hematology, neonatology, surgery, and interventional radiology.

Currently, there are two main treatment modalities for perioperative management of placenta percreta. The first involves cesarean delivery with subsequent removal of the placenta and hysterectomy. A more conservative therapeutic option is to leave the placenta *in situ* after cesarean delivery of the fetus with subsequent administration of chemotherapeutics. Regardless of the obstetrician's treatment algorithm, interventional radiology has come to play a pivotal role in both the prevention and treatment of hemorrhagic complications.

Predelivery prophylactic catheterization is a relatively new approach to help prevent hemorrhage and can be performed via an axillary or femoral approach. Advantages of an axillary approach include technical ease and a reduced likelihood of contaminating the abdominal incision. In the operating room, the working environment around the left axillary artery is often unconfined, whereas surgical drapes and instruments commonly obscure the femoral artery. Another reported advantage is decreased radiation exposure to the fetus (74). In the first report of prophylactic catheter placement, the patient was brought to the angiography suite, and the gravid uterus was shielded with a lead apron. A catheter was passed from the left axillary artery to the level of the first lumbar vertebra, just above the patient's shielded uterus. Subsequently, the patient was transferred to the operating room and underwent cesarean section. When hemorrhage occurred, the catheter was advanced into the bleeding vessel and subsequently embolized. However, Dubois et al. (75) maintain that although this technique may be successful in cases of placenta accreta, it is inadequate for treatment of placenta percreta. This conclusion was based on a single experience where the blood loss was so great that the treating radiologists were unable to selectively catheterize the uterine arteries in the operating room. Therefore, Dubois et al. maintain that subselection of the anterior division of the hypogastric arteries prior to delivery is imperative in cases of placenta percreta. Additionally, Hansch et al. (46), who used the femoral artery approach, reported that such subselection could usually be done in less than 5 to 8 minutes of fluoroscopy time, which equates to minimal radiographic exposure to the fetus in most cases. At a deep exposure of 2 rad per minute, the exposure to the fetus is estimated to be approximately 10 to 16 rad (76). Although it is believed that there is no threshold dose below which there is no risk to the fetus, analysis of the available data suggests an absolute risk of approximately 0.06% per rad (77).

In 1993, Mitty et al. (74) first investigated prophylactic arterial catheterization prior to delivery in nine obstetric patients who were at high risk for bleeding due to abnormal placental insertion. Their study compared the delivery outcome and operative blood loss between patients undergoing prophylactic catheterization and those undergoing emergent catheterization. Study patients included those with placenta previa and placenta accreta, uterine leiomyomas, twin fetal death, and ectopic pregnancy. In the prophylactic group, prior to cesarean section, a 5-French headhunter (HIH) catheter was passed from the left axillary artery to the aorta at the level of the first lumbar vertebra. After delivery, four of these patients required selection of the uterine arteries and embolization with Gelfoam pledgets because of hemorrhage. The estimated blood loss was less than 1 L in patients who had prophylactic catheterization, compared to 4.5 L in the group who had undergone emergency embolization for postpartum bleeding. These findings were later supported in a technically similar study of nine patients, five of whom received prophylactic catheter placement. In the four patients who eventually required embolization to control blood loss, the estimated blood loss was 1.2 L in the prophylactic catheterization group compared to 4.4 L in the emergency group (78).

Dubois et al. (75) used balloon occlusion as well as embolization to minimize intraoperative blood losses in two cases. In their study, the axillary arteries were accessed through 6-French vascular sheaths, and the anterior divisions of bilateral hypogastric arteries were selected. Two 5-French occluding balloon catheters (inflated 8.5 mm)

were inserted. Both the catheters and the sheaths were then connected to perfusion lines and secured in place. If hemorrhage occurred after delivery, small (2 × 2 × 2 mm) pieces of Gelfoam sponge were used to embolize the anterior branch of the hypogastric arteries through the balloon occlusion catheters. The balloons were then deflated in a controlled fashion and removed. Less than 2,000 mL of blood loss was documented in the two cases, and neither required a blood transfusion. The authors emphasized that the balloons were only inflated after the delivery, minimizing the hazard of uteroplacental insufficiency. One advantage of this procedure is a reduced risk of Gelfoam reflux into the posterior division of the hypogastric artery with its potential for sciatic nerve injury.

In 1999, Hansch et al. (46) recommended the use of balloon catheters after a failed embolization attempt in a patient with placenta accreta. In this case, the bleeding was so brisk that the time to catheterize and completely embolize the individual uterine arteries was insufficient. Hansch et al. maintain that the inflation balloon achieves a temporary hemostasis, which in turn allows for complete selective embolization.

This limited experience suggests a place for the prophylactic use of hypogastric or uterine artery catheterization in high-risk patients. Additional experience is needed before the efficacy and safety of this approach can be firmly established.

CONCLUSION

The full potential of arterial transcatheterization is being explored in patients identified as being at high risk for peripartum hemorrhage. With good clinical history and modern imaging techniques, many conditions such as placenta previa, placenta accreta, and ectopic cervical and abdominal pregnancies can be diagnosed. Early diagnosis allows for prophylactic, presurgical embolization or prophylactic, presurgical placement of catheters or balloons, thus enabling rapid treatment of hemorrhage should it arise.

Although embolization is becoming the treatment modality of choice for preventing and controlling PPH, its use depends on the availability of interventional radiologists, staff, and angiographic equipment. These cases represent true emergencies, and it is important that each institution have protocols for the prompt treatment of these patients. With rapid intervention, significant morbidity and mortality associated with PPH can become a thing of the past.

REFERENCES

1. Kaunitz AM, Hughes JM, Grimes DA, et al. Causes of maternal mortality in the United States. *Obstet Gynecol* 1985;65:605–612.
2. Pritchard JA, Baldwin RM, Dickey JC, et al. Blood volume changes in pregnancy and the puerperium. Red blood cell loss

and changes in apparent blood volume during and following vaginal delivery, cesarean section, and cesarean section plus total hysterectomy. *Am J Obstet Gynecol* 1962;84:1271–1282.

3. Combs CA, Murphy EL, Laros RK Jr. Factors associated with postpartum hemorrhage with vaginal birth. *Obstet Gynecol* 1991;77:69–76.

4. Combs CA, Murphy EL, Laros RK Jr. Factors associated with hemorrhage in cesarean deliveries. *Obstet Gynecol* 1991;77:77–82.

5. Dildy GA. Post partum hemorrhage. *Contemp Ob Gynecol* 1993;August:21–29.

6. Fahmy K, el Gazar A, Sammour M, et al. Post-partum colposcopy of the cervix: injury and healing. *Int J Gynaecol Obstet* 1991;34:133.

7. Pritchard JA, Cunningham FG, Mason RA. Coagulation changes in eclampsia: their frequency and pathogenesis. *Am J Obstet Gynecol* 1976;124:855.

8. Sibai BM, Ramadan MK, Usta I, et al. Maternal morbidity and mortality in 442 pregnancies with hemolysis, elevated liver enzymes, and low platelets (HELLP syndrome). *Am J Obstet Gynecol* 1993;169:1000–1006.

9. Sibai BM. The HELLP syndrome (hemolysis, elevated liver enzymes and low platelets): much ado about nothing? *Am J Obstet Gynecol* 1990;162:311–316.

10. Sibai BM, Soinnato JA, Watson DL, et al. Pregnancy outcome in 303 cases with severe preeclampsia. *Obstet Gynecol* 1984:64: 319–325.

11. Sibai BM, Anderson GD, McCubbin JH. Eclampsia II: clinical significance of laboratory findings. *Obstet Gynecol* 1982;59: 153–157.

12. Van Dam PA, Renier M, Baekelandt M, et al. Disseminated intravascular coagulation and the syndrome of hemolysis, elevated liver enzymes, and low platelets in severe preeclampsia. *Obstet Gynecol* 1989;73:97–102

13. Sibai BM, Taslimi MM, el-Nazer A, et al. Maternal-perinatal outcome associated with the syndrome of hemolysis, elevated liver enzymes, and low platelets in severe preeclampsia-eclampsia. *Am J Obstet Gynecol* 1986;155:501–509.

14. Pockros PJ, Perers RL, Reynolds TB. Idiopathic fatty liver of pregnancy: findings in ten cases. *Medicine (Baltimore)*1984; 63:1–11.

15. Riely CA. Acute fatty liver of pregnancy. *Semin Liver Dis* 1987;7:47–54.

16. Usta IM, Barton JR, Amon EA, et al. Acute fatty liver of pregnancy: an experience in the diagnosis and management of fourteen cases. *Am J Obstet Gynecol* 1994;171:1342–1347.

17. Rolfes DB, Ishak GK. Acute fatty liver of pregnancy: a clinico-pathologic study of 35 cases. *Hepatology* 1985;5:1149–1158.

18. Kaplan MM. Acute fatty liver of pregnancy. *N Engl J Med* 1985;313:367–370.

19. Ockner SA, Brunt EM, Cohn SM, et al. Fulminant hepatic failure caused by acute fatty liver of pregnancy treated by orthotopic liver transplantation. *Hepatology* 1990:11:59–64.

20. Pritchard JA. Fetal death in utero. *Obstet Gynecol* 1959;14:393.

21. Pritchard JA. Haematological problems associated with deliver, placental abruption, retained dead fetus, and amniotic fluid embolism. *Clin Haematol* 1973;2:256.

22. Pahlavan P, Nezhat C, Nezhat C. Hemorrhage in obstetrics and gynecology. *Curr Opin Obstet Gynecol* 2001;13:419–24.

23. Burchell RC. Internal iliac artery ligation: hemodynamics. *Obstet Gynecol* 1964;24:737–739.

24. Evans S, McShane P. The efficacy of internal iliac artery ligation in obstetric hemorrhage. *Surg Gynecol Obstet* 1985;160:250–253.

25. Clark SL, Phelan JP, Yeh S, et al. Hypogastric artery ligation for obstetric hemorrhage. *Obstet Gynecol* 1985;66:353–356.

26. Thavarasah AS, Sivalingam N, Almohdzar SA. Internal iliac and ovarian artery ligation in the control of pelvic haemorrhage. *Aust N Z J Obstet Gynecol* 1989;29:22–25.

27. Chattopadhyay SK, Deb Roy B, Edrees YB. Surgical control of obstetric hemorrhage: hypogastric artery ligation or hysterectomy? *Int J Gynecol Obstet* 1990;32:345–351.

28. Likeman MA. The boldest procedure possible for checking the bleeding: a new look at an old operation, and a series of 13 cases from an Australian hospital. *Aust N Z J Obstet Gynecol* 1992;32:256–262.

29. Paris SO, Glickman M, Schwartz PE, et al. Embolization of pelvic arteries for control of postpartum hemorrhage. *Obstet Gynecol* 1980;55:754–758.

30. Vedantham S, Goodwin SC, McLucas B, et al. Uterine artery embolization: an underused method of controlling pelvic hemorrhage. *Am J Obstet Gynecol* 1997;176:938–948.

31. Waters EG. Surgical management of postpartum hemorrhage with particular reference to ligation of uterine arteries. *Am J Obstet Gynecol* 1952:64:1143–1148.

32. AbdRabbo SA. Stepwise uterine devascularization: a novel technique for management of uncontrollable postpartum hemorrhage with preservation of the uterus. *Am J Obstet Gynecol* 1994;171:694–700.

33. O'Leary JA. Uterine artery ligation in the control of post-cesarean hemorrhage. *J Reprod Med* 1995;40:189–193.

34. Baum S, Nusbaum M, Clearfield Hr, et al. Angiography in the diagnosis of gastrointestinal bleeding. *Arch Intern Med* 1967;119: 16–24.

35. Nusbaum M, Baum S, Blakemore WS. Clinical experience with the diagnosis and management of gastrointestinal hemorrhage by selective mesenteric catheterization. *Ann Surg* 1969;170: 506–514.

36. Matalon TSA, Athanasoulis CA, Waltman AC, et al. Hemorrhage with pelvic fractures: efficacy of transcatheter embolization. *AJR Am J Roentgenol* 1979;133:859–864.

37. Brown BJ, Heaston DK, Poulson AM, et al. Uncontrollable postpartum bleeding: a new approach to hemostasis through angiographic embolization. *Obstet Gynecol* 1979;54:361–365.

38. Mitty HA, Sterling KM, Alvarez M, et al. Obstetric hemorrhage; prophylactic and emergency arterial catheterization and embolotherapy. *Radiology* 1993;188:183–187.

39. Yamashita Y, Takashi M, Ito M, et al. Transcatheter arterial embolization in the management of postpartum hemorrhage due to genital tract injury. *Obstet Gynecol* 1991;77:160–163.

40. Pelage JP, Le Dref O, Soyer P, et al. Arterial anatomy of the female genital tract: variations and relevance to transcatheter embolization of the uterus. *AJR Am J Roentgenol* 1999;172:989–994.

41. Cottier JP, Fignon A, Tranquart F, et al. Uterine necrosis after arterial embolization for postpartum hemorrhage. *Obstet Gynecol* 2002;100[Suppl]:1074–1077.

42. Yamashita Y, Harada M, Yamamoto H, et al. Transcatheter arterial embolization of obstetric and gynecological bleeding: efficacy and clinical outcome. *Br J Radiol* 1994;67:530–534.

43. Abbas FM, Currie JL, Mitchell S, et al. Selective vascular embolization in benign gynecological condition. *J Reprod Med* 1994;39:492–496.

44. Pelage JP, Le Dref O, Mateo J, et al. Life-threatening primary postpartum hemorrhage: treatment with emergency selective arterial embolization. *Radiology* 1998;208:359–362.

45. Oei PL, Chua S, Tan L, et al. Arterial embolization for bleeding following hysterectomy for intractable postpartum hemorrhage. *Int J Gynaecol Obstet* 1998;62:83–86.

46. Hansch E, Chitkara U, McAlpine J, et al. Pelvic arterial embolization for control of obstetric hemorrhage: a five year experience. *Am J Obstet Gynecol* 1999;180:1454–1460.

47. Dildy GA. Postpartum hemorrhage: new management options. *Clin Obstet Gynecol* 2002;45:330–344.

48. Bakri YN, Linjawi T. Angiographic embolization for control of pelvic genital tract hemorrhage. *Acta Obstet Gynecol Scand* 1992;71:17–21.

49. Gilbert WM, Moore TR, Resnik R, et al. Angiographic embolization in the management of hemorrhagic complications of pregnancy. *Am J Obstet Gynecol* 1992;166:493–497.

50. Greenwood LH, Glickman MG, Schwartz PE, et al. Obstetric and non-malignant bleeding; treatment with angiographic embolization. *Radiology* 1987;164:155–159.

51. Chin HG, Scott DR, Resnik R, et al. Angiographic embolization of intractable puerperal hematomas. *Am J Obstet Gynecol* 1989;160:434–438.

52. Pirard C, Squifflet J, Gilles A, et al. Uterine necrosis and sepsis after vascular embolization and surgical ligation in a patient with post partum hemorrhage. *Fertil Steril* 2002;78:412–413.

53. Mengert WF, Burchell RC, Blumstein RW, et al. Pregnancy after bilateral ligation of the internal iliac and ovarian arteries. *Obstet Gynecol* 1969;34:664–666.

54. Pelage JP, Le Dref O, Jacob D, et al. Selective arterial embolization of the uterine arteries in the management of intractable post-partum hemorrhage. *Acta Obstet Gynecol Scand* 1999;78:698–703.

55. Poppe W, Van Assche FA, Wilms G, et al. Pregnancy after transcatheter embolization of a uterine arteriovenous malformation. *Am J Obstet Gynecol* 1987;156:1179–1180.

56. Ornan D, White R, Pollak J, et al. Pelvic embolization for intractable post partum hemorrhage: long-term follow-up and implications for fertility. *Obstet Gynecol* 2003;102:904–910.

57. Kivikoski AL, Marin C, Weyman P, et al. Angiographic arterial embolization to control hemorrhage in abdominal pregnancy: a case report. *Obstet Gynecol* 1988;71:456–459.

58. Kerr A, Trambert J, Mikhail M, et al. Preoperative transcatheter embolization of abdominal pregnancy: report of three cases. *J Vasc Interv Radiol* 1993;4:733–35.

59. McCaul MJ. Emergent management of abdominal pregnancy. *Clin Obstet Gynecol* 1990;33:438–447.

60. Ratten GJ. Cervical pregnancy treated by libation of the descending branch of the uterine arteries. Case report. *Br J Obstet Gynaecol* 1983;90:367–371.

61. Lobel SM, Meyerovitz MF, Benson CC, et al. Preoperative angiographic uterine artery embolization in the management of cervical pregnancy. *Obstet Gynecol* 1990;76:938–941.

62. Frates MC, Benson CB, Doubiliet PM, et al. Cervical ectopic pregnancy: results of conservative treatment. *Radiology* 1994;191:773–775.

63. Breen JL, Neubecker R, Gregori CA, et al. Placenta accreta, increta, and percreta: a survey of 40 cases. *Obstet Gynecol* 1977;49:43–47.

64. Lloyd-Jones R, Winterton WR. Spontaneous rupture of the uterus due to placenta percreta: a case report. *J Obstet Gynaecol Br Commonw* 1961;68:273–276.

65. Clark SL, Koonings PP, Phelan JP. Placenta previa/accreta and prior cesarean section. *Obstet Gynecol* 1985;66:89–92.

66. Fineberg G, Williams J. Placenta accreta: prospective sonographic diagnosis in patients with placenta previa and prior cesarean section. *J Ultrasound Med* 1992;11:333–343.

67. Catanzarite V, Stanco L, Schrimmer S, et al. Managing placenta previa/accreta. *Cont Obstet Gynecol* 1996;41:66–95.

68. Price F, Resnik E, Heller K, et al. Placenta previa/percreta involving the urinary bladder: a report of two cases and review of the literature. *Obstet Gynecol* 1991;78:508–511.

69. de Mondoca LK. Sonographic diagnosis of placenta accreta. *J Ultrasound Med* 1988;7:211–215.

70. Hoffman-Tretin F, Koenigsberg M, Rabin A, et al. Placenta accreta: additional sonographic observations. *J Ultrasound Med* 1992;11:29–34.

71. Clark SL, Yeh SY, Phelan JP, et al. Emergency hysterectomy for obstetric hemorrhage. *Obstet Gynecol* 1984;64:376–380.

72. O'Leary JA, Steer CM. A 10 year review of cesarean hysterectomy. *Am J Obstet Gynecol* 1964;20:227–231.

73. Stanco LM, Schrimmer DB, Paul RH, et al. Emergency peripartum hysterectomy and associated risk factors. *Am J Obstet Gynecol* 1993;168:879–883.

74. Mitty HA, Sterling KM, Alvarez M, et al. Obstetric hemorrhage: prophylactic and emergency arterial catheterization and embolotherapy. *Radiology* 1993;188:183–187.

75. Dubois J, Garel L, Grignon A, et al. Placenta percreta: balloon occlusion and embolization of the internal iliac arteries to reduce intraoperative blood losses. *Am J Obstet Gynecol* 1997;176:723–726.

76. Huda W, Stone R. *Review of radiation physics.* Baltimore: Williams & Williams, 1995:85.

77. Doll R, Wakeford R. Risk of childhood cancer from fetal irradiation. *Br J Radiol* 1997;70:130–139.

78. Alvarez MA, Lockwood CJ, Ghidini A, et al. Prophylactic and emergent arterial catheterization for selective embolization in obstetric hemorrhage. *Am J Perinatol* 1992;9:441–444.

15

EMBOLIZATION FOR THE MANAGEMENT OF GYNECOLOGIC MALIGNANCIES AND VASCULAR MALFORMATIONS

ANTOINETTE ROTH
SCOTT C. GOODWIN
SURESH VEDANTHAM
MICHAEL L. DOUEK
JAMES B. SPIES

INTRODUCTION

Just as with postpartum hemorrhage, interventional therapies play a key role in the management of patients with gynecologic hemorrhage. Most of the reports in the literature have been in the setting of gynecologic malignancy, but the same principles apply in the management of benign conditions such as congenital and acquired arteriovenous malformations (AVMs) and pseudoaneurysms. Similarly, embolization has long been established as the treatment modality of choice when vessel rupture is encountered secondary to trauma. This chapter discusses in detail the pathophysiology and use of transcatheter arterial embolization in the treatment of hemorrhage due to malignancy and vascular malformations and discusses in brief its use in the trauma patient.

PELVIC HEMORRHAGE FROM MALIGNANCY

Pelvic malignancies include a wide range of cancers. The most common gynecologic malignancy in developed countries is endometrial cancer, which accounts for 13% of all cancers in women (1). The majority of women present with stage I disease, which is clinically confined to the uterus. Women with stage I disease have an overall unadjusted 5-year survival of approximately 75% (2,3). The preferred treatment of stage I disease is total hysterectomy with bilateral salpingo-oophorectomy and staging pelvic/aortic lymphadenectomy (3). Patients with high-risk disease, including those with positive retroperitoneal lymph nodes and high histologic grade, may receive adjuvant radiotherapy (3–5). The prognosis for patients with more advanced (stages II–IV) or recurrent disease is poor, with a

median survival being less than 1 year (3). Treatment for these patients is usually limited to systemic chemotherapy.

The second most common gynecologic malignancy worldwide and the third most common in the United States is cervical cancer. In the United States alone, there are approximately 12,200 new cases each year and 4,100 deaths (6). The disease distribution is bimodal, with peaks at ages 35 to 39 years and 60 to 64 years. The molecular biology of cervical cancer is well understood. The human papillomavirus (HPV) is the causative agent in a large majority of cervical cancers, with the prevalence of HPV in cervical tumors being approximately 99.7% (7). The prognosis for patients with cervical cancer depends on the stage of disease at diagnosis (8). Preinvasive disease is conventionally managed with ablative or excision procedures such as loop electrosurgical excision, conization, or cryosurgery. Early invasive disease (stages IA, IB, and small stage IIA with no parametrial involvement) is treated with radical hysterectomy or radiotherapy, resulting in a 5-year survival rate of 80% to 90% (9). Advanced disease (stage IIB to IV) is treated with radiotherapy or a combination of chemotherapy and radiotherapy.

Malignancy-related vaginal hemorrhage most commonly results from carcinoma of the cervix, carcinoma of the endometrium, and choriocarcinoma (10). Hemorrhage from these malignancies is usually slow and chronic and occasionally intractable. Bleeding usually arises from small capillaries and veins as a result of ulceration or necrosis of the tumors. Massive bleeding from tumors invading into large vessels is rare. However, massive bleeding can occur as a complication of conventional therapies such as radiation or surgery. These treatments may lead to friability, inflammation, and/or necrosis of surrounding tissues and major vessels, which can result in massive hemorrhage

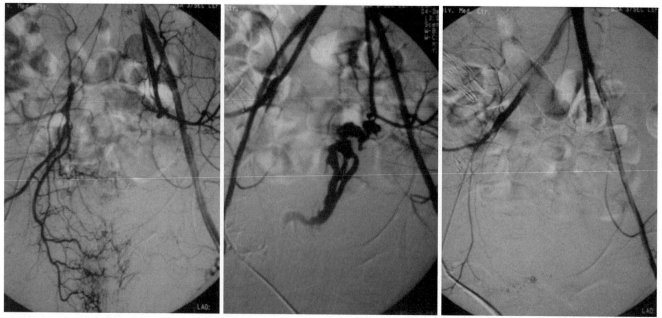

A, B   C

FIGURE 15-1. Massive hemorrhage from neoplastic erosion or radiation injury to the left hypogastric artery. **A:** Initial bilateral hypogastric arteriogram reveals postoperative changes in the left hypogastric artery, intact vessels on the right, without a clear site of bleeding. It was elected to proceed with embolization on the right, using polyvinyl alcohol particles. After the embolization on the right, the patient suddenly became tachycardic. Blood pressure was maintained, and the cause of the tachycardia was not immediately clear. Because of the patient's instability, it was decided to perform a final arteriogram with the anticipation of terminating the procedure. **B:** Repeat arteriogram reveals massive bleeding from the left hypogastric artery stump. The anterior division of the right hypogastric artery was occluded. **C:** After embolization of the left bleeding site with Gelfoam and coils, bleeding was controlled.

(Fig. 15-1). Additionally, the tumors may extend into adjacent organs, such as the bladder or rectosigmoid colon, creating fistulas, eroding into large vessels of the involved organs, and causing massive hematuria or hematochezia.

From this discussion, it is apparent that the mainstay of treatment for most pelvic malignancies remains surgical excision with adjuvant measures such as chemotherapy and radiation therapy. However, embolotherapy has an increasingly important role in treating bleeding complications arising from both the malignancy itself and the various treatment modalities. Originally, angiography was used purely as a diagnostic tool to delineate blood supply prior to surgery. Diagnostic arteriography of the pelvis is still sometimes used if variant anatomy is suspected or if the patient has undergone multiple previous surgeries. However, pelvic hemorrhage is now the primary indication for angiography in the oncology patient.

Embolization is the treatment of choice to control bleeding for many of the same reasons discussed in Chapter 14. Similar to cases of postpartum hemorrhage, angiography has been found to be effective in identifying the bleeding vessel. In cases where bleeding from a tumor is suspected but a bleeding vessel cannot be identified, embolization of the neovasculature as well as of the anatomic source of the blood supply has proven stabilizing (Fig. 15-2) (11).

There are additional advantages of embolization unique to the oncology patient. Frequently, surgical control of bleeding is extremely difficult, as extensive prior surgery or radiotherapy destroys normal anatomic relationships and makes identifying the source of bleeding difficult. Even if the source is known, access to the vessels to control the hemorrhage may be difficult for the same reasons. Finally, oncology patients commonly have multiple medical problems and are frequently hemodynamically unstable, making anesthesia and major surgery a high risk.

EMBOLIZATION TECHNIQUE IN THE ONCOLOGY PATIENT

Embolization can be more complicated in cases of malignancy compared to embolization in the postpartum setting. The vessels that cause bleeding from the female genital tract are usually predictable. The uterine artery supplies the uterus and cervix and accounts for the majority of bleeding. However, often the tumor extends outside of these structures into the pelvis, and other anterior division vessels are recruited to supply the tumor. Thus, the embolization may need to be more extensive than a typical postpartum embolization in order to be effective.

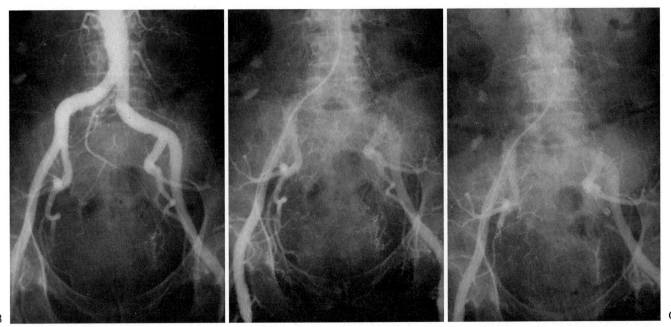

A, B   C

FIGURE 15-2. Recurrent bleeding from recurrent cervical cancer without identification of the bleeding site. **A:** Patient with a history of cervical cancer and chronic recurrent vaginal bleeding. Pelvic arteriogram in early arterial phase reveals minor hypervascularity in the left lower pelvis but no identifiable bleeding source. **B:** Late arterial phase confirms that there is no active bleeding. Embolization undertaken bilaterally with polyvinyl alcohol particles and coils. **C:** Postembolization with partial devascularization of the anterior division.

A variety of materials have been used in the oncology patient throughout the years and have included, but are not limited to, Gelfoam (11–14), polyvinyl alcohol particles (15–17), and wire coils (12,14). Different materials are chosen for transcatheter embolization, depending on the size of the vessel to be embolized and whether permanent, semipermanent, or short-term occlusion is desired. As stated previously, it is not uncommon for the specific site of bleeding to be inconspicuous in the oncology patient. Under these circumstances, all branches of the hypogastric artery may require embolization. The choice of embolic material is therefore critical. Particle size and consistency must be such that the embolics lodge in arterioles proximal to the precapillary collaterals to safeguard against ischemic necrosis of the target organ (18–20). Gelfoam is a readily available substance suitable for temporary occlusion. Usually it is used in pledget or slurry form. Although the cubes can fragment, collateral flow via the precapillary collaterals is maintained. Gelfoam powder, conversely, embolizes the capillary bed and can cause infarction (18,19). In patients with extensive parasitic tumor neovascularity, polyvinyl alcohol particles have several advantages (Fig. 15-3). They are not prone to fragmentation and retain their position once lodged in the vessel by expanding when exposed to liquid, thereby effectively embolizing the precapillary arterioles and maintaining precapillary collateral flow. For permanent occlusion of larger arteries, such as the hypogastric, wire coils can be used (Fig. 15-2). Concomitant occlusion at the level of the capillary bed can be obtained by combining coils with other embolic agents.

OUTCOME OF EMBOLOTHERAPY FOR PELVIC MALIGNANCY

Although large series have not been reported, smaller published case series suggest that embolization can be both safe and effective in controlling hemorrhage secondary to pelvic malignancy. In 1981, Lang (12) reported on a total of 23 patients with pelvic neoplasms, 12 of whom had cervical cancer and developed life-threatening hemorrhage. The causes of hemorrhage varied from tumor invading the bladder (seven patients) or vagina (three patients) or secondary to radiation cystitis (two patients). Gelfoam was the embolic agent used in all patients, and the addition of wire coils was required in one patient. There was 100% immediate cessation of bleeding. However, among the total 23 patients, five (21.7%) developed delayed complications that were probably due to tumor progression. Two patients with cervical cancer invading the bladder developed fistulas approximately two months later, and three patients had reduced bladder capacity.

In 1993, Yamshita et al. (14) reported on 17 patients with cervical cancer who developed malignancy-related hemorrhage. Of these patients, 12 had advanced primary cervical cancer and five had recurrent cervical cancer. Emergency embolotherapy was performed after uncontrollable massive vaginal bleeding. Angiography initially performed using standard techniques demonstrated definite extravasation from the uterine artery in only two of the 17 patients, but neovascularity was demonstrated in 12 of 17 patients. The presence of neovascularity is not uncommon

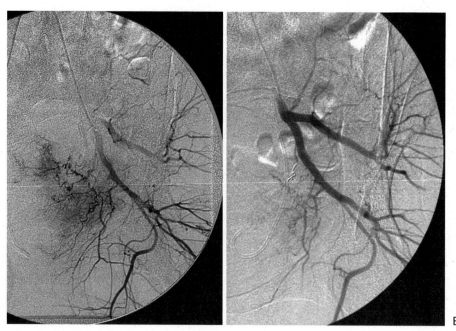

FIGURE 15-3. Recurrent cervical cancer with hemorrhage. **A:** Patient with recurrent cervical cancer and vaginal bleeding. Parasitized vessels from the left hypogastric artery supply a recurrent cervical cancer. **B:** Initial embolization with polyvinyl alcohol particles did not completely occlude the vessels, and supplementary microcoils were used. There is minimal residual hypovascularity.

and is largely due to malignant tumors being supplied by multiple small branches of the internal iliac arteries (Fig. 15-3). Therefore, multiple branches or main trunks of the anterior division of the internal iliac arteries required embolization. All patients were initially treated with Gelfoam particles (1 mm), and four required the supplemental use of steel coils. The authors noted that coils are not usually recommended because they preclude any further attempt at vessel access; however, they were used in these four cases when extravasation occurred in the larger arteries, and embolization could not be achieved despite the use of large quantities of gelatin sponge. In these cases, it was presumed that the small particles had been swept into the extravascular space due to the massive hemorrhage. The immediate response rate was 100%. However, seven patients (41.1%) had recurrent bleeding after 2 weeks, three of whom required repeat embolization. After the control of hemorrhage by embolization, all patients underwent treatment with radiation therapy, chemotherapy, or surgery. In total, two complications were reported. One patient had temporary numbness of the lower extremity, and a second had a skin ulcer on her buttock.

UTERINE VASCULAR ABNORMALITIES

Uterine curettage and surgical trauma have been associated with different vascular abnormalities, including pseudoaneurysms, acquired AVMs, and rupture of vessels. Recognition of these entities as causes of hemorrhage is imperative,

because these abnormalities can be treated safely and effectively with transcatheter arterial embolization.

Hemorrhage is one of the principal complications of uterine curettage and pelvic surgery, developing in 0.05% to 4.9% of abortion procedures (21,22). Hemorrhage refractory to conservative measures may potentially be attributed to arterial injury. In a recent study of 14 patients, the three patients who underwent transcatheter arterial embolization for intractable delayed postpartum hemorrhage had uterine vascular abnormalities as the underlying cause (Fig. 15-4) (23). Uterine vascular abnormalities have been reported sporadically following uterine curettage or surgical trauma (23–32). These vascular abnormalities include pseudoaneurysms (23–27), arteriovenous fistulas (28–31), and direct vessel rupture (32). These abnormalities may cause massive uterine bleeding and may be aggravated by dilation and curettage (D&C), in contrast to the more common causes of excessive uterine bleeding.

Pseudoaneurysms

A pseudoaneurysm results from inadequate sealing of a laceration or puncture of the arterial wall during surgery or trauma. Due to the sustained arterial pressure, blood dissects into the tissues around the damaged artery and forms a perfused sack that communicates with the artery. Pseudoaneurysms have been reported after D&C, cesarean section, and other surgeries on the uterus (23–27).

The diagnosis is usually made with color and duplex Doppler ultrasound that demonstrates a blood-filled cystic

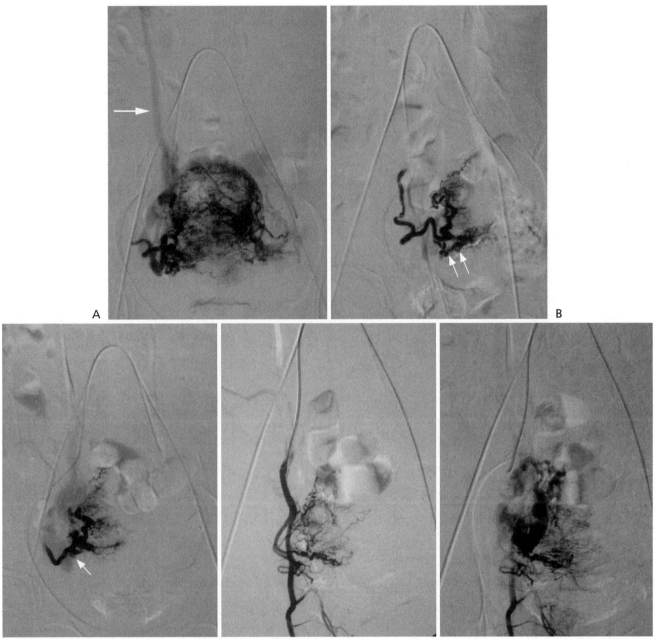

A

B

C, D

E

FIGURE 15-4. Uterine and adnexal arteriovenous malformation. **A:** Twenty-four-year-old woman with recent miscarriage and D&C complicated by severe bleeding and subsequent recurrent hemorrhage. Ultrasound examination showed hypervascular lesion in the right cervical area, with a differential diagnosis of either cervical pregnancy or arteriovenous fistula. Bilateral simultaneous anteroposterior arteriographic image reveals increased vascularity of the right uterus with an early-filling right ovarian vein *(arrow)*. **B:** Right uterine arteriogram, early arterial phase, in the left anterior oblique position. There is an enlarged cervicovaginal branch *(arrows)*, which on subsequent images is seen to supply a hypervascular nidus. The position correlated with the cervical abnormality on duplex ultrasound (not shown). **C:** Right uterine arteriogram in the left anterior oblique position after embolization. The cervicovaginal branch is occluded *(arrow)*, and arterial flow is diminished. For uncertain reasons there is faint early opacification of the veins in the right adnexa. **D:** Arteriogram of the anterior division of the right hypogastric artery after embolization reveals additional branches to the adnexa from other pelvic branches. **E:** Late-phase arteriogram shows markedly enlarged veins extending laterally from the margin of the uterus into the adnexa. Uterine bleeding was controlled by limited embolization of the cervicovaginal branch. The larger asymptomatic portion of the vascular malformation was asymptomatic and not treated.

structure with swirling arterial flow. Angiography will also demonstrate pseudoaneurysms supplied by one or more feeding arteries. In general, urgent intervention is required because pseudoaneurysms are at high risk for rupture.

The technique of embolization of pseudoaneurysms is discussed later in this chapter, but two important causes of procedure failure should be noted. When retained villi are present within a pseudoaneurysm associated with placenta accreta (33), rapid recruitment of collateral vessels following arterial embolization may occur from pelvic arteries, resulting in recanalization of the pseudoaneurysm (34,35). Ultrasound is insensitive in demonstrating retained villi; therefore, attention should be made to serum β-human chorionic gonadotropin levels.

A second cause of embolization failure is inadequate embolization of a pseudoaneurysm supplied by extrauterine feeding arteries, such as the internal pudendal artery, ovarian artery, inferior epigastric artery, or contralateral uterine artery (23,24,34). It is imperative to perform a meticulous search for other feeding arteries, including detection of simultaneous cross filling of the sac by two or more arteries.

Arteriovenous Malformations

AVMs are characterized by multiple communications between arteries and veins centered at a vascular nidus. An arteriovenous fistula is similar but contains fewer or, in some cases, only one abnormal direct passage between an artery and adjoining vein. Uterine AVMs are traditionally classified as either congenital or acquired. Congenital AVMs occur secondary to an abnormality in the embryologic development of primitive vascular structures resulting in multiple abnormal communications between arteries and veins (30). They tend to have multiple feeding arteries and draining veins, in addition to an intervening nidus (Fig. 15-4). Acquired AVMs, on the other hand, are multiple small arteriovenous communications between intramural arterial branches and the myometrial venous plexus. They appear as a vascular tangle, thus mimicking congenital AVMs. However, acquired AVMs typically have a single or bilateral feeding uterine arteries without being supplied by extrauterine arteries and do not have a nidus.

Endometrial carcinoma, cervical carcinoma, gestational trophoblastic disease, and maternal diethylstilbestrol exposure have all been implicated in acquired uterine AVMs (28,36–38) (Fig. 15-5). However, they more commonly occur as a result of trauma, because there is usually a history of D&C, uterine surgery, or trauma to the uterus in cases of AVMs (28–30). These conditions have the potential for development of abnormal fistulous communication between arteries and veins within the uterine wall, which may develop and persist as an AVM. The patient's history, coupled with the angiographic findings, help in differentiating between congenital and acquired AVMs. The pattern of bleeding is commonly intermittent and torrential, consistent with arterial hemorrhage. Bleeding is thought to occur

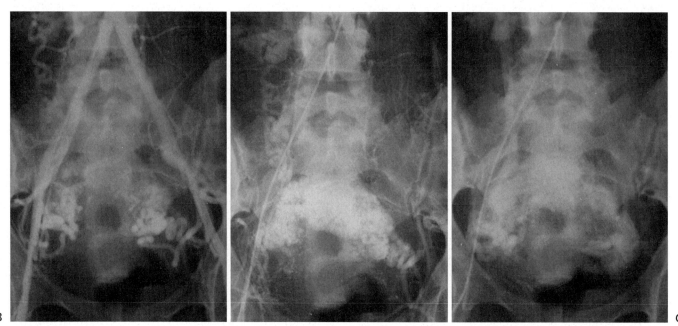

A, B   C

FIGURE 15-5. Molar pregnancy. **A:** Patient diagnosed with molar pregnancy treated with methotrexate but with persistent high serum β-human chorionic gonadotropin hormone levels. Early arterial phase of pelvic arteriogram with midaortic injection reveals enlarged uterine and ovarian arteries and a markedly vascular mass in the pelvis at the site of the molar pregnancy. **B:** Late arterial phase confirms intense vascular mass. **C:** Venous phase shows markedly enlarged draining veins.

when the vessels of the AVM are exposed from sloughing of the endometrium, which can be iatrogenic in a D&C or physiologic during menses (30).

As with pseudoaneurysms, ultrasound is the diagnostic tool of choice for vascular malformations. The details of diagnosis are beyond the scope of this text; however, in brief, color Doppler ultrasound shows an intense vascular tangle with duplex Doppler demonstrating low-resistance, high-velocity arterial flow. Transcatheter arterial embolization is the therapy of choice in treating these lesions.

EMBOLIZATION TECHNIQUE

Embolization is performed via catheterization of the uterine artery on the side of the presumed defect determined by ultrasound. Embolic materials are then introduced into the uterine artery or other feeding arteries until stasis of flow is confirmed angiographically. Ipsilateral internal iliac angiography is repeated to exclude the possibility of additional feeding arteries, which occasionally become conspicuous only after the major feeding artery is occluded. The contralateral internal iliac and uterine arteries should next be examined, with subsequent embolization of the uterine artery. Embolization of the contralateral uterine artery is performed in order to decrease the likelihood of cross filling. If bleeding does not stop or the vascular abnormality does not disappear, it is imperative to examine other possible feeding arteries such as the ovarian artery, inferior epigastric, or middle sacral artery.

Although a multitude of different embolic agents have been used, most uterine vascular abnormalities are safely and effectively treated with Gelfoam (23,39). Gelfoam is usually the material of choice for acquired AVMs, pseudoaneurysms arising from small branches, and direct arterial rupture because of the ease of embolic delivery and the duration of effect. Occlusion for 3 to 5 weeks is typical of Gelfoam and is sufficient to stop hemorrhage while permitting development of collateral vessels (40). Occasionally, occlusion of the proximal vessel is required in cases of pseudoaneurysms arising from larger branches or large arteriovenous fistulas. In these cases, metallic coils are preferred because of the risk of shunting of particulate embolic materials via the fistula in the systemic circulation or into the pseudoaneurysm.

CONCLUSION

Transcatheter arterial embolization is a safe and effective treatment for pelvic hemorrhage in a wide range of clinical settings. The advantages of embolotherapy over surgical approaches include the enhanced ability to detect the bleeding vessel, the ability to control bleeding even in the absence of specific bleeding vessel identification, the ease of access to reembolize multiple vessels if needed, the lack of need for general anesthesia, and the ability to more distally occlude vessels, thereby limiting the contribution of collateral circulation in perpetuating hemorrhage. Although these cases are much less frequent than fibroids, the ability to rapidly control hemorrhage via embolization is often dramatic and very gratifying. The success rates in bleeding control are very high, and the complication rates for embolization have been low. In circumstances with few other treatment options, this therapy is often life saving and represents a key tool in the armamentarium of physicians treating these often desperately ill patients.

REFERENCES

1. Lewis E, Zornoza J, Jing B, et al. Radiologic contributions to the diagnosis and management of gynecologic neoplasms. *Semin Roentgenol* 1982;17:251–268.
2. Martin-Hirsch PL, Jarvis G, Kitchener H, et al. Progestogens for endometrial cancer (Cochrane review). In: *The Cochrane library. Issue 2*. Oxford: Update Software, 2002.
3. Elit L, Hirte H. Current status and future innovations of hormonal agents, chemotherapy and investigation agents in endometrial cancer. *Curr Opin Obstet Gynecol* 2002:14:67–73.
4. Barakat, RR, Park RC, Grigsby PW, et al. *Principles and practice of gynecologic oncology*. Philadelphia: Lippincott Williams & Wilkins, 1997:880.
5. Bristow RE. Endometrial cancer. *Curr Opin Oncol* 1999;11: 338–393.
6. Parkin DM. Global cancer statistics in the year 2000. *Lancet Oncol* 2001;2:533–545.
7. Walboomers JM, Jacobs MV, Manos MM, et al. Human papillomavirus in cervical cancer: a worldwide perspective. *J Natl Cancer Inst* 1995;87:796–802.
8. Fiorica JV. Update on the treatment of cervical and uterine carcinoma: focus on topotecan. *Oncologist* 2002;7[Suppl 5]: 36–45.
9. Cannistra SA, Niloff JM, Cancer of the uterine cervix. *N Engl J Med* 1996;334:436–442.
10. Worthington-Kirsch RL, Scott ME, Charnsangavej C. Pelvic embolotherapy. In: Tareras JM, Ferracci JT, eds. *Radiology diagnosis-imaging-interpretation*. Philadelphia: Lippincott Williams & Wilkins, 2002:9
11. Mann WJ, Jander HP, Partridge EE, et al. Selective arterial embolization for control of bleeding in gynecologic malignancy. *Gynecol Oncol* 1980;10:279–289.
12. Lang EK. Transcatheter embolization of pelvic vessels for control of intractable hemorrhage. *Radiology* 1981;140:331–339.
13. Lin YC, Kudelka AP, Lawrence D, et al. Transcatheter arterial embolization for the control of life-threatening pelvic hemorrhage in a patient with locally advanced cervix carcinoma. *Eur J Gynaecol Oncol* 1996;6:480–483.
14. Yamashita Y, Harada M, Yamamoto H, et al. Transcatheter arterial embolization of obstetric and gynaecological bleeding: efficacy and clinical outcome. *Br J Radiol* 1994;67:530–534.
15. Mihamali I, Cantasdemir, Kantarci F, et al. Percutaneous embolization in the management of intractable vaginal bleeding. *Arch Gynecol Obstet* 2001;264:211–214.
16. Yalvac S, Kayikcioglu F, Boran N, et al. Embolization of uterine artery in terminal stage cervical cancers. *Cancer Invest* 2002;20: 754–758.

17. Takemura M, Yamasake M, Tanaka F, et al. Transcatheter arterial embolization in the management of gynecological neoplasms. *Gynecol Oncol* 1989;34:38–42.
18. Hietala SO. Urinary bladder necrosis following selective embolization of the internal iliac artery. *Acta Radiol* 1978;19:316–320.
19. Braf ZF, Koontz WW Jr. Gangrene of bladder. Complication of hypogastric artery embolization. *Urology* 1977;9:670–671.
20. Hald T, Mygind T. Control of life threatening hemorrhage by unilateral hypogastric artery muscle embolization. *J Urol* 1974;112:60–63.
21. Grimes DA. Management of abortion. In: Rock JA, Thompson JD, eds. *Te Linde's operative gynecology,* 8th ed. Philadelphia: Lippincott-Raven, 1997:477–499.
22. Hern WM. The epidemiologic foundation of abortion practice. In: Hern WM, ed. *Abortion practice.* Philadelphia: Lippincott, 1984:1–62.
23. Pelage JP, Soyer P, Repiquet D, et al. Secondary postpartum hemorrhage: treatment with selective arterial embolization. *Radiology* 1999;212:385–389.
24. Bromley PJ, Clark T, Weir IH, et al. Radiologic diagnosis and management of uterine artery pseudoaneurysm: case report. *Can Assoc Radiol J* 1997;48:119–122.
25. Zimon AE, Hwang JK, Principe DL, et al. Pseudoaneurysm of the uterine artery. *Obstet Gynecol* 1999;94:827–830.
26. Langer JE, Cope C. Ultrasonographic diagnosis of uterine artery pseudoaneurysm after hysterectomy. *J Ultrasound Med* 1999;18:711–714.
27. Ball RH, Picus D, Goyal RK, et al. Ovarian artery pseudoaneurysm: diagnosis by Doppler sonography and treatment with transcatheter embolization. *J Ultrasound Med* 1995;14:250–252.
28. Fleming H, Ostor AG, Pickel H, et al. Arteriovenous malformation of the uterus. *Obstet Gynecol* 1989;73:209–213.
29. Flynn MK, Levine D. The noninvasive diagnosis and management of a uterine arteriovenous malformation. *Obstet Gynecol* 1996;88:650–652.
30. Huang MW, Muradali D, Thurston WA, et al. Uterine arteriovenous malformations: gray-scale and Doppler US features with MR imaging correlation. *Radiology* 1998;206:115–123.
31. Itoh H, Keitoku M, Fukuoka M, et al. Spontaneous resolution of postcesarean arteriovenous fistula of the uterine cervix: the usefulness of transvaginal color Doppler scanning. *J Obstet Gynaecol Res* 1997;23:439–444.
32. Hasteltine FP, Glickman MG, Marchesi S, et al. Uterine embolization in a patient with postabortal hemorrhage. *Obstet Gynecol* 1984;63:78–80.
33. Kwon JH, Kim GS. Obstetric iatrogenic arterial injuries of the uterus: diagnosis with US and treatment with transcatheter arterial embolization. *Radiographics* 2002;22:35–46.
34. Pelage JP, Le Dref O, Mateo J, et al. Life-threatening primary postpartum hemorrhage: treatment with emergency selective arterial embolization. *Radiology* 1998;208:359–362.
35. Greenwood LH, Glickman MG, Schwartz PE, et al. Obstetric and nonmalignant gynecologic bleeding; treatment with angiographic embolization. *Radiology* 1987;164:155–159.
36. Cockshott WP, Hendrickse JP. Persistent arteriovenous fistulae following chemotherapy of malignant trophoblastic disease. *Radiology* 1967;88:329–333.
37. Vogelzang RL, Nemcek AA, Skrtic Z, et al. Uterine arteriovenous malformations; primary treatment with therapeutic embolization. *J Vasc Interv Radiol* 1991;2:517–522.
38. Follen MM, Fox HE, Levine RU. Cervical vascular malformation as a cause of antepartum and intrapartum bleeding in three diethylstilbestrol-exposed progeny. *Am J Obstet Gynecol* 1985;153:890–891.
39. Vandantham S, Goodwin SC, McLucus B, et al. Uterine artery embolization: an underused method of controlling pelvic hemorrhage. *Am J Obstet Gynecol* 1997;176:938–948.
40. Novak D. Embolization materials. In: Dondelinger RF, Rossi P, Kurdziel JC, et al., eds. *Interventional radiology.* New York: Thieme, 1990:295–313.

INDEX

Expulsion of fibroid
transcervical
fertility and, 130
vaginal discharge and, 124
vaginal, 47, 47f

F

Failure of embolization, 95–105
adenomyosis and, 102–103
cause of, 95–101
arterial spasm, 98–99
failed catheterization, 95–96,
98f, 99f
false endpoint, 96
ovarian blood supply, 99–101,
100f–102f
definition of, 95, 96f, 97f
leiomyosarcoma and, 103–104
Failure, ovarian, 122–123
False endpoint for embolization, 96–98
Family history, 28
Fatigue, postprocedural, 75–76
Fatty liver of pregnancy, 140
Femoral artery catheterization
for fibroids, 82
for hemorrhage, 143
Fentanyl
for conscious sedation, 75
patient-controlled analgesia with, 78
Fertility
embolic agents and, 91–92
embolization and, 71
fibroids affecting, 10
myomectomy and, 55
of uterine artery embolization, 131
Fetal death, 140–141
Fever, 123
Fibroid
abnormal uterine bleeding with, 10
classification of, 34–35, 35f
development of, 7–8
diagnosis of, 10
epidemiology of, 9–10
found on ultrasound, 38–40, 39f, 40f
genetic basis of, 8–9
growth of, 7–8
image-guided approaches for, 13–14
incidence of, 6
infertility and, 129
macroscopic features of, 6–7
medical therapy for, 12–13
microscopic features of, 7
nomenclature for, 7f
ovarian artery and, 100–101, 100f
pain caused by, 10
pathophysiology of, 8–9
position of, 101–102, 102f
presentation of, 10
pressure effects of, 10
reproduction and, 10
steroid hormones affecting, 8
transcervical expulsion of, 124
treatment of, 10–14
embolization for. *See* Embolization
surgical, 11–12. *See also* Surgery.
uterine artery anatomy and, 22

Fibrosis, 8
Financial issues, 116
Flumazenil, 75
Fluoroscopy, 92, 130
Follow-up, postprocedural, 80
Fragment, retained placental, 140
Fumarase hydratase, 9

G

Gadolinium enhancement, 43
Ganirelix acetate, 13
Gelatin sponge
characteristics of, 86
outcome with, 112
pregnancy after embolization with, 131
pregnancy and, 91–92
Gelfoam
for arteriovenous malformation, 157
in malignancy, 153
for postpartum hemorrhage embolization, 143
Genetics in growth of fibroids, 8–9
Genital tract laceration, 139–140
Gonadotropin-releasing hormone
(GnRH), 7
Gonadotropin-releasing hormone agonist
advantages and disadvantages of, 12–13
spasm and, 84, 84f
Gonadotropin-releasing hormone
analogue, 57
Gonadotropin-releasing hormone
antagonist, 13
Goserelin acetate implant, 12
Granulocyte colony-stimulating factor, 8
Granulocyte-macrophage colony-stimulating
factor, 8
Growth factor
growth of fibroids and, 8
therapy with, 13
Gynecologic examination
of asymptomatic patient, 29–30
family history in, 28
physical examination in, 28–29
Gynecologic intervention, subsequent, 112

H

Health-related quality of life assessment,
113–114
HELLP syndrome, 140
Hemolytic anemia, 140
Hemorrhage
malignancy causing, 151–152
postpartum, 139–150. *See also*
Postpartum hemorrhage.
High-density focused ultrasound, 14
History, family, 28
HMGA1 gene, 9
HMGA2 gene, 9
Hormonal therapy, 70
Hormone evaluation, 33
Human papillomavirus, 151
Hyaline degeneration, 7
Hypercoagulability, 125
Hypogastric artery
arterial anatomy of, 19–22, 19f–22f, 21t
in postpartum hemorrhage, 141–142

Hysterectomy, 71
abdominal, 11
for adenomyosis, 70
alternatives to, 4
blood loss during, 29
cost analysis of, 116
after embolization, 76, 112
indications for, 130
for leiomyosarcoma, 126
myomectomy compared with, 55
outcome evaluation of, 114–115, 114t
quality of life assessment and, 114
traditional, 52–54
Hysterosalpingography, 33
Hysteroscopic myomectomy, 12
Hysteroscopy, 56
for abnormal uterine bleeding, 34, 34f
after embolization, 112

I

Iatrogenic uterine bleeding, 31–32
Ibuprofen, 79
Iliac artery, internal
anatomy of, 19–22, 19f–22f, 21t
catheterization of, 82–83
Iliac vein, drainage into, 24, 24f
Imaging, 37–51
in abnormal uterine bleeding, 33–34
leiomyosarcoma and, 126
magnetic resonance, 41–49. *See also*
Magnetic resonance imaging.
in outcome analysis, 112
for pelvic pressure evaluation, 35
in physical examination, 29
in predicting outcome, 113
in transcervical fibroid expulsion, 124
ultrasound. *See* Ultrasound
in uterine infarction, 124
Inapsine, 75
Incision
for hysterectomy, 53
for myomectomy, 55
Indomethacin, 79
Infarction, uterine, 124
Infection
abnormal uterine bleeding in, 32
as complication, 123–124
embolization in patient with, 70
papillomavirus, 151
prophylactic antibiotic for, 74
Infertility, 10, 129–130
Instruction, discharge, 80
Insufflation, 54
Insulin-like growth factor, 8
Intermenstrual bleeding, 65
Internal iliac artery
anatomy of, 19–22, 19f–22f, 21t
catheterization of, 82–83
Internet, 63
Interventional radiologist, 63–64
Intraarterial nitroglycerin, 99
Intramural fibroid
fertility and, 129, 130
imaging of, 39
location of, 6, 7f
symptoms of, 65